USMLE® Steps 2 & 3
In Your Pocket

ALSO FROM KAPLAN MEDICAL

Books

Master the Boards USMLE® Step 2 CK

USMLE® Step 2 CK Qbook

USMLE® Step 2 CS Core Cases

Dr. Pestana's Surgery Notes:
Top 180 Vignettes for the Surgical Wards

Master the Boards Internal Medicine Clerkship:
Survive Clerkship & Ace the Shelf

Master the Boards USMLE® Step 3

USMLE® Step 3 Qbook

Master the Boards USMLE® Medical Ethics

Flashcards

USMLE® Diagnostic Test Flashcards:
The 200 Questions You Need to Know for the Exam for Steps 2 & 3

USMLE® Examination Flashcards:
The 200 "Most Likely Diagnosis" Questions You Will See on the
Exam for Steps 2 & 3

USMLE® Pharmacology and Treatment Flashcards:
The 200 Questions You're Most Likely to See on Steps 1, 2 & 3

USMLE® Physical Findings Flashcards:
The 200 Questions You're Most Likely to See on the Exam

USMLE® Steps 2 & 3
In Your Pocket

Carla McWilliams, MD
Daniel Giaccio, MD, FACP

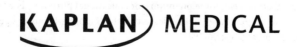

© 2013, 2010 Daniel Giaccio and Carla McWilliams

Published by Kaplan Publishing, a division of Kaplan, Inc.
385 Hudson Street, 4th Floor
New York, NY 10014

Printed in the United States of America

10 9 8 7 6 5 4 3 2 1

ISBN-13: 978-1-60978-898-8

Kaplan Publishing books are available at special quantity discounts to use for sales promotions, employee premiums, or educational purposes. For more information or to purchase books, please call the Simon & Schuster special sales department at 866-506-1949.

DEDICATION

I must thank my family for providing me with the opportunity to fulfill my dreams; my countless friends and colleagues for their continuing encouragement; and to my greatest contributor, my husband, for his never-ending love and support.

For all of you, Carla

To Hugh J. Carroll, MD, for having inspired so many of us with his knowledge, clarity, commitment, enthusiasm, generosity, patience, and humor.

Dr. Carroll is Professor of Medicine, Director Emeritus, Fluid and Electrolytes, SUNY Downstate Medical Center.

For Test Changes or Late-Breaking Developments

kaptest.com/publishing

The material in this book is up-to-date at the time of publication. However, the Federation of State Medical Boards (FSMB) and the National Board of Medical Examiners (NBME) may have instituted changes in the test after this book was published. Be sure to carefully read the materials you receive when you register for the test. If there are any important late-breaking developments—or any changes or corrections to the Kaplan test preparation materials in this book—we will post that information online at *kaptest.com/publishing*.

Contents

FOREWORD

When I was studying for the USMLE® Step 3 exam while working a very busy full-time job, I wished there was a concise review book available, something designed to use my time efficiently by learning on the go. Years later, when I was a medical intern in New York City, I had the good fortune to write my dreams into reality by producing this book with the help of my Internal Medicine residency program director, Dr. Daniel Giaccio.

This book is designed to supplement your study for the USMLE exams while in the clinical setting. It is concise, to the point, and filled with helpful tidbits *you must know* before exam day. It also features original algorithms illustrating the key concepts involved in some of the most important management decisions in clinical medicine. You can easily review 2 to 3 topics in this pocket-sized guide in only a few minutes.

Students studying for the USMLE® Step 2 CK exam who are aiming for a score above the 90th percentile will find this book particularly valuable. Although Step 2 emphasizes pathophysiology and diagnosis, you cannot excel on the exam without a thorough understanding of basic patient management, the focus of this book.

Finally, this guide is useful for residents who want a quick reference on how they should care for their patients. We therefore encourage you to keep this guide in your white coat throughout your clinical clerkships as well.

We wish you the very best on your exams and we hope you enjoy using this book as much as we did creating it!

> Sincerely,
> Carla McWilliams
> Daniel Giaccio
> and the Kaplan Medical Team

1

ETHICAL AND LEGAL PRINCIPLES

AUTONOMY AND BENEFICENCE

- Autonomy—an individual's fundamental right to **make his or her own health-care decisions**
  - ▸ A patient has the **right to refuse** any medical therapy or lifesaving intervention, even if this means that the patient may die, **as long as the patient understands the potential outcome of his/her refusal**

- Beneficence—"do no harm"
  - ▸ Physicians are bound by the oath of Hippocrates to "do no harm" to their patients
  - ▸ This often conflicts with autonomy, because a patient's refusal of lifesaving therapy may ultimately lead to his/her death
  - ▸ **Autonomy always trumps beneficence.** In other words, in the eyes of U.S. law, a person's right to freedom of choice is more powerful than any potentially lethal outcome.

INFORMED CONSENT

- This is a legal term whereby patients are considered to have consented to a medical therapy or procedure after they have been provided with a full, detailed, and clear explanation of the risks, benefits, and expected future outcome(s) of the intervention

- Any **impairment of cognitive function** due to organic medical illness or psychiatric disease **prohibits informed consent** because the patient is **not capable of understanding the intervention**

1

- If a patient is not capable of giving informed consent, the decision-making process is handed down in a stepwise fashion:
  1. Health-care proxy (this trumps any wishes the family may have; legally speaking, the health-care proxy carries total power over medical decisions)
  2. Spouse
  3. A son or daughter 18 years of age or older
  4. The patient's mother or father
  5. A sister or brother 18 years of age or older
  6. A close friend, if the patient has no family

LEGAL APPOINTMENT OF HEALTH-CARE PROXIES

- Power of attorney—signed by the patient, this legally designates an agent who makes financial, business, and/or legal decisions on the patient's behalf. A power of attorney may be specific or generalized, and may or may not include the ability to make medical decisions. It does not necessarily meet legal requirements as a health-care proxy.

- Health-care proxy—designates an agent appointed by the patient to make health-care decisions **only** in the event that the patient is incapable of making them due to coma or lack of competency

- Living will—states the patient's health-care wishes, including the desire for (or against) resuscitative measures, artificial feeding, etc., **in the patient's own words**
  - ▸ The level of detail with respect to the patient's health-care wishes is dependent upon the person writing the document; it may be generalized or extremely detailed
  - ▸ Although a living will states the patient's known wishes, **it does not appoint a health-care agent or proxy**
  - ▸ The consenting party (i.e., the person making decisions on the patient's behalf) should be encouraged to follow the patient's known wishes

1

▶ The hospital ethics committee should be consulted and involved if there is significant conflict

COMPETENCE AND EMANCIPATION

- Competence—a legal term whereby a patient is considered mentally capable of making his/her own decisions
- Only a court can deem a person "incompetent"; any patient deemed incompetent is not capable of making his/her own medical and/or legal decisions
- All patients should be considered competent unless an underlying disorder makes you (the physician) suspicious that they cannot comprehend what you are telling them
- Physicians often use the word "capacity" when it comes to whether they think a patient is capable of making his or her own decisions
  - ▶ If a physician thinks a patient lacks capacity, then it is appropriate to ask the proxy or the next of kin to make the decisions for that patient
- Minors (i.e., persons less than 18 years of age) are considered **legally incompetent** unless they obtain "emancipated minor" status. There are only three circumstances under which a person younger than age 18 years can be considered emancipated:
  - ▶ The minor is legally married
  - ▶ The minor can demonstrate to the court that he or she lives and provides for her/himself independent of her/his legal guardian or parent(s)
  - ▶ The minor is currently enlisted in the U.S. military
- Exceptions—minors who are seeking oral contraceptives, prenatal care, or treatment of sexually transmitted diseases (STDs) or communicable disease such as HIV **do not require consent** from their parents. This is because leaving the minor untreated for the amount of time it takes to ask for and obtain parental permission may create too great a public health risk.

1

PHYSICIAN RELATIONSHIPS— PATIENTS AND FELLOW PHYSICIANS

- A physician has the right to terminate the patient-physician relationship provided the physician allows adequate time and notice for the patient to obtain alternate medical care. Until the patient obtains this alternate care, the physician is legally responsible for providing routine medical follow-up.

- In the hospital, the physician is **not allowed to withhold lifesaving treatment** because the patient has no money to pay for it

- Physicians are prohibited from having any sexual relations with their patients

- If you suspect that a fellow physician is impaired from either substance abuse or psychosocial matters **and** this is directly affecting **patient care**, you should report it

  ▸ If the fellow physician is in private practice—contact the state medical board

  ▸ If the fellow physician is employed by a hospital—report to the department chair

CONFIDENTIALITY

- Physicians have the right to violate confidentiality **only** when a **third party** is at risk of harm; this includes instances of tuberculosis, HIV and other STDs, and intent of homicide or rape

- Medical records are confidential (i.e., not available to any third party) **unless** the patient has consented to their release

REPORTING ABUSE

- All health-care providers are **required** to report suspected child (Child Protective Services) or elder (Adult Protective Services) abuse

  ▸ Elder abuse differs from child abuse because some elderly patients may still be legally competent and may decide not to press charges, even if they understand that they are being abused

- Abuse is considered "willful mental, physical/bodily injury or sexual violation"
- Provided the report of abuse was made in **good faith**, the health-care provider **is immune from prosecution** by the court even if the claim is found to be false

ETHICS IN OBSTETRICS AND GYNECOLOGY AND SEXUALLY TRANSMITTED DISEASE

- Autonomy in pregnancy—all pregnant women have the right to refuse lifesaving medical care for themselves and their unborn children provided the mothers are competent and fully understand the potential outcome of their choice
  - ▸ In other words, the physician **cannot** force a pregnant woman to undergo any medical or surgical intervention she does not want even if this means she and/or her fetus may die

- There are several STDs that must be reported (this is **mandatory** at a national level) to the public health department: HIV infection, syphilis, gonorrhea, chlamydia, chancroid, and hepatitis B and C
  - ▸ Encourage the patient to notify anyone at risk of infection
  - ▸ If the patient is unwilling to do so, the physician may offer to notify the patient's sexual contacts without disclosing the patient's name
  - ▸ If this is not possible, the department of health will take the notification initiative by creating "contact tracings"; the infected patient's identity is not revealed when potentially infected persons are contacted

TUBERCULOSIS (TB)

- Any patient with confirmed pulmonary TB **must be placed on respiratory isolation** in a negative-pressure unit until sputum is free of acid-fast bacilli
- TB lock-up—this means the physician and state board of health have the right to detain any individual with pulmonary TB who

1

refuses treatment. Such patients are considered to be a serious threat to public health.

▶ Patients can be detained indefinitely until they consent to treatment; overall, about 2% of cases will require detention

HIV AND AIDS

- **Consent is required** to screen for HIV infection
- If there is a known third party at risk (boyfriend, girlfriend, spouse, intravenous drug abusers [IVDAs], etc.), then:
  - ▶ First, encourage the patient to tell the potential victim(s)
  - ▶ If this fails, you (the physician) must either:
    - ▷ Warn the potential victim yourself (if known), or
    - ▷ Contact the public health department in your district to start "contact tracings"
- **Tip:** The laws that govern how a third party at risk of HIV exposure should be notified vary from state to state and *probably will not be tested*. In clinical practice, many physicians will leave disclosure issues in the hands of the local public health department.

ORGAN DONATION

- Even if a patient's driver's license says he or she is an organ donor, the patient's health-care proxy or family must still consent to the donation after terminal illness or brain death has occurred
- There is no monetary compensation for organ donation, with the exception of egg donation, sperm donation, and blood donation

MALPRACTICE

In order to prove malpractice, the disputing party must be able to prove either medical negligence or that the physician deviated from the standard of care.

EMERGENCY MEDICINE AND TOXICOLOGY

CARDIAC RESUSCITATION

With any patient who is unresponsive, the **next step** in management is to **call for help**.

TRAUMA

Trauma is the leading cause of death in those age <35 in the United States.

1. **ABCs/primary survey**

   A: Airway maintenance with cervical spine control

   B: Breathing and ventilation

   C: Circulation with hemorrhage control

   D: Disability—neurologic status (brief neurologic examination)

   E: Exposure/Environmental control—completely undress the patient, but prevent hypothermia

2. **Resuscitation/secondary survey**

   ► Does not begin until the primary survey is completed, resuscitative efforts are well established, and the patient has normal vital functions

   ► Includes a complete evaluation—past medical history (PMH), allergies, medications, last meal, events and environment related to the injury

Glasgow Coma Scale (GCS)

Area	Score
EYE opening	
• Spontaneous	4
• To speech	3
• To pain	2
• None	1
VERBAL response	
• Oriented	5
• Confused conversation	4
• Inappropriate words	3
• Incomprehensive sounds	2
• No response	1
MOTOR response	
• Obeys commands	6
• Localizes pain	5
• Withdraws to pain	4
• Abnormal flexion (decorticate)	3
• Abnormal extension (decerebrate)	2
• No response (flaccid)	1

GLASGOW COMA SCALE (GCS)

- **Most valuable when multiple other assessments are taking place**

- Mild brain injury: GCS 14–15
    - ▶ Consider CT scan if loss of consciousness, amnesia, severe headache, GCS <15, or focal neurologic deficits
    - ▶ If evidence of abnormalities on CT scan, or if the patient remains symptomatic or neurologically abnormal → admit patient and obtain neurosurgical/trauma consultation
    - ▶ If the patient is asymptomatic and neurologically intact (negative CT scan), you may observe for several hours, then reexamine, and if no changes → discharge to the care of a companion who can stay with/observe the patient for the next 24 hours

- Moderate brain injury: GCS 9–13
    - ▶ Obtain immediate CT scan of the head, then neurosurgical/ trauma consultation

  ▸ Close observation/frequent neurologic reassessment/admission to intensive care unit (ICU) are all required

- Severe brain injury: GCS 3–8
  ▸ Requires immediate admission to ICU, neurosurgical/trauma consultation, and imaging studies
  ▸ GCS ≤8 → intubate the patient

HEAD-TO-TOE EVALUATION

- Head
  ▸ Evaluation—inspect pupils (reactive/nonreactive and equal/unequal) and look for signs of basilar skull fracture → hemorrhage around the mastoid (Battle sign), the eyes (raccoon eyes), and tympanic membrane (hemotympanum); also inspect nose for cerebrospinal fluid (CSF) leakage (clear rhinorrhea)
  ▸ Management—maintain airway and ventilation, imaging studies (CT scan of head and/or facial bones), intubate if necessary based on the GCS score

- Neck
  ▸ Evaluation—palpate trachea; check midline for local tenderness or deformities
  ▸ Management—maintain **in-line immobilization with hard cervical collar**, then obtain imaging to rule out fracture
    ▹ Lateral x-rays—80% are negative for injury
    ▹ Must have three views—lateral, anteroposterior (AP), and odontoid (open-mouth view)
    ▹ Spiral CT scan is now most commonly used if readily available, particularly in those at high risk of cervical fracture (e.g., postcervical spine tenderness or high-velocity injury)
    ▹ Collar may be removed when all of the following are present: negative imaging studies, GCS score of 15, ability to follow commands, ability to move head side-to-side, and ability to perform head flexion without neurologic symptoms or pain
    ▹ If there are findings consistent with spinal cord injury, MRI is indicated (in stable patients)

- Chest
  - ► Inspect—multiple rib fractures present with irregular/ paradoxical breathing (flail chest)
  - ► Auscultate
    - ▷ For bilateral breath sounds—if unilateral → suspect pneumothorax
      - – Management—chest tube for pneumothorax; if tension pneumothorax → needle thoracostomy **first**, then chest tube placement
    - ▷ If muffled heart sounds plus jugulovenous distention (JVD) → suspect cardiac tamponade
      - – Management—immediate pericardiocentesis for decompression
- Abdomen
  - ► Palpate for signs of peritoneal irritation
  - ► Palpate pelvis for tenderness/instability → obtain pelvic x-rays if either is present, and immobilize with sandbags or tie a sheet to secure
  - ► Arrange for abdominal ultrasound—bedside FAST (focused assessment with sonography in trauma)/CT if indicated
    - ▷ CT scan **only** if patient hemodynamically **stable**
    - ▷ If initial FAST exam is negative and patient remains stable, may repeat serial FAST exams or perform CT scan
  - ► Consider **diagnostic peritoneal lavage (DPL)** if hemodynamically **unstable** and **equivocal** abdominal exam/ultrasound
  - ► Management—aggressive fluid resuscitation; take patient to the operating room (OR) if patient is hemodynamically unstable and/or has significant bleeding, has penetrating wound to the abdomen deeper than the fascia, or has evidence of bowel injury (free air or feces on DPL)
- Assess for urethral bleeding in males and females; and for vaginal trauma/bleeding in females
- Rectal exam—assess for rectal tone, blood, and prostate position

- Musculoskeletal
  - ▸ Evaluation—look for contusions, lacerations, and deformities
  - ▸ Management—x-rays; immobilize thoracic and lumbar spine (in addition to cervical spine)
  - ▸ Apply splint if indicated
  - ▸ Consult orthopedics if suspected fractures; all open fractures and compartment syndromes require prompt intervention
  - ▸ Tetanus immunization if indicated
- Pregnant patients
  - ▸ There are some minor changes in procedures, but the overall management in blunt trauma with no acute injury to the mother requires a minimum of 4 hours of fetal monitoring
    - ▹ If positive for abnormalities/change in condition, then emergent obstetrical consultation and an additional 24 hours of monitoring are indicated
    - ▹ Place the mother in the **left lateral decubitus** position to optimize uterine blood flow to the fetus

ADVANCED CARDIAC LIFE SUPPORT

- Call for help
- Start ABCs + D (drugs)
- Give oxygen
- Attach monitor/defibrillator when available
- Always identify and treat possible contributing factors— remember the H's and the T's:
  - ▸ **H**ypovolemia, **H**ypoxia, **H**ydrogen ion (acidosis), **H**ypo-**H**yperkalemia, **H**ypoglycemia, **H**ypothermia
  - ▸ **T**oxins, **T**amponade (cardiac), **T**ension pneumothorax, **T**hrombosis (coronary or pulmonary), **T**rauma
- **Asystole**
  - ▸ Definition—complete absence of electrical activity in the heart

- ► Management—cardiopulmonary resuscitation (CPR), obtain IV/IO access, prepare patient for intubation
- ► Epinephrine 1 mg every 3–5 minutes up to 3 doses
- ► Atropine 1 mg every 3–5 minutes up to 3 doses
- ► Consider high-dose epinephrine or continue epinephrine 1 mg IVP every 3–5 minutes

- **Bradycardia**
  - ► Heart rate <60 beats/minute
  - ► Treatment
    - ▷ Asymptomatic bradycardia, first-degree atrioventricular (AV) block, and second-degree AV block Mobitz-type I (Wenckebach)—**no** specific therapy
    - ▷ Symptomatic bradycardia—atropine every 3–5 minutes up to 3 doses; transcutaneous pacemaker if no response to atropine
    - ▷ Second-degree AV block Mobitz-type II and third-degree AV block—transcutaneous pacemaker must be placed (even if patient is asymptomatic), then arrange for permanent pacemaker
    - ▷ Epinephrine and dopamine may also be used if no response to atropine

- **Pulseless electrical activity (PEA)**
  - ► Definition—patient with hypotension and absent pulse, but with some type of electrical activity on the ECG strip
  - ► Management—the most important step is to find the cause of the PEA and treat it
  - ► Epinephrine 1 mg every 3–5 minutes up to 3 doses
  - ► Atropine 1 mg every 3–5 minutes up to 3 doses if slow PEA

- **Ventricular fibrillation/pulseless ventricular tachycardia**
  - ► Give 1 shock (or a precordial thump until a defibrillator is available) and resume CPR immediately
  - ► Check for rhythm and pulse; give 1 shock and resume CPR immediately if no pulse is present

- ▶ Epinephrine 1 mg IV/IO (intravenous/intraosseous) every 3–5 minutes up to 3 doses
- ▶ May give 1 dose of vasopressin 40 U IV/IO instead of first or second dose of epinephrine
- ▶ Give drugs during active CPR
- ▶ Give 1 shock after drug administration and resume CPR immediately
- ▶ Consider amiodarone, procainamide, lidocaine, or magnesium (if evidence of torsade de pointes)
- ▶ Remember: shock → CPR + drug → shock

CPR Pearls

- Push hard: ≥2 inches
- Push fast: ≥100 compressions/minutes
- Change compressions every 2 minutes
- Rate of 30:2 compressions, bag mouth ventilation

- **Tachycardia with pulses**
  - ▶ ABCs; give oxygen
  - ▶ Identify reversible causes
  - ▶ Obtain IV access
  - ▶ Monitor ECG and identify rhythm (see Arrhythmias, page 42)
    - ▷ If patient is unstable → altered mental status/signs of shock → synchronized cardioversion
  - ▶ **Ventricular tachycardia (with pulse)**
    - ▷ Wide complex tachycardia (QRS >0.12 second)
    - ▷ Uniform pattern on ECG
    - ▷ No P waves
    - ▷ Drugs
      - – Amiodarone 150 mg over 10 minutes (may repeat to maximum dose of 2.2 g/24 hours)
      - – May use lidocaine or consider cardioversion if no initial response to amiodarone

► **Torsade de pointes**
  ▷ Give magnesium initial bolus 1–2 g, then continuous infusion

► **Pre-excitation/Wolff-Parkinson-White syndrome**
  ▷ Short PR interval and wide QRS
  ▷ Delta waves (slurred upstroke in the QRS complex)
  ▷ Associated with supraventricular tachycardia
  ▷ Management
    – Synchronized cardioversion if unstable
    – Procainamide best alternative
    – Avoid calcium-channel blockers (CCBs), beta-blockers, and adenosine

● **Supraventricular arrhythmias**
  ► Includes paroxysmal supraventricular tachycardia, multifocal atrial tachycardia, atrial fibrillation (A-fib)/flutter
  ► If unstable → synchronized cardioversion
  ► Use with caution/avoid beta-blockers or CCBs in acute congestive heart failure (CHF)/severe left ventricular dysfunction
  ► Avoid beta-blockers in patients with reactive airway disease or acute shortness of breath
  ► Consider digoxin if history of heart failure
  ► **Paroxysmal supraventricular tachycardia**
    ▷ Narrow QRS (<0.12 second)
    ▷ Absent P wave
    ▷ Regular rhythm
    ▷ Start with maneuvers to decrease vagal tone: Valsalva, carotid massage (avoid massage in patients with carotid bruits or the elderly; may cause strokes)
    ▷ Adenosine (drug of choice [DOC]) 6 mg IV push initial dose; may give a second and third dose (12 mg IV)
      – Warn patients they will have a sensation of impending doom or severe pain, which is self-limited and resolves quickly
      – The push **must be rapid**
    ▷ Consider beta-blockers, CCBs, or digitalis if adenosine fails

- **Multifocal atrial tachycardia (MAT)**
  - Irregular rhythm
  - Narrow QRS
  - Morphology of P waves **varies**
  - Treatment—CCBs, especially diltiazem, are preferred by most ER physicians; may also try beta-blockers

- **Atrial flutter**
  - Narrow QRS
  - Regular rhythm; **sawtooth** waves
  - Absent P wave
  - Treatment—same as MAT; may try digoxin but takes several hours for response to occur

- **Atrial fibrillation**
  - Narrow QRS
  - Absent P wave
  - **Irregularly irregular** rhythm
  - Associated with thromboembolic events and **new** myocardial infarction
  - Treatment
    - First: same as A-flutter
    - If there is no spontaneous conversion to sinus rhythm, consider cardioversion
    - If A-fib <48 hours → immediate cardioversion
    - Pharmacologic cardioversion may be attempted with procainamide, sotalol, amiodarone, ibutilide, dofetilide
    - If unsuccessful, consider elective electrical cardioversion
    - If >48 hours → must anticoagulate before cardioversion is attempted
    - Cardioversion must always be followed by anticoagulation (see Atrial Fibrillation, page 42) if no contraindication

TOXICOLOGY

- Determine what toxin the patient was exposed to, when the exposure occurred, and the extent of exposure

- Obtain history and physical examination

- Obtain urine and blood samples

- For topical exposure, remove all contaminated clothing and thoroughly rinse/wash skin

- **General approach**

  ▸ **Gastric lavage** (note that induced vomiting is **no longer recommended** due to **high risk of aspiration**)

    ▷ Indicated in cases of serious and recent ingestion only (<30–60 minutes)

    ▷ Performed only if the patient is already intubated with a nasogastric tube in place

    ▷ Contraindicated if ingestion of any caustic agent is known or suspected

  ▸ **Activated charcoal**

    ▷ First-line treatment

    ▷ Dose: 1 gram per kilogram of patient body weight (g/kg) every 2–4 hours

    ▷ Not effective with ingestion of ethylene glycol, methanol, or iron

    ▷ Do not use if patient is at risk of aspiration

  ▸ **Whole-bowel irrigation**

    ▷ Indicated for ingestions of sustained-release drugs, large numbers of pills, body-packers (cocaine), iron, heavy metals, or lithium

    ▷ Place a gastric tube and infuse a high volume of polyethylene glycol (1,000–2,000 mL/hour)

    ▷ Requires ICU admission and observation

  ▸ **Dialysis**

    ▷ Used in cases of hemodynamic or respiratory compromise, or altered mental status (coma), especially if renal insufficiency

> ▷ May be necessary in cases of ingestion of salicylates, lithium, ethylene glycol, methanol, or theophylline

- ▶ **Diuresis/alkalization methods**
  - ▷ Useful in cases of salicylate, phenobarbital, or chlorpropamide ingestion
  - ▷ Useful as a temporary measure until dialysis can be performed, which is the standard of care

- **Acetaminophen**
  - ▶ Clinical presentation: nausea, vomiting, abdominal pain, elevation of liver function tests (LFTs), followed by signs of hepatic and renal failure
  - ▶ Diagnosis—drug levels and nomogram plotting
  - ▶ Treatment—DOC is N-acetylcysteine (NAC); charcoal may be given in between the doses of NAC

- **Alcohol**
  - ▶ Clinical presentation
    - ▷ Methanol poisoning is associated with **visual disturbances**, including blindness (from formic acid metabolites), and **anion gap** metabolic acidosis
    - ▷ Ethylene glycol poisoning is associated with **oxalate crystals** seen on urinalysis (UA), kidney stones, **anion gap** metabolic acidosis, and **renal failure**
    - ▷ Isopropyl alcohol (rubbing alcohol) is characterized by metabolic acidosis **without** evidence of an elevated anion gap
  - ▶ Diagnosis
    - ▷ Alcohol levels via serum gas chromatography, if available
    - ▷ Arterial blood gas will reveal acidosis and increased lactate
    - ▷ Urine test (oxalate crystals may be seen); urine fluorescence may be positive in ethylene glycol poisoning
    - ▷ Chemistry (BUN/creatinine)

▶ Treatment
  ▷ Fomepizole (alcohol dehydrogenase inhibitor) is the DOC
  ▷ When fomepizole is not available, methanol and ethylene glycol intoxication may be treated with an ethanol infusion. Hemodialysis may be necessary if there is evidence of metabolic acidosis or end organ damage.

- **Opiates**
  - ▶ Clinical presentation
    - ▷ Miosis, constipation, bradycardia, hypotension, hypothermia, respiratory depression, and respiratory acidosis
  - ▶ Treatment
    - ▷ Naloxone is the DOC

- **Cocaine**
  - ▶ Clinical presentation
    - ▷ Hypertension, tachycardia, cardiovascular accident (CVA; i.e., stroke, subarachnoid hemorrhage [SAH]), arrhythmia, seizures, and pulmonary edema
  - ▶ Treatment
    - ▷ Supportive
    - ▷ May control agitation with **benzodiazepines**
    - ▷ Alpha-blockers (phentolamine), or combined alpha/beta-blockers (labetalol) can be used to control hypertension
    - ▷ **Avoid using pure beta-blockers**. They can cause unopposed alpha-stimulatory effects.

- **Digoxin**
  - ▶ Clinical presentation
    - ▷ Nausea, vomiting, diarrhea, blurred vision, altered color vision (especially **yellowing of vision**), cardiac arrhythmias, hallucinations, and altered mental status
    - ▷ Paroxysmal atrial tachycardia—most common arrhythmia
    - ▷ Lab—hyperkalemia usually occurs. Order digoxin levels.

- ▶ Treatment
  - ▷ Charcoal
  - ▷ DOC: digoxin-specific antibodies/digitalis Fab fragments/ digoxin immune fab (Digibind®)
  - ▷ Correct arrhythmias: lidocaine
  - ▷ Correct electrolyte abnormalities
  - ▷ Dialysis

- **Benzodiazepines**
  - ▶ Clinical presentation
    - ▷ Somnolence, confusion, respiratory depression
  - ▶ Treatment
    - ▷ DOC: flumazenil
    - ▷ Must exercise extreme caution in patients with history of chronic abuse—may induce withdrawal seizures

- **Barbiturates**
  - ▶ Clinical presentation
    - ▷ Altered mental status, severe respiratory and central nervous system (CNS) depression, and loss of reflexes
    - ▷ Absent activity in EEG
  - ▶ Treatment
    - ▷ Mainly supportive; there is no specific antidote
    - ▷ May alkalinize urine with bicarbonate to increase urinary excretion of the drug

- **Carbon monoxide**
  - ▶ Clinical presentation
    - ▷ Nausea, vomiting, dizziness, altered mental status, dyspnea, headache, impaired judgment
    - ▷ In severe cases, arrhythmias, chest pain, hypotension, and coma
  - ▶ Labs
    - ▷ Carboxyhemoglobin levels—up to 10% is considered normal; anything above this is strongly suggestive of CO poisoning

2

▷ Arterial blood gas (ABG): metabolic acidosis from anaerobic metabolism, PO_2 is normal

▷ Do not use or rely on pulse oximetry (cannot differentiate between oxyhemoglobin and carboxyhemoglobin)

▷ Must use **co-oximetry** to measure carboxyhemoglobin

► Treatment

▷ Be cautious if patient is pregnant (fetal hypoxemia may occur)

▷ 100% oxygen administration by either face mask or ET tube depending on mental status

▷ In severe cases, consider hyperbaric oxygen (decreases carbon monoxide half-life from 90 min to 30 min) if carboxyhemoglobin is >20% in pregnant women or >25% in nonpregnant adults

- **Lead**
  ► Clinical presentation
    ▷ Abdominal pain, anemia, headache, memory loss, constipation (children), altered mental status, and renal dysfunction
    ▷ Children with chronic exposure may present with mental retardation and poor cognitive function (see Lead Poisoning, page 370)
  ► Labs
    ▷ CBC and blood lead levels, chemistry (BUN/creatinine)
  ► Treatment
    ▷ In the acute setting, charcoal may be used
    ▷ Chelation therapy: calcium, EDTA, dimercaprol (BAL), succimer, penicillamine

- **Salicylates**
  ► Clinical presentation
    ▷ Nausea, vomiting, epigastric pain, **tinnitus** (specific symptom), altered mental status, seizures, hyperthermia, pulmonary edema, and encephalopathy
  ► Labs
    ▷ ABG: combined **respiratory alkalosis** with **elevated anion gap metabolic acidosis**

▷ Low glucose levels
▷ Aspirin levels—most specific test
- Treatment
  ▷ Charcoal if early detection
  ▷ Alkalization of urine
  ▷ Aggressive fluid resuscitation
  ▷ Dialysis in severe cases

2

- **Tricyclic antidepressants (TCAs)**
  - Clinical presentation
    ▷ Tachycardia, **mydriasis, flushed skin, dry mouth**, altered mental status, seizures, cardiac arrhythmias (**wide QRS and prolonged QT interval**); may progress to ventricular arrhythmias or cause heart blocks
  - Labs
    ▷ ECG
    ▷ Drug levels
  - Treatment
    ▷ Charcoal
    ▷ If signs of cardiac toxicity, DOC is bicarbonate (protects the heart from TCA effects)

- **Organophosphate poisoning**
  - Clinical presentation
    ▷ **Miosis, salivation**, bronchospasm, **diarrhea**, bradycardia, anxiety, **fasciculations, lacrimation**, altered mental status, seizures, and pulmonary edema
  - Labs
    ▷ Specific test—red blood cell cholinesterase level
  - Treatment
    ▷ Respiratory support
    ▷ Must remove patient's clothes (a source of further exposure)
    ▷ Atropine
    ▷ Pralidoxime

Must-Know Drugs and Antidotes

Drug	Antidote
Opioids	Naloxone
Phenothiazines	Diphenhydramine, benztropine
Lead	EDTA, BAL, succimer
Acetaminophen	N-acetylcysteine
Salicylates	Bicarbonate
Carbon monoxide	100% oxygen
Tricyclic antidepressants	Bicarbonate
Warfarin	FFP, vitamin K
Organophosphates	Atropine, pralidoxime
Anticholinergics	Physostigmine
Arsenic, mercury	BAL, succimer
Benzodiazepines	Flumazenil
Beta-blockers	Glucagon
Atropine	Physostigmine
Cyanide	Sodium nitrite, thiosulphate
Heparin	Protamine sulfate
Methanol/ethylene glycol	Fomepizole
Nitrites	Methylene blue
Digoxin	Digoxin-specific antibodies
Iron	Deferoxamine

Abbreviations: dimercaprol, BAL; fresh frozen plasma, FFP

PREVENTIVE MEDICINE

ABDOMINAL AORTIC ANEURYSM (AAA) SCREENING

The U.S. Preventive Services Task Force advises that only **men** who are **65–75 years old** and have a history of smoking **100 cigarettes in their lifetimes** be screened with **abdominal ultrasound**.

COLONOSCOPY

See Guidelines for Colon Cancer Surveillance, page 106.

HYPERTENSION (HTN)

Diagnosis of Hypertension

Stage	Systolic (mm Hg)		Diastolic (mm Hg)
Normal	<120	and	<80
Pre-HTN	120–139	or	80–89
Stage 1 HTN	140–159	or	90–99
Stage 2 HTN	≥160	or	≥100

Abbreviation: hypertension, HTN

Important Points of HTN

- Systolic pressure increases with age in most (74% of patients age >80 years have HTN)

- Diastolic typically increases until about age 50, then either stabilizes or decreases

- HTN is a risk factor for stroke, myocardial infarction (MI), chronic kidney disease (CKD), progressive atherosclerosis, and dementia

- Systolic HTN **predicts cardiovascular events** better than diastolic hypertension

- Treatment of HTN reduces the incidence of stroke, coronary artery disease, and congestive heart failure (CHF), and all of these conditions cause cardiovascular morbidity and mortality

White-Coat HTN

Responsible for 10–15% of patients with elevated office blood pressures; associated with a lower cardiovascular risk, but may be a precursor to sustained HTN.

Essential HTN (Primary HTN)

- More than 90% of cases

- Polygenic, heterogenous disorder with a small component of genetic defect

- No secondary cause can be identified

Secondary HTN

- Risk factors—consider working up a patient for secondary HTN when:
  - ▶ HTN is severe/resistant (i.e., not controlled with 3 agents)
  - ▶ There is acute, rapid rise in blood pressure
  - ▶ Patient is age ≤30, not obese, not African American
  - ▶ Onset is prior to pubescence
  - ▶ HTN is malignant

- Etiology—most common cause is renovascular disease
- Primary aldosteronism
  - ► Suspect this in a patient with **resistant HTN, hypokalemia, and metabolic alkalosis**
  - ► Etiology—solitary autonomous adenoma (referred to as Conn syndrome and often <1 cm in diameter), bilateral or unilateral adrenal hyperplasia, and glucocorticoid-remediable hyperaldosteronism
  - ► Diagnosis—best initial test is an aldosterone-renin ratio (ARR; normal ARR is 2–17) → plasma aldosterone level usually >15 ng/dL in a volume-expanded patient with either IV or oral salt loading
    - ▷ Ratio is usually >25–34 in primary hyperaldosteronism
    - ▷ Ratio is usually <10 in secondary hypertension (think of diuretics and renovascular disease)
  - ► Confirmatory test—24-hour urinary excretion for aldosterone (>12 μg/24 hours)
  - ► Best next step is a high-resolution CT scan when increased
  - ► Management
    - ▷ Solitary adenomas → surgical removal
    - ▷ Bilateral adrenal hyperplasia → aldosterone blockade
- Pheochromocytoma—chromaffin cell tumor of the adrenal medulla or extra-adrenal paraganglia (see Pheochromocytoma, page 82)
- Renovascular HTN—unilateral or bilateral renal artery stenosis stimulates the renin-angiotensin system → **refractory** HTN
  - ► Two main case scenarios
    - ▷ Fibromuscular dysplasia—usually **females <35 years of age**, rare azotemia
    - ▷ Atherosclerotic disease—usually **older males or females**, with azotemia (this is most common)
  - ► Diagnosis—best initial test is magnetic resonance angiography (MRA) or spiral CT with contrast; gold-standard test is angiography

3

▶ Management
  ▷ Fibromuscular dysplasia—**revascularization** with stents improves or cures the HTN
  ▷ Atherosclerotic renal artery disease—revascularization **not** recommended (rarely improves HTN, and a higher risk of complications with significant loss of renal function and atheroembolic disease)

- Obstructive sleep apnea—apneic episodes increase sympathetic activation → diastolic HTN and failure of blood pressure to decrease during sleep

- Cushing syndrome, thyroid or parathyroid disease, alcohol

- Drug-induced—oral contraceptive pills (OCPs), sympathomimetics, nonsteroidal anti-inflammatory drugs (NSAIDs), erythropoietin, calcineurin inhibitors (cyclosporine, tacrolimus)

- Low-renin, hypertensive syndromes associated with specific genetic mutations—Liddle syndrome, Gordon syndrome, mineralocorticoid excess, corticosteroid-remediable hyperaldosteronism

Clinical Evaluation of the Hypertensive Patient

- Measure all vital signs, examine the optic fundi, calculate the body mass index (BMI), auscultate the major arteries for bruits, perform a careful heart and lung examination, examine the abdomen for masses, examine the extremities for edema and circulatory abnormalities, and perform a complete neurologic examination

- Laboratory tests for secondary examination: urinalysis, complete blood count (CBC), serum chemistries, and ECG (left ventricular hypertrophy)

Treatment of HTN

- First-line therapy—therapeutic lifestyle changes (TLCs) including low-salt (2 g/day) diet, weight reduction, limit alcohol consumption to two drinks a day for men, one for women

- If first-line therapy is not effective, pharmacologic treatment is indicated
  - ▸ Best initial choice depends on **the patient's medical history** (see Choosing the Right Antihypertensive Medication table)
  - ▸ Monotherapy controls 40% of cases
- Combination therapy usually needed to control stage II or higher

3

Choosing the Right Antihypertensive Medication

Medication	Indications	Contraindications	Side Effects
Diuretics	• Advanced age, CHF, systolic HTN • Thiazides useful in **osteoporosis** (increases Ca^{2+} reabsorption)	Gout	Hypokalemia, **hyperuricemia**
Beta-blockers (-lol)	Angina, CHF	Asthma, COPD, heart block	**Asthma,** bradycardia, CHF, hypertri-glyceridemia
ACE-I (-pril)	CHF when LV dysfunction shows **EF <40%, post-MI** (decreases cardiac remodeling), diabetic nephropathy (slows progression of disease, start when positive for **proteinuria**), any other process resulting in positive proteinuria	Pregnancy, hyperkalemia	**Cough, angioedema,** hyperkalemia, loss of taste, leukopenia
CCB	Advanced age, systolic HTN, cyclosporine-induced HTN, angina	Heart block (verapamil, diltiazem)	Headache, flushing, gingival hyperplasia, **peripheral edema, constipation**

(continued)

Choosing the Right Antihypertensive Medication (continued)

Medication	Indications	Contraindications	Side Effects
Alpha-blockers (-ozin)	BPH	Orthostatic hypotension	Headache, **postural hypotension**, fatigue
ARBs	**Cough with ACE-I**, diabetic nephropathy, CHF	Pregnancy, hyperkalemia	Hyperkalemia

Abbreviations: angiotensin-converting enzyme, ACE; angiotensin receptor blocker, ARBs; benign prostatic hypertrophy, BPH; calcium-channel blocker, CCB; congestive heart failure, CHF; chronic obstructive pulmonary disease, COPD; ejection fraction, EF; hypertension, HTN; left ventricular, LV; myocardial infarction, MI

HYPERCHOLESTEROLEMIA

- The Adult Treatment Panel (ATP III) of the National Cholesterol Education Program recommends obtaining a fasting (9–12 hours) serum lipid profile starting at **age 20** and repeated **every 5 years**

- Major cardiovascular heart disease (CHD) risk factors—smoking, hypertensive and taking antihypertensive medication, low HDL cholesterol (<40 mg/dL), family history of premature CHD (in male first-degree relatives age <55 years or in female first-degree relatives age <65 years), and patient age ≥45 years in males or ≥55 years in females
  - ▸ An HDL level >60 mg/dL counts as a **negative risk factor** (subtract 1 point)

- Coronary artery disease (CAD) equivalents—diabetes mellitus (DM), CKD (creatinine clearance <60 mL/minute or serum creatinine >1.5 mg/dL), peripheral vascular disease (PVD), symptomatic carotid artery disease, AAA

ATP III Goals

Risk Category	LDL Goal*	Initiate TLCs	Consider Drug Therapy
High risk: includes CAD, CAD equivalents, with 10-year risk >20%	<100 mg/dL (optional goal: <70 mg/dL	≥100 mg/dL	≥100 mg/dL (<100 mg/dL: consider drug options)
Moderately high risk: two or more risk factors with 10-year risk 10–20%	<160 mg/dL	≥130 mg/dL	≥130 mg/dL (100–129 mg/dL: consider drug options)
Moderate risk: two or more risk factors with 10-year risk <10%	<160 mg/dL	≥130 mg/dL	≥160 mg/dL
Lower risk: no or one risk factor	<160 mg/dL	≥160 mg/dL	≥190 mg/dL (160–189 mg/dL: consider drug options)

Abbreviations: coronary artery disease, CAD; therapeutic lifestyle changes, TLCs
*If history of diabetes mellitus, the LDL goal should be <**70 mg/dL**.

Framingham Risk Table

- 10-year risk of 10–20%

- Management—TLCs are first-line

  ▸ Diet: total fat 25–35% of total calories, saturated fat <7% of total calories, cholesterol <200 mg/dL, carbohydrates 50–60% of total calories, protein 15% of total calories, fiber 20–30 g/day, plant stanols/sterols 2 g/day

  ▸ Weight reduction and increased physical activity

- If TLCs are ineffective or if LDL >100 mg/dL in high-risk groups, medical intervention is indicated

  ▸ **HMG-CoA reductase inhibitors** (-statins, e.g., lovastatin, pravastatin) are the most **potent LDL-lowering drugs and are proven to decrease mortality from cardiac events** (West of Scotland Coronary Prevention Study [WOSCOPS])

    ▹ Measure **creatinine kinase** levels prior to starting, and again if muscle pain occurs—may cause **myositis** or progressive **rhabdomyolysis**

3

▷ Measure **transaminase** levels prior to starting, and again in 3 months, then annually—may cause drug-induced hepatitis

▶ Cholesterol absorption inhibitor: **ezetimibe** used to **lower LDL cholesterol** → can be **added to statin therapy** if LDL goals are not met with monotherapy, but now used only as a last resort. Shown in 2 trials (2008, 2009) not to improve clinical outcomes.

▶ **Bile acid sequestrants**: cholestyramine and colestipol used to **lower LDL cholesterol** → can also be **added to statin or nicotinic acid** therapy if LDL goals are not met with monotherapy

▶ **Nicotinic acid increases HDL cholesterol** but is often poorly tolerated—look for a patient with **flushing** → may try **aspirin** for symptomatic relief or give at bedtime

▶ **Fibric acids derivatives**: gemfibrozil, fenofibrate, and clofibrate **lower serum triglycerides** and **increase serum HDL**

▷ **Tip: Do not combine therapy with statins; leads to high risk of rhabdomyolysis.**

▶ Omega-3 fatty acids lower serum triglycerides and increase serum HDL

IMMUNIZATIONS FOR ADULTS

- Influenza → yearly for those >65 years of age and those <65 years with risk factors: chronic heart disease, COPD, DM, CKD, immunosuppression, employment in health-care field, and pregnancy

  ▶ Killed inactivated vaccine—IM injection

  ▶ Live attenuated vaccine—intranasal; avoid using in the immunosuppressed, pregnant women, those <5 years or >50 years of age, asthmatics, or those with chronic medical illness(es)

  ▶ Avoid vaccination in those with history of **egg allergy** (killed or live vaccine)

- Pneumococcal (PPSV23)—indicated in those >65 years of age and <65 years with risk factors: chronic heart disease, COPD, DM

  ▶ Revaccination with a second dose is indicated in adults >65 years of age who were previously vaccinated >5 years ago and immunocompromised persons who were previously vaccinated >5 years ago

- ▷ PCV13 and PPSV23 is recommended in the following patients age >19:
  - – Immunocompromised with HIV, cancer, asplenia, or solid organ transplant
  - – Chronic kidney disease or nephrotic syndrome
  - – CSF leak or cochlear implants

- Hepatitis A vaccination recommended in occupational exposure (travelers, food handlers), chronic liver disease, men who have sex with men (MSM), and intravenous drug abusers (IVDAs)

- Hepatitis B vaccination recommended in sexually active young adults and high-risk groups: health-care workers, public safety workers, IVDAs, MSM, people with recent sexually transmitted diseases (STDs)
  - ▸ Given at 0, 1, and 6 months or 0, 1, 2, and 6 months (series of three or four vaccines)
  - ▸ Assess serologic response—successful vaccination yields anti-Hbs (HBsAb) >10 IU/mL (95% of patients)
  - ▸ Nonresponders have anti-Hbs (HBsAb) <10 IU/mL—recommendations are to repeat vaccination up to three additional doses; if there is still failure to respond, further vaccination is unlikely to result in appropriate titers

- Tetanus, diphtheria, acellular pertussis (Tdap) in all age 11–18, then booster age 19–64 and age >65 if not previously immunized (ACIP 2012 guidelines)

- Measles, mumps, rubella (MMR)—all adults born after 1956 should receive a second vaccination

- Varicella—high-risk groups, including health-care workers, family contacts of immunosuppressed persons, teachers, child-care providers, and residents and staff in institutional settings

- Inactivated polio vaccination (IPV, intramuscular) recommended only if primary series was not completed in those traveling to endemic areas during times of outbreak, and in high-risk groups (health-care workers)

3

- Meningococcal vaccination containing serogroup A, C, Y, and W135 antigens (Menactra®) is recommended for persons who:
  - ▸ were exposed during a recent outbreak
  - ▸ have history of complement deficiency
  - ▸ have functional asplenia
  - ▸ are travelers to the meningitis belt of sub-Saharan Africa
  - ▸ are college dormitory residents

INTERNATIONAL TRAVEL PROPHYLAXIS

Malaria

- Travel to Asia, Oceania, and Africa—incidence of chloroquine-resistant malaria is high, so prophylaxis requires other medications, such as mefloquine or atovaquone-proguanil
- Travel to the Caribbean, Mexico, and Central America—low incidence of resistance, so chloroquine is still the drug of choice

Mosquito-Borne Flavivirus (Dengue Fever or "Breakbone Fever")

- Causes 50–100 million cases a year, especially in the tropics (Caribbean, and Central and South America)
- Symptoms—fever, **severe myalgias**, headache with **retro-orbital pain**, macular or **petechial rash**, lymphadenopathy, leukopenia, and thrombocytopenia → most serious form is dengue hemorrhagic fever, which occurs only with reinfection (look for platelet count <100,000 and a positive tourniquet test)
- No specific therapy or vaccine, so treatment is symptomatic and supportive

Hepatitis A

- Due to fecal-oral transmission of a picornavirus found in contaminated food and water
- Vaccination with inactivated killed virus (Havrix®) is highly effective if given 2 weeks **before** exposure (live vaccine rarely used)

- If travel is sooner than 2 weeks or the patient is a close contact of a confirmed case, polyvalent **serum immune globulin** is most effective

SMOKING CESSATION

- Quitting smoking is a two-step process that includes:
  - ► Overcoming the physical addiction to nicotine
  - ► Breaking the smoking habit

- Combined behavioral and pharmacologic therapy is proven most effective in cessation
  - ► Support groups
  - ► Nicotine preparations include gum, patch, cigarette, and inhaler; the patch is the easiest to use and provides the most controlled release of nicotine
  - ► Bupropion is the best initial choice in a patient who has symptoms of depression and also desires to quit smoking
  - ► Varenicline is also highly effective pharmacotherapy, but use caution if history of psychiatric disease or cardiovascular disease
  - ► Nortriptyline is second-line pharmacotherapy (higher side-effect profile)

INTERNAL MEDICINE

I. CARDIOLOGY

CORONARY ARTERY DISEASE

Major Risk Factors

- Diabetes (probably greatest risk factor)
- Smoking (most preventable risk factor)
- Family history
- Hypertension
- HDL cholesterol <40 in males or <50 in females

Minor Risk Factors

- Age
- Obesity
- Estrogen deficiency
- Homocysteinemia

Emerging Risk Factors

- Highly sensitive test is C-reactive protein (CRP) → predictor of myocardial infarction (MI) and stroke but should be used only for those at intermediate risk of CAD (10–20% Framingham risk)
- Cardiac CT to determine coronary artery calcium score is also being utilized in intermediate-risk patients

Stable Angina/Chronic Stable Coronary Artery Disease

- Pathophysiology—atherosclerotic disease of the epicardial coronary arteries due to **fixed stenosis** of the epicardial coronary arteries → unable to supply increased myocardial O_2 demand during exertion

- Clinical—**precordial pain**, usually with a **predictable** amount of exertion and pain, is usually relieved by a **predictable** amount of time or nitroglycerin; may or may not radiate to the left arm or jaw

- Diagnostic tests—ECG may show **ST depression, asymmetry, or flattening of T waves** during periods of chest pain

  ‣ If the ECG is negative (usually during rest) → best next step is a stress test

- Labs—cardiac enzymes (troponin, creatinine phosphokinase-MB [CPK-MB]) are **negative**

- Management—best next step is **stress test**

  ‣ Outpatient treatment with aspirin, long-acting nitroglycerin, beta-blocker plus a statin

> Acute coronary syndrome (ACS) is a term that describes both unstable angina and MI.

Unstable Angina

- Pathophysiology—caused by **transient clotting** of atherosclerotic coronary arteries

- Clinical—chest pain may be **more severe**, or of **greater frequency** with less exertion or **at rest**, or require **more time or nitroglycerin** for relief

- Diagnostic tests—ECG may show **ST depression** or **flattening of T waves**

  ‣ If ECG progresses to ST elevation, *infarction is occurring*

- Labs—cardiac enzymes **negative** unless actively infarcting or troponin "leak" from increased left ventricular (LV) wall tension

- Management—if chest pain relieved and enzymes negative, best next step is stress test
- If stress test positive → percutaneous transluminal coronary angiography (PTCA) or coronary artery bypass graft (CABG)
- Management
  ‣ Hospitalize
  ‣ Physician must give some form of heparin (if no active bleeding)—choice between IV heparin vs. low molecular-weight heparin (LMWH) is dependent on whether cardiac intervention is planned in the near future
    ▷ No angioplasty is planned—LMWH (effect lasts 12 hours or more)
    ▷ If angioplasty is planned—IV heparin (effect lasts 6 hours after drip is stopped)
  ‣ Aspirin (decreases mortality)
  ‣ Clopidogrel
  ‣ Nitroglycerin to increase O_2 delivery
  ‣ Beta-blockers to decrease O_2 demand (and decreases mortality)

Coronary Revascularization

Percutaneous coronary intervention (PCI)

- PCI techniques include angioplasty, atherectomy, and stenting
- Drug-eluting stents have a significantly decreased rate of in-stent restenosis as compared to bare-metal stents

Indications for coronary artery bypass graft (CABG)

- The ACC/AHA guidelines recommend **CABG** be performed over PCI in the following settings (diagnosed via coronary angiography):
  ‣ Evidence of **significant left main coronary artery disease**
  ‣ Greater than **70% stenosis** of the **proximal** left anterior descending (**LAD**) and **proximal left circumflex** arteries

4

> ▸ Three-vessel coronary artery disease
> ▸ Significant **proximal LAD disease with one- or two-vessel disease** plus ejection fraction (EF) <50% and/or a large area of myocardium at risk on noninvasive testing (hypokinesia or akinesia)
> ▸ One- or two-vessel disease with a large area of at-risk myocardium and high-risk criteria on noninvasive testing

Myocardial Infarction

- Pathophysiology—usually due to **complete thrombosis** of coronary arteries; plaque rupture 70–80%, plaque erosion 20%

- Clinical—chest pain not relieved by rest; chest pain may feel like pressure, heaviness, or squeezing, but can also be dull, burning, or sharp
  - ▸ May radiate to shoulders, arms, neck, throat, jaw, teeth
  - ▸ Can have associated symptoms: nausea, vomiting, dyspnea, diaphoresis, palpitations, lightheadedness

- ECG
  - ▸ **Q waves, new left bundle branch block (LBBB), ST-segment elevation ≥1-mm in two or more limb leads or ≥2-mm in two or more chest leads** → ST elevation MI (STEMI)
  - ▸ If **no** ST elevation but **T-wave changes (usually inversions or flattening)** and/or **≥1-mm ST-segment depression** → non-ST elevation MI (NSTEMI)

- Labs—cardiac enzymes **positive**
  - ▸ Troponin very sensitive, rises within 4 hours and may remain detectable for 2 weeks
    - ▹ Best serum marker for **recent MI**
    - ▹ Artificially increased in renal disease → less reliable
  - ▸ Creatinine kinase (CK)-MB rises within 4 hours, peaks at 12–24 hours, and returns to baseline in 2 or 3 days
    - ▹ Best serum marker for **reinfarction**

- Management—hospitalize

- All patients should receive:
  - ► Aspirin—improves survival
  - ► Nitroglycerin to reduce preload and afterload
  - ► Beta-blockers to decrease O_2 demand—improves survival
  - ► Angiotensin-converting enzyme-I (ACE-I) to prevent remodeling
  - ► O_2
  - ► Morphine for severe pain

- NSTEMI
  - ► Immediate coronary catheterization → PTC is the best next step in management if it can be performed within **90 minutes** of presentation but may be delayed for 48 hours while the patient is being stabilized (PTC is much more important to be done early in STEMI)
  - ► Add either **IV heparin** (preferred if procedures are planned) **or LMWH** (preferred if no plan for invasive procedures)

- STEMI
  - ► Immediate coronary catheterization → PTC is the best next step in management if it can be performed within **90 minutes** of presentation

    OR

  - ► Thrombolysis with tissue plasminogen activator (tPA) if cath lab not available (no benefit in NSTEMI); tPA is most effective if given within 6 hours of symptom onset, effective **up to 12 hours**
    - ▷ Then, IV heparin for 48 hours if tPA was given
    - ▷ Absolute contraindications for tPA: history of hemorrhagic stroke, brain tumor, head trauma or ischemic stroke within 3 months, any serious bleeding, aortic dissection
    - ▷ Relative contraindications for tPA: pregnancy, blood pressure >180/110 mm Hg, ischemic stroke within <3 months, active peptic ulcer disease (PUD), international ratio (INR) >2.0, surgery within 3 weeks
    - ▷ Hemoccult-positive stool with no evidence of active bleeding is **not a contraindication** to tPA

4

Complications of MI

Diagnosis	Time Frame	Symptoms	Management
Myocardial aneurysm	1 month post-MI	**Persistent ST-elevation on ECG** or found on echocardiogram or other routine studies	Empiric anticoagulation with warfarin (most have mural thrombus) → surgical repair
Papillary muscle rupture (MCC is inferior wall MI)	2–7 days post-MI	Acute hemodynamic compromise + new **pansystolic systolic murmur in the cardiac apex radiating to the axilla**	Emergent 2-D echo confirms diagnosis → emergent surgical repair
Rupture of the interventricular septum (MCC is anterior wall MI)	3–5 days post-MI	New, sudden heart failure (predominantly right-sided) + **harsh holosystolic murmur along LLSB + a thrill**	Emergent balloon catheterization → surgical repair, if possible
Free wall rupture (MCC is lateral wall MI)	5 days–2 weeks post-MI	**Sudden chest pain, heart failure →** hemopericardium **→ cardiac tamponade →** PEA → death (90% mortality)	Emergent pericardiocentesis → confirms hemopericardium → emergent thoracotomy

Abbreviations: left lower sternal border, LLSB, most common cause, MCC; myocardial infarction, MI; pulseless electrical activity, PEA

CHOOSING THE RIGHT STRESS TEST

- **Question:** Should asymptomatic patients with multiple risk factors for coronary artery disease be stress tested?
    - ▶ **Answer:** No. Only symptomatic patients or those with an abnormal resting ECG. A good general rule is: **"Don't try to make an asymptomatic patient better."**

- Patients who are able to walk, exercise, and exert themselves
  - **Exercise stress test** is the best of all methods to evaluate stable ischemic heart disease (IHD)
    - ▷ Positive when there is a ≥2-mm ST-segment depression and/or a drop of more than 10 mm of systolic blood pressure
    - ▷ Contraindications—unable to exercise for any reason (disabled, amputee, etc.); significant valvular disease (places patient at risk of syncope); arrhythmias, unstable coronary artery disease (CAD), or severe congestive heart failure (CHF)

- Patients who are unable to walk, exercise, and/or exert themselves
  - Dobutamine or dipyridamole (Persantine®) stress test will chemically induce tachycardia and should show evidence of ischemia
    - ▷ Criteria for being positive is the same as for exercise stress test

- Patients with baseline ECG abnormalities (LBBB, ST-segment depression)
  - Nuclear stress test with thallium or a sestamibi scan will show myocardial perfusion patterns on imaging
    - ▷ Areas with decreased uptake are likely ischemic

Approach to Chest Pain after Acute MI Has Been Ruled Out with Cardiac Enzymes

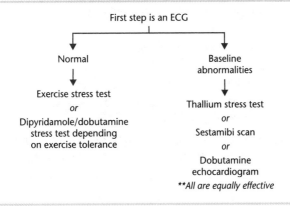

4

ARRHYTHMIAS

Premature Ventricular Contractions (PVCs)

Most common abnormal event, not clinically worrisome if there is no sign of hypotension or chest pain.

Atrial Fibrillation (A-fib)

- Most common abnormal rhythm

- Pathophysiology—chaotic atrial depolarizations → grossly irregular ventricular response → **irregularly irregular** pulse

  ▸ Irregular ventricular response is usually **100–160 bpm**; it can be <100/min with atrioventricular (AV) node disease or certain medications

- Etiology—three most common causes: heart failure, IHD, hypertensive heart disease

  ▸ Others—valvular disease, hyperthyroidism, pulmonary embolism, alcohol, Wolff-Parkinson-White syndrome (WPW)

- Clinical—approximately 90% of patients do not experience palpitations or symptoms; **stroke** from cardiac stasis and clot formation is most feared complication

- Management

  ▸ Rate control **preferred** with calcium-channel blockers (CCBs; verapamil or diltiazem), beta-blockers, digoxin

  ▸ Rhythm control (convert to normal sinus rhythm)

  ▹ Chemical—IV procainamide (first-line), sotalol (normal LV function), amiodarone (CHF)

  ▹ Electrical—synchronized cardioversion first at 100 joules, then at 200 or 360 if necessary

  – If A-fib >48 hours—anticoagulate for 3 weeks before electrical cardioversion

  – If A-fib for <48 hours or signs of hemodynamic instability—immediate electrical cardioversion

- Long-term management—always consider long-term anticoagulation
  - CHADS$_2$ score
    - CHF, hypertension (HTN), Age >75 years, diabetes mellitus (DM)—1 point for each
    - Stroke or TIA—2 points
  - If no points = lone A-fib; no anticoagulation necessary, but must start aspirin (81 mg) if no contraindications for therapy
  - If 1 point = intermediate risk; discuss risks and benefits of anticoagulation (aspirin or warfarin)
  - If 2 or more points = high risk; should anticoagulate with warfarin (goal INR 2.0–3.0), dabigatran (direct thrombin inhibitor), or rivaroxaban (factor Xa inhibitor)
  - In those who are not candidates for the above therapies, you can add clopidogrel to aspirin

ECG: Atrial Fibrillation

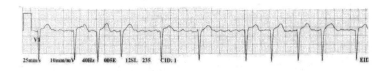

ECG: Atrial Flutter

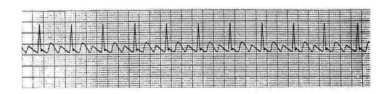

Supraventricular Tachycardia (SVT)

- Several types of tachyarrhythmias which originate **above the ventricles**—the pacer can be in the atrium or the AV junction
- Results in **narrow QRS complexes**, unless aberrantly conducted; may be difficult to distinguish from ventricular tachycardia if the QRS complexes are wide
- If **P waves** are present, the origin is definitely supraventricular
- Management
  - ▸ If unstable—immediate electrical cardioversion
  - ▸ If stable:
    - ▹ First, may attempt mechanical cardioversion (carotid massage)
    - ▹ Then, IV adenosine (avoid in patients with history of bronchospasm) or IV verapamil are the drugs of choice; also may use beta-blockers or digoxin
  - ▸ Correct electrolyte imbalances

ECG: Supraventricular Tachycardia

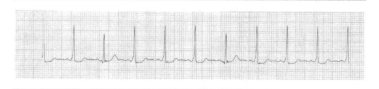

Multifocal (Chaotic) Atrial Tachycardia

- A type of supraventricular arrhythmia with **multiple concurrent pacemakers** in the atria
- Clinical—irregularly irregular rhythm (like A-fib) seen in **chronic obstructive pulmonary disease (COPD)** patients
- ECG—**three or more distinctly different P waves and rate >100 bpm**
- Management—always start oxygen first (hypoxemia can induce the arrhythmia); then CCBs are first-line drug therapy (do not induce vasospasm), correct electrolytes, and treat COPD or underlying causes

ECG: Multifocal Atrial Tachycardia

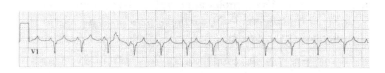

Wandering Pacemaker

- Almost identical to multifocal atrial tachycardia but **rate is 60–100 bpm**
- No treatment indicated

Ventricular Tachycardia

- ECG—three or more consecutive PVCs with **wide and regular QRS complexes**; sustained ventricular tachycardia (V-tach) lasts **>30 seconds** and is at high risk of converting to ventricular fibrillation (V-fib)
- Management
  - ▸ If asymptomatic and **stable—IV amiodarone** to convert to normal rhythm is the drug of choice; may also use lidocaine
  - ▸ If **unstable**, confused, or pulseless—immediate electrical **cardioversion**

ECG: Ventricular Tachycardia

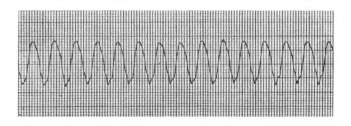

Torsade de Pointes ("Twisting of the Spikes")

- ECG—a **wide QRS complex appears to twist around the baseline** (i.e., "spindle-shaped"), common in those with **congenital prolonged QT syndrome**

- Etiology—may be drug-induced, familial, or from severe electrolyte abnormalities

- Management—**remember: if signs of hemodynamic instability, immediate electrical cardioversion is first-line**

  ▸ Drug-induced or acquired
    ▹ Immediately stop offending drug (antiarrhythmic, antipsychotics, tricyclic antidepressants [TCAs], and quinolones are most common)
    ▹ **IV magnesium sulfate** bolus
    ▹ Acute pacing and/or isoproterenol
    ▹ May try IV lidocaine or phenytoin

  ▸ Congenital prolonged QT syndrome
    ▹ Beta-blockers
    ▹ Acute pacing if needed
    ▹ If recurrent, pacemaker and automatic implanted cardiac defibrillator (AICD) recommended

  ▸ Especially common with hypomagnesemia and hypokalemia—must check electrolytes!

ECG: Torsade de Pointes

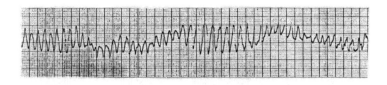

Ventricular Fibrillation

- ECG—complete absence of P waves, and presence of **irregular, bizarre QRS complexes**

- Clinical—hypotension → syncope → sudden death
- Management—immediate electrical defibrillation

ECG: Ventricular Fibrillation

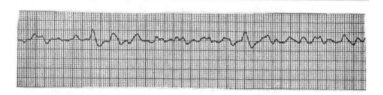

Rhythms by Heart Rate

<60/min (Bradyarrhythmias)	60–100/min	>100/min (Tachyarrhythmias)
Sinus bradycardia	Normal sinus rhythm	Sinus tachycardia
Junctional rhythm	Sinus arrhythmia	Atrial fibrillation (rapid VR)
Complete heart block	Ectopic atrial rhythm	Atrial flutter
	Atrial tachycardia with block	Multifocal (chaotic) atrial tachycardia
	Accelerated junctional rhythm	Supraventricular tachycardia
	Atrial fibrillation (moderate VR)	Atrioventricular nodal reentrant tachycardia
	Wandering atrial pacemaker	Paroxysmal atrial tachycardia
		Ventricular tachycardia
		Torsade de pointes
		Ventricular fibrillation

Abbreviations: ventricular response, VR

Diagnosis of Beat Characteristics

Dropped Beats	Extra Beats
Sinus arrest (pause)	Atrial premature contractions
Sinoatrial block	Premature ventricular contractions
Second-degree Mobitz type I	
Second-degree Mobitz type II	

4

Diagnosis and Management of Heart Block

Type	Characteristics	Etiology	Prognosis	Treatment
First-degree	• Prolonged AV conduction (PR interval >**0.20** seconds) • All atrial impulses are conducted (no blocks)	Normal due to **increased vagal tone or digitalis effect**	• Good • No change in survival	None
Second-degree Mobitz type I or Wenckebach	• **Progressively longer PR intervals until a P wave is not conducted** • After the nonconducted P wave, the rhythm resumes with the baseline PR interval	Can be normal or due to beta-blockers, CCBs, or digoxin	Good	Stop beta-blockers, CCBs, digoxin
Second-degree Mobitz type II	• **Fixed PR intervals** do not have to be prolonged • Low grade = a single nonconducted P wave • High grade = consecutive nonconducted P waves	Usually **His bundle defect** due to: MI, degenerative conduction system, viral myocarditis, acute rheumatic fever, Lyme disease	• Poor • **May progress to third-degree heart block**	**Permanent pacemaker**
Third-degree complete heart block	• **All atrial impulses are blocked** • Atrial activity (P-P intervals) is faster and independent of the slower ventricular activity (R-R intervals)	MI, digitalis, degenerative conduction system	Poor	**Permanent pacemaker** *except* if associated with inferior MI or asymptomatic congenital heart block

Abbreviations: atrioventricular, AV; calcium-channel blocker, CCB; myocardial infarction, MI

ECG: First-Degree Block

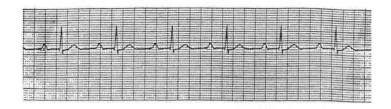

ECG: Mobitz Type I Second-Degree Block

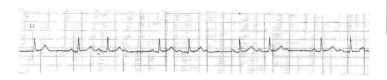

ECG: Mobitz Type II Second-Degree Block

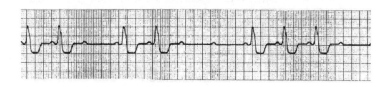

ECG: Third-Degree Block

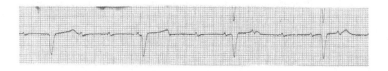

CONGESTIVE HEART FAILURE

- Pathophysiology—cardiac output insufficient to meet systemic demands, results in compensatory responses with sodium and water retention
  - ▸ Heart failure (HF) can be left-sided, right-sided, or both
  - ▸ 50% of cases are systolic HF → impaired ability of the ventricle to eject blood
    - ▹ Have **dilated left ventricle**, ejection fraction low, **<50%**
  - ▸ 50% of cases are diastolic HF → impaired ability of the ventricle to fill with blood
    - ▹ **Normal** size **left ventricle**, ejection fraction **>50%**

- Signs and symptoms
  - ▸ Fatigue, exertional and resting dyspnea, orthopnea, paroxysmal nocturnal dyspnea, wheezing, cough, early satiety, nausea/vomiting, cardiomegaly, crackles, S3 gallop, peripheral edema, increased jugulovenous distension (JVD), A-fib (risk of stroke)
  - ▸ Chronic HF patients can suddenly decompensate (acute HF) with worsened symptoms due to myocardial ischemia, volume overload, excess dietary salt, or tachycardia (rapid A-fib, sepsis, etc.)

- Diagnosis
  - ▸ **Echocardiogram** is first-line, to evaluate structure and function (systolic versus diastolic dysfunction)
  - ▸ **B-type natriuretic peptide (BNP)** useful to diagnoses **acute CHF** exacerbation and **decompensation**. Levels <100 pg/mL exclude decompensated HF
  - ▸ Chest x-ray shows cardiomegaly, acute bilateral infiltrates (especially in acute CHF), Kerley B lines
  - ▸ ECG may reveal the etiology of HF (e.g., Q waves show evidence of prior MI, etc.). In general, the wider the QRS interval, the greater the systolic dysfunction.

- Management—control hypertension
  - ▸ Loop diuretics (furosemide)—helps decrease edema and improve symptoms; use in high doses during acute decompensation
  - ▸ ACE-I—reduces preload and afterload and has been shown to **decrease mortality** in patients with **EF <40%**; use angiotensin receptor blocker (ARB) instead if patient develops cough or angioedema
    - ▹ If patients are unable to tolerate ACE-I or ARBs or have renal failure, use hydralazine plus isosorbide dinitrate
      - – Stop ACE-I in any patient if: >**30% increase in creatinine above baseline** 8 weeks after therapy is begun, or **hyperkalemia**
  - ▸ Beta-blockers (carvedilol or long-acting metoprolol succinate)—shown to improve myocardial function, decrease myocardial demand, and **decrease mortality**; be cautious in acute decompensation
  - ▸ Spironolactone—shown to **decrease mortality** in those with NYHA (New York Heart Association) Class III or IV CHF
  - ▸ Digoxin—has been shown to improve symptoms and **decrease rate of hospitalizations**, but no demonstrable effect on reducing mortality
  - ▸ If patient is African American, add hydralazine and isosorbide dinitrate; both have been shown to **decrease mortality** in this patient population. You may also use this regimen in those who are unable to tolerate an ACE inhibitor or ARB.
  - ▸ AICD if EF <35% shown to **decrease mortality**
  - ▸ Cardiac resynchronization therapy (CRT)—biventricular pacing reduces mortality in patients with mild to moderate systolic HF with an EF ≤30% and a prolonged QRS complex on ECG
- Cardioversion or rate control of A-fib
- Anticoagulation for A-fib—if indicated
- Overall, management of HF focuses on treatment of HTN, tachycardia, and ischemia

4

VALVULAR HEART DISEASE

Valvulopathies are categorized as stenotic, regurgitant, or combined. All valvulopathies → **cardiac remodeling** → clinical sequelae. The **compensatory changes** help to delay the development of symptoms, unless the valvulopathies occur suddenly before compensatory changes can develop (e.g., acute MR → sudden dyspnea).

4

Etiology of Valvular Heart Disease

MS	**Rheumatic heart disease**, annular calcification		
AS	**<30 years** Congenital AS (unicuspid)	**40–60 years** Bicuspid aortic rheumatic heart disease	**>70 years** Senile degenerative* (calcific aortic stenosis)
MR	**Myxomatous degeneration** of the valves (e.g., flail or prolapse) 68% Ischemic MR (inferior wall ischemia which retracts the posterior leaflet) 23% Chordae tendinae rupture (ischemic or endocarditis) 6% Rheumatic disease (usually associated with MS) 1%		
AR	Congenital— hereditary bicuspid valve Direct valve disease—endocarditis, rheumatic heart disease Proximal ascending aorta dissection: hypertension-associated ectasia, marfan syndrome, ankylosing spondylitis, reactive arthritis, syphilis		
TR	RV overload from LV failure (most common cause) RV and inferior wall MIs Tricuspid valve endocarditis (IV drug abusers) Pulmonary HTN, carcinoid syndrome, SLE, myxomatous degeneration		
PS	Congenital Carcinoid syndrome		
PR	Pulmonary HTN Endocarditis Carcinoid syndrome		

Abbreviations: aortic regurgitation, AR; aortic stenosis, AS; hypertension, HTN; left ventricular, LV; mitral regurgitation, MR; mitral stenosis, MS; myocardial infarction, MI; pulmonary regurgitation, PR; pulmonary stenosis, PS; systemic lupus erythematosus, SLE; tricuspid regurgitation, TR

* Same risk factors as atherosclerotic coronary artery disease (dyslipidemia, chronic kidney disease, diabetes mellitus, HTN, old age, etc.). Treatment of these risk factors does not prevent the progression of the aortic valve disease.

Initial Evaluation of Valvular Disease

- History
  - ▸ Patient's symptoms?
  - ▸ History of RF?
  - ▸ Family history of bicuspid aortic valve?

- Physical examination (S1, S2, murmurs, S3, OS)

- CXR, ECG

The best next step in the diagnosis of any valvular heart disease is a 2-D echocardiogram; the gold standard is angiography. Angiography is indicated **only in those patients who have indications for valve replacement surgery**. If evidence of CAD is found, it must be addressed before valve repair takes place.

Aortic Stenosis (AS)

- Etiology—see table on previous page

- Subtype—aortic valve sclerosis is an early-phase calcific valve stenosis, present in 20% of people **≥65 years of age**
  - ▸ The systolic murmur is very similar to AS and is associated with a 50% risk for MI and death over a 5½-year period

- Signs and symptoms—see table on page 57

- Diagnosis—clinical, ECG (LV hypertrophy or suggestive repolarization changes), echocardiography (valve calcification, valve opening, LV thickness, LV function, aortic valve gradient with Doppler)
  - ▸ Cardiac catheterization is definitive (showing valve area **<0.8 cm^2**) and **must** also assess coronary arteries for atherosclerotic disease

- Management—aortic valve replacement if symptomatic **plus** CABG **if** significant cardiac stenosis during catheterization
  - ▸ **Warning:** Beta-blockers and afterload reducers (vasodilators and ACE-I) increase ventricular filling time but must be used

with extreme caution initially; may result in shock because peripheral circulation is maximally constricted to maintain blood pressure

▸ Do not order an exercise stress test if AS is suspected; the test could result in syncope

▸ **Tip:** In general, emphasis is now on repairing or replacing heart valves **before LV dysfunction** starts.

Aortic Regurgitation (AR)

- Etiology—see table on page 52
- Signs and symptoms—see table on page 57
- Diagnosis—clinical, ECG (LV hypertrophy), echocardiography (determine LV size and function), cardiac catheterization (quantify AR severity, coronary artery assessment, and preoperative aortic root anatomy)
- Management
  ▸ Asymptomatic mild-moderate AR—periodic follow-up with 2-D echo
  ▸ Asymptomatic AR with HTN or LV dilation—vasodilators, ACE-I are the drugs of choice; also may use hydralazine or nifedipine
  ▸ Symptomatic AR or if significant LV dysfunction, i.e., EF <55% or left ventricular end-systolic pressure (LVESD) >55 mm—aortic valve replacement

Mitral Regurgitation (MR)

- Etiology—see table on page 52
- Signs and symptoms—see table on page 57
- Diagnosis—clinical, ECG (left atrial enlargement), echocardiography (measure LV dimensions and function); cardiac catheterization for pre-op assessment of regurgitation, LV function, and pulmonary artery pressure; and assess coronary arteries for atherosclerotic disease

- Management
  - ► Acute MR → emergency surgery
  - ► Chronic MR → surgical repair or replacement when symptoms develop or when asymptomatic patients have LVEF (left ventricular ejection fraction) <60% or LVESD (left ventricular end-systolic diameter) >45 mm
  - ► MR caused by myxomatous degeneration with flail or prolapsed noncalcified leaflets → annuloplasty rings or suturing the opposing leaflets is indicated
  - ► Benefit from vasodilators in chronic MR is controversial

Mitral Stenosis

- Etiology—see table on page 52
- Signs and symptoms—see table on page 57
- Diagnosis—clinical, ECG (left atrial enlargement), echocardiography (measure left atrial dimensions, mitral valve area, and decay of transvalvular gradient)
- Management
  - ► Symptomatic or asymptomatic with evidence of pulmonary HTN (pulmonary artery pressure >50 at rest or >60 during exercise)
    - ▷ Balloon valvotomy is preferred if no evidence of MR, valve calcification is not excessive and no evidence of left atrial thrombi
    - ▷ If any of the previous are present or disease is congenital → open surgical commissurotomy is preferred
  - ► Rate or rhythm control of A-fib
    - ▷ If A-fib present, anticoagulation should be started and continued even if sinus rhythm is restored because risk of systemic embolization is 20–30% if untreated
  - ► Diuretics are usually effective for mild symptoms

4

- ▶ Pregnant patients with MS
    - ▷ If asymptomatic before the pregnancy → beta-blockers help the patient through the pregnancy
    - ▷ If symptomatic before the pregnancy → the MS should be corrected prior to the pregnancy
    - ▷ Remember that pregnancy increases blood volume by 50%—the ultimate stress test. **They will get worse!**

Tricuspid Regurgitation

- Etiology—see table on page 52
- Signs and symptoms—see table on following page
- Diagnosis—ECG (right atrial enlargement = P pulmonale, right ventricular hypertrophy [RVH], right bundle branch block [RBBB]), echocardiography (severity of tricuspid regurgitation)
- Management—tricuspid valve annuloplasty or, if not amenable, valve replacement

Pulmonary Stenosis

- Etiology—see table on page 52
- Signs and symptoms—see table on following page
- Management—balloon valvotomy in symptomatic patients with peak systolic gradient >30 mm Hg or in asymptomatic patients with peak systolic gradient >40 mm Hg

Pulmonary Regurgitation

- Etiology—see table on page 52
- Signs and symptoms—see table on following page
- Management—balloon valvuloplasty or, if not amenable, valve replacement

Valvular Heart Disease Symptoms, Murmurs, and Other Physical Findings

	Symptoms	Signs
MS	• **History of plateaus** every **10 years** (→) • Rheumatic fever → first signs → Class II HF symptoms → A-fib → Class III-IV HF • **Tachycardia of any etiology** reduces cardiac output and increases pulmonary pressure **(exertional dyspnea, orthopnea, paroxysmal nocturnal dyspnea)** • Some experience **palpitations** (A-fib), **hemoptysis, hoarseness**, and right-sided heart failure symptoms: **pedal edema, early satiety**	• **Loud S1** • Early diastole • **Opening snap (OS)** • Mid-**diastolic rumble** at the apex • **Loud P2** • <u>Severe MS</u> (very elevated LA pressures): **OS** is louder **interval** between A2 and OS is **shorter;** diastolic rumble is softer • If both MS and MR, the systolic murmur of MR may dominate with little or no diastolic murmur and a delayed OS
AS	• **Angina** (average 3 years to death) • **Syncope** • **Exertional dyspnea**	<u>Mild to moderate AS:</u> **early peaking** crescendo-decrescendo systolic murmur at right second intercostal space, radiating to the carotids <u>Severe AS:</u> systolic murmur **peaks later** in systole and extends to a **weak to absent A2** with a weak carotid pulse = **pulsus parvus et tardus**
MR	<u>Determined by the rapidity of the MR</u> • Acute MR: **sudden pulmonary edema** • Chronic MR: asymptomatic many years → pulmonary congestive symptoms **(exertional dyspnea)** and low cardiac output symptoms **(fatigue)**	1. **Holosystolic murmur** maximal at apex, radiates to the axilla 2. Prominent **S3** (due to large volume of blood flowing from LA into the LV at the start of diastole) **If both loud holosystolic murmur and S3 are heard = severe MR**

4

(continued)

Valvular Heart Disease Symptoms, Murmurs, and Other Physical Findings (continued)

	Symptoms	Signs
AR	Determined by the rapidity of the AR • Acute AR: **dyspnea** • Chronic AR: may be asymptomatic for years while LV dilatation compensates → ultimately LV decompensates: **fatigue, exertional dyspnea, paroxysmal nocturnal dyspnea and chest pain** (syncope is uncommon)	Three types of murmurs 1. Aortic **diastolic** murmur: blowing, decrescendo in early diastole at the left third intercostal space 2. **Midsystolic** flow murmur: at base 3. **Austin Flint murmur** (seen in severe AR) mid to late **diastolic** **Rumble** (like MS) caused by regurgitant flow partially obstructing normal mitral flow Many signs are due to the **widened pulse pressure**
TR	**Severe disease:** RV failure symptoms: edema, early satiety, ascites	Murmur (LSB) that increases in inspiration (Carvallo sign)
PS	**Severe disease:** RV failure symptoms: edema, early satiety, ascites	Crescendo-decrescendo midsystolic murmur
PR	**Severe disease:** RV failure symptoms: edema, early satiety, ascites	Decrescendo Diastolic murmur at LSB

Abbreviations: aortic regurgitation, AR; aortic stenosis, AS; atrial fibrillation, A-fib; heart failure, HF; left atrium, LA; left ventricle, LV; mitral regurgitation, MR; mitral stenosis, MS; pulmonary regurgitation, PR; pulmonary stenosis, PS; right ventricle, RV; tricuspid regurgitation, TR

Murmur Characteristics During the Cardiac Cycle

Valve Disease	Systole	Diastole	Characteristics
MR	Holosystolic / Blowing @ apex	S3	Loud P2
TR	Holosystolic / Blowing @ lower LSB		Increases with inspiration (Carvallo sign)
ASclerosis	Peaks earlier		
AStenosis	Mid (mild) / Late (severe) / Harsh @ Right second ICS / Radiates to carotids & apex		A2 absent in severe disease / Pulsus parvus et tardus
AR	@ Base / Radiates to axilla	Blowing @ aorta / Austin Flint (Severe AR)	Wide pulse pressure / Pulsus bisferiens
ASD			Fixed split S2
Adolescence Anemia Pregnancy			Flow murmurs
PS	@ Second Left ICS		With inspiration
HSS			Increases with Valsalva
PR		Graham Steell @ upper LSB	Increases with inspiration
MS		OS Rumbling	No change with inspiration
TS			Louder with inspiration
PDA			Loudest in back
Coarctation of aorta			Lower pulses weaker

4

Abbreviations: aortic regurgitation, AR; aortic sclerosis, Asclerosis; aortic stenosis, AStenosis; atrial septal defect, ASD; hypertrophic subaortic stenosis; HSS; intercostal space, ICS; left sternal border, LSB; mitral regurgitation, MR; mitral stenosis, MS; patent ductus arteriosus, PDA; pulmonic regurgitation, PR; pulmonary stenosis, PS; tricuspid regurgitation, TR; tricuspid stenosis, TS

Evaluating Physical Findings for Valvular Heart Disease

- **TTE (transthoracic echocardiography)** is used to assess the **natural history of valvulopathies** and to follow parameters for the **optimal timing of valve replacement** (i.e., before LV dysfunction occurs)
- Parameters include mean gradient across the valve, EF, end diastolic volume. You do not need to memorize the parameters for the USMLE exam, but you do need to know that ordering an echo is the next best step if you suspect symptomatic valvular heart disease.

- It is strongly advised to **compare the physical examination to the results of Doppler echocardiography.** If the clinical exam suggests severe disease, while the echo suggests only mild to moderate disease, another procedure must be performed (e.g., cardiac catheterization). **The opportunity to replace a valve before LV dysfunction starts should not be missed.**

ENDOCARDITIS

- Pathophysiology—infection of the endothelial surface of the heart results in vegetations of platelet, fibrin, and microorganisms; usually on the heart valves

- Subtypes
  - ▸ **Acute** bacterial endocarditis progresses over **days to weeks,** typically due to *Staphylococcus aureus, Streptococcus pneumoniae,* and *Neisseria gonorrhoeae;* more common in **IV drug abusers**
  - ▸ **Subacute** bacterial endocarditis progresses over **weeks to months,** due to less virulent organisms (*Strep. viridans,* coagulase-negative staphylococci, enterococci, and gram-negative rods); more common in those with **native valve disease**
  - ▸ **Libman-Sacks endocarditis** in SLE is due to autoantibody damage of valves, but is usually asymptomatic

- Culture negative endocarditis historically due to **HACEK** organisms
  - ► *Haemophilus parainfluenzae,* **A**ctinobacillus, **C**ardiobacterium, **E**ikenella, *Kingella kingae*
  - ► Modern culture media are now 97% sensitive for these organisms
  - ► "Culture negative" endocarditis is now a result of fastidious organisms and some fungi

- Signs—splenomegaly, **splinter hemorrhages** in fingernails, **Osler nodes** (painful red nodules on fingers), **Roth spots** (retinal hemorrhages with clear central areas), **Janeway lesions** (dark macules on palms/soles), **conjunctival petechiae**, brain/kidney/splenic **abscesses**

- Diagnosis
  - ► Best initial test is **transthoracic echocardiogram (TTE)**
  - ► If TTE is **not diagnostic**, get **transesophageal echocardiogram** (TEE; more sensitive)

- Management is 4–6 weeks of IV antibiotics targeted to the specific organism

- Empiric therapy is generally not recommended before culture results except in an acutely ill patient in whom withholding therapy might be lethal or harmful
  - ► Native valve empiric regimen—IV penicillin or ampicillin *plus* nafcillin or oxacillin *plus* gentamicin; alternative is IV vancomycin *plus* gentamicin
  - ► Prosthetic valve empiric regimen—IV vancomycin *plus* gentamicin *plus* rifampin
  - ► **Valve replacement** for severe disease; for large, expanding **abscesses**; or if endocarditis infects a **prosthetic valve**

Marantic Endocarditis

- Sterile vegetation due to metastatic seeding of the valves due to cancer
- Malignant emboli can result in cerebral infarcts

4

PERICARDIAL DISEASE

Pericardial Effusion

- Etiology
    - ▶ Transudates—any disease that can cause systemic edema (CHF, cirrhosis, nephrotic syndrome, hypoalbuminemia)
    - ▶ Exudates—infection, neoplastic process, inflammatory effusions due to autoimmune disease, hypothyroidism
    - ▶ Frank blood or hemopericardium—seen in trauma, metastatic cancer, tuberculosis
    - ▶ Uremia may cause either a transudative effusion or hemopericardium
    - ▶ Some drugs may also cause pericarditis and pericardial effusions, including procainamide, hydralazine, isoniazid, minoxidil, phenytoin, and some anticoagulants

- Clinical
    - ▶ If slowly occurring—onset of symptoms insidious as pericardium slowly expands
    - ▶ If rapid onset—development of cardiac tamponade
        - ▷ Beck triad—distant heart sounds, JVD, and hypotension
        - ▷ Pulsus paradoxus is a fall of >10 mm Hg in blood pressure during inspiration
        - ▷ Kussmaul sign—sharp increase in jugulovenous pressure with inspiration

- Diagnosis—best initial test is echocardiogram showing free fluid in pericardial space; if massive amount of fluid collects, the ECG will show **decreased QRS voltage** and **electrical alternans** as the heart beats freely in the pericardial space

- Management—if evidence of tamponade, immediate pericardiocentesis followed by pericardial window is required; otherwise, may aspirate fluid for diagnostic purposes

Acute Pericarditis

- Etiology—most common cause is **viral infections**; others include bacterial and fungal infections, rheumatoid arthritis, SLE, scleroderma, and uremia

- Signs—early **pericardial friction rub** (85%), then decreased heart sounds

- Symptoms—**pleuritic** retrosternal chest pain, **worse when supine, improved with sitting up**

- Diagnosis—ECG is the best initial test showing **concave ST elevation across all leads**, usually with **PR depression early**, then isometric T waves progressing to ST depression; echocardiography may show pericardial effusion

- Management
  - ▸ Aspirin or NSAIDs for 3–4 weeks plus colchicine for 3 months for viral, postsurgical, or idiopathic disease
  - ▸ Steroids for refractory cases
  - ▸ Antibiotics for more severe disease and evidence of infection
  - ▸ Pericardiocentesis if any evidence of pericardial tamponade

Constrictive Pericarditis

- Etiology—widespread fibrotic changes of the pericardium as a result of prior pericarditis causes decreased elasticity and decreased filling of all chambers

- Clinical—fatigue, exertional dyspnea, and signs of right heart failure with characteristic **"pericardial knock"** during auscultation
  - ▸ **Tip: No signs of pulmonary congestion.**

- Diagnosis—best initial test is **TTE** showing increased pericardial thickness with or without calcifications; chest x-ray may show a ring of calcification around the heart; CT or MRI is the most sensitive test for evaluation of pericardial thickness

- Management
  - ▸ If mild disease, try diuretics plus ACE-I but be careful to not overtreat (delicate balance to maintain cardiac output)
  - ▸ Pericardiectomy required if severe symptoms or right heart failure (RHF) (i.e., ≥ class II HF)

CARDIOMYOPATHY

Hypertrophic Obstructive Cardiomyopathy

- Etiology—majority are autosomal dominant defect resulting in **diffuse thickening of the intraventricular septum**

- Clinical—dyspnea, syncope, and high risk of **sudden cardiac death** in young **athletes**

- Features—systolic murmur **improves with handgrip** and **worsens with standing**

- Diagnosis—best initial test is an ECG showing left ventricular hypertrophy (LVH); gold standard is TTE showing the thickened septum

- Management—placement of an **AICD** indicated in all patients with **history of syncope or with family history of sudden death**

Stepwise Management of Hypertrophic Obstructive Cardiomyopathy (HOCM)

Beta-blockers or verapamil are first-line medical therapy
Increases diastolic filling → decreasing outflow tract obstruction

↓ *Fails*

Injection of pure alcohol into septal perforator arteries
Should decrease wall thickness

↓ *Fails*

Surgical myomectomy

Dilated Cardiomyopathy

- Etiology—diffusely dilated heart most often due to **IHD,** but important causes are **alcohol, peripartum, doxorubicin** (after chemotherapy), **viral-induced**, idiopathic, and some heavy metals

- Clinical—symptoms of CHF, right- and left-sided

- Diagnosis—best test is echocardiogram showing chamber dilation, valvular regurgitation, and diffuse wall motion abnormalities

- ▸ Doxorubicin-induced cardiomyopathy is most accurately diagnosed with a MUGA scan before and after therapy
- Management—treat as CHF

Restrictive Cardiomyopathy

- Etiology—rigid, noncompliant ventricles due to infiltrative process including **sarcoidosis, amyloidosis, hemochromatosis** or **rheumatologic diseases** (diffuse scleroderma), radiation exposure, and **diabetes** (thought to be the most common cause)
- Clinical—exertional dyspnea and signs of heart failure; diastolic dysfunction greater than systolic dysfunction
- Diagnosis—amyloidosis has characteristic **granular and sparkling appearance of the myocardium** during echocardiography, other findings are RHF > left heart failure (LHF)
- Management—treat as CHF

MYOCARDITIS

- Etiology—most common cause is viral infection, especially **coxsackie B virus**; in South American immigrants you should be suspicious of parasitic infiltration, i.e., **Chagas disease**; many other causes include fungi, radiation, drugs, rheumatic diseases
- Clinical—exertional dyspnea, fatigue, signs of CHF
- Diagnosis—**increased cardiac enzymes** (troponin, CK-MB) are most characteristic to suspect myocarditis
  - ▸ ECG (diffuse ST changes or PVCs) and echo findings (systolic dysfunction) are nonspecific
  - ▸ Gold-standard test is **myocardial biopsy**
  - ▸ If you suspect Chagas disease, first send *Trypanosoma cruzi* serologies; or if you suspect viral infections, send polymerase chain reaction (PCR)-DNA serologies (e.g., for coxsackie B virus)
  - ▸ Diagnosis is often based on clinical presentation alone
- Management
  - ▸ If viral, supportive treatment
  - ▸ If Chagas disease, benznidazole

II. ENDOCRINOLOGY

PITUITARY DISEASE

Normal physiology—hypothalamus communicates with pituitary via releasing hormones (to anterior pituitary via portal system) and via nerves (to posterior pituitary).

Hypothalamic-Pituitary Axis

Anterior Pituitary Hormones	Controlled by Hypothalamic Release of:
ACTH	CRH stimulates
GH	GHRH stimulates
TSH	TRH stimulates
LH	GnRH stimulates
FSH	GnRH stimulates
PRL	Dopamine *inhibits*

Abbreviations: adrenocorticotropic hormone, ACTH; corticotropin-releasing hormone, CRH; follicle-stimulating hormone, FSH; growth hormone, GH; growth hormone-releasing hormone, GHRH; gonadotropin-releasing hormone, GnRH; luteinizing hormone, LH; prolactin, PRL; thyrotropin-releasing hormone, TRH; thyroid-stimulating hormone, TSH

Pituitary Tumors

Note: Pituitary adenomas often grow slowly and exist for years before diagnosis.

Null cell tumors

Have no measurable hormonal activity, but alpha chains (inactive portion of thyroid-stimulating hormone [TSH], luteinizing hormone [LH], follicle-stimulating hormone [FSH]) may be produced. Symptoms related to mass effect: seizures, visual field changes, headaches.

Hyperpituitarism

Prolactinoma

- Most common secretory pituitary tumor
- Diagnosis and clinical presentation—prolactin level (PRL) should correlate with size of tumor (>1 cm usually have PRL **>200 ng/mL**)
  - ▸ Elevated PRL decreases secretion of gonadotropin-releasing hormone (GnRH), leading to decreased LH and FSH and their target organ functions
    - ▹ Men → impotence and hypogonadism
    - ▹ Women → **amenorrhea, galactorrhea**, hirsutism
    - ▹ **Tip:** Serum prolactin level is the best initial step in any young male or female with symptoms of hypogonadism **and** galactorrhea.
- Microadenomas are <1 cm in size; macroadenomas are >1 cm in size
- Management—best initial step is drug therapy with bromocriptine or cabergoline; monitor response to therapy with periodic serum PRL levels
- If failure to respond to medical therapy → transsphenoidal surgery is the best next step in management (may not always provide long-term relief)

Secondary causes of hyperprolactinemia

- Usually have levels **<150 ng/mL** (normal PRL is usually <20 ng/mL)
- Any mass or infiltrative process that interrupts normal hypothalamic-pituitary axis
- Drugs—metoclopramide, amitriptyline, phenothiazines, antipsychotics, antidopaminergics, opioids, calcium channel blockers, protease inhibitors
- Normal pregnancy (high endogenous estrogens)
- **Hypothyroidism—always check serum TSH if prolactin levels are elevated!** Increased circulating TRH inhibits dopamine release and stimulates lactotropes.

4

Acromegaly

- Due to growth hormone (GH)-secreting pituitary macroadenoma
  - ▸ **May** secrete **prolactin** too!
- Pathophysiology—stimulates production of insulin-like growth factor (IGF) in the liver stimulating hepatic gluconeogenesis, inhibiting the peripheral action of insulin
- Clinical—**large hands and feet**, frontal **bossing, deep voice**, excessive sweating, skin tags, colonic polyps, **carpal tunnel syndrome** (bony overgrowth compresses the tunnel), **HTN**
  - ▸ **Tip:** Compare the patient's current appearance to an old photograph; facial features will be **dramatically different**.
- Labs—hyperglycemia
- Diagnosis—screen with **serum IGF-1** → will be elevated in most (best initial test)
  - ▸ Best confirmatory test—serum GH level with an **oral glucose tolerance test** → glucose normally suppresses GH levels (0.5–1.0 ng/dL in normal subjects), but not in acromegaly (85% will have levels >2 ng/dL)
  - ▸ Next step would be CT scan of the head or MRI to determine tumor size and pre-op planning
- Management—**transsphenoidal surgical resection** is the best initial step in management
  - ▸ Repeat IGF-1 post-op → should be normal
  - ▸ If still high, then medical therapy is the next step—**octreotide** or **lanreotide** is the drug of choice (long-acting somatostatin analogues available in SQ or IM forms). They suppress **normal + neoplastic** sources of GH and cause tumor shrinkage in some patients.
    - ▷ Pegvisomant (GH receptor blocker) is a new treatment but is used as a last resort
    - ▷ Cabergoline and bromocriptine **are no longer recommended**
- Monitor response to medical management with serum IGF-1

Empty sella syndrome

- Etiology—pituitary tissue is pushed to the side by invaginating diaphragm of the subarachnoid space superior to the sella. Although the sella appears not to contain pituitary tissue, its pituitary function remains intact.

- **Tip:** Look for an **overweight female** complaining of continuous **headaches** whose MRI or CT reveals an **empty sella**.

- No treatment is necessary

Hypopituitarism

- Etiology—pituitary tumors, pituitary surgery, head trauma, radiation, Sheehan syndrome, pituitary apoplexy

Signs and Symptoms of Hypopituitarism	Hormone Deficiency
Loss of muscle mass	Growth hormone
Amenorrhea, loss of libido, erectile dysfunction	FSH/LH
Cold intolerance, weight gain, or constipation	TSH
Fatigue, nausea, vomiting, weight loss, abdominal pain	ACTH
Polyuria, polydipsia	ADH

  ► When related to **mass effect**, generally predictable **progression** of symptoms and signs: GH decreases first → then prolactin **increases** → then FSH/LH decreases → then TSH decreases → finally, ACTH decreases

Sheehan syndrome

- Etiology—postpartum infarction (1 in 10,000 deliveries) of pituitary with hemorrhagic necrosis usually due to **severe postpartum hemorrhage**

- Clinical—can cause panhypopituitarism or just one hormone deficiency; typical case scenario is a postpartum woman with sudden onset of **fatigue, weight loss**, and **inability to lactate** days to weeks after delivery

Pituitary apoplexy

- Etiology—sudden hemorrhagic infarction of a pituitary tumor; patients with DM, taking warfarin, or with recent radiation therapy are at highest risk

- Symptoms—sudden onset of **severe headache, nausea and vomiting**, meningismus, vertigo, altered consciousness, and **diplopia**

- Diagnosis—CT scan or MRI (more sensitive) shows evidence of bleeding into the pituitary

- Management—emergency surgery to decompress is best if presentation is severe; mild cases can be treated with steroids

4

GH deficiency

- Etiology—most common cause is mass effect of pituitary adenoma

- Clinical—hyperlipidemia, central obesity, increased waist-to-hip ratio, decreased lean body mass

- Diagnosis—best initial test is serum IGF-1 → will be low
  - ▸ Best confirmatory test is a low GH level with induced hypoglycemia (insulin tolerance test) **or** low IGF-1 with confirmed deficiencies of three other pituitary hormones

- Management—human recombinant GH

Diabetes insipidus (DI)

- Clinical—**polydipsia** (especially for cold liquids), **polyuria**, and **nocturia** (note that patients with psychogenic polydipsia **do not urinate at night because they are not drinking!**)

- Initial diagnosis—get serum and urine osmolarity and electrolytes
  - ▸ Serum sodium is usually >142 mEq/L
  - ▸ Extremely dilute urine—despite high serum osmolality (a hyperosmolar patient should maximally **concentrate** the urine to preserve water)
  - ▸ Hyperosmolar patients with no evidence of glucosuria and with dilute urine have, by definition, DI or solute diuresis
  - ▸ Best next test is the water deprivation test

Neurogenic (central) DI

- Deficiency of antidiuretic hormone (ADH) **production**
- Water deprivation test: restrict fluids and perform the following:
  1. Plasma vasopressin (AVP) level → inappropriately **low**
  2. Administer SQ vasopressin or intranasal desmopressin; if urine osmolality increases >50% of baseline **within 1–2 hours**, diagnosis is confirmed (central DI)
  3. Next, get MRI of brain—will show lack of a posterior pituitary "bright spot" and a "thickened pituitary stalk"
- Management—desmopressin (DDAVP®) and fluids is the treatment of choice

4

Nephrogenic DI

- Kidneys are **unable to respond** to ADH, so the urine stays dilute despite high ADH levels (be sure to exclude hypercalcemia and lithium-induced DI)
  1. Diagnosis—plasma vasopressin → **normal to elevated**
  2. After administering SQ vasopressin or intranasal desmopressin → no change in urine osmolarity
- Management—thiazide diuretics are first-line agents (includes hydrochlorothiazide, amiloride, or chlorthalidone); they act by decreasing urine flow to the distal tubule; water can be absorbed by the distal collecting duct.

Differential diagnosis of polyuric, polydipsic patients

- Those with DM plus symptoms of primary polydipsia usually maintain a **normal serum sodium + plasma osmolality**; urine will be positive for glucose
- In DM, water intake is adequate to keep up with urinary losses
- In primary polydipsia, renal excretion of water keeps up with oral intake so patients do not become hyperosmolar
- Sodium level rarely helpful unless at extremes
  - ▸ Very low sodium suggests primary polydipsia
  - ▸ Very high sodium suggests DM

THYROID DISEASE

Hypothyroidism

- Primary—disease affects the **thyroid gland**
  - ► Hashimoto thyroiditis (chronic lymphocytic thyroiditis) due to loss of thyroid gland function from **antithyroglobulin and antithyroperoxidase antibodies** against the TSH receptor
    - ▷ Most common cause of hypothyroidism, and affects women 7 times more often than men
    - ▷ **Painless goiter** on physical exam
  - ► Other causes include previous surgery, radiation, iodine deficiency, use of propylthiouracil (PTU)/methimazole, iodine load known as the Wolff-Chaikoff effect

- Secondary—**pituitary** disease

- Signs and symptoms—dementia, **fatigue**, CHF, pericardial effusions, pleural effusions, respiratory depression, chronic **constipation**, ascites, **amenorrhea, galactorrhea** (high circulating TSH), muscle cramps, hyperlipidemia, anemia, **depression**, arthralgia, **dry skin, hair loss, hypertension**, coarse hair, periorbital swelling, hoarse voice, large tongue, cold intolerance, weight gain, carpal tunnel syndrome
  - ► **Tip:** If a patient presents with a **large, diffuse goiter** and **dysphagia**, the best next step is a CT scan of the head, neck, and chest; if the goiter extends into the superior mediastinum, surgical debulking is required.

- Diagnosis—best initial test is serum TSH (high) and free T4 (low)

- Management—oral levothyroxine
  - ► If heart disease, start with a low dose and titrate slowly; otherwise you may precipitate CHF or MI
  - ► Titrate dose to achieve a target TSH of 2; in elderly patients, titrate to a TSH of 6
  - ► **Tip:** Levothyroxine replacement **does not** cause weight loss!
  - ► **Tip:** Celiac disease is associated with poor levothyroxine assorption!

Myxedema coma

- Etiology—due to severe hypothyroidism
- Clinical—**altered mental status, hypothermia**, hyponatremia, hypoventilation
- Diagnosis—clinical
- Management—treat aggressively with **IV T4 or IV T3** (peripheral conversion of T4 may be poor) and hydrocortisone IV until adrenal insufficiency is ruled out

Subclinical hypothyroidism

- Clinical—asymptomatic
- Diagnosis—TSH is mildly depressed with a normal free T4; may also occur with incomplete treatment of primary hypothyroidism
- Treatment with levothyroxine indicated if: TSH >10, positive antithyroperoxidase antibodies, menstrual changes, pregnant or planning to become pregnant

Hyperthyroidism

- Clinical syndromes
  - ► Graves disease
    - ▷ Etiology—autoimmune production of thyroid-stimulating antibodies
    - ▷ Clinical—diffuse goiter, **ophthalmopathy**, and **dermopathy** are hallmarks; look for other autoimmune disorders in the history
    - ▷ Diagnosis—decreased TSH, increased free T4, increased radioactive iodine uptake (RAIU), and **antimicrosomal and antithyroglobulin antibodies**
  - ► Toxic multinodular goiter (Plummer disease)
    - ▷ Etiology—autonomously functioning thyroid nodules
    - ▷ Clinical—look for an enlarged, nodular thyroid gland
  - ► Excessive iodine (Jod-Basedow effect) from IV contrast, amiodarone, and kelp
  - ► Excessive exogenous thyroid hormone ingestion

4

- Signs and symptoms—CHF, **emotionally unstable with anxiety and panic attacks,** irregular menses, weakness, fatigue, **hair loss, weight loss, polyphagia,** excessive **sweating, palpitations, diarrhea,** conjunctivitis, diplopia, **osteopenia,** and gynecomastia
  - ► **Tip:** Always check thyroid function tests (TFTs) in any patient with new onset **A-flutter** or **A-fib.**

- Labs—anemia, thrombocytopenia, elevated alkaline phosphatase, mild hypercalcemia, low cholesterol, low HDL

- Management—**first,** start **beta-blockers** to control the B-adrenergic symptoms; then start a **thionamide** (either PTU or methimazole); if the patient is pregnant, PTU is the drug of choice
  - ► Once disease is controlled, may schedule radioactive iodine ablation if desired—the patient may need oral levothyroxine for life (gland destruction usually results in hypothyroidism)
  - ► Subtotal thyroidectomy is preferred over ablation in pregnant women and should be done after the second trimester; it is also indicated in failure of medical therapy or in massive goiter causing compression of neck/thoracic structures

Subclinical hyperthyroidism

- Clinical—no symptoms but at increased risk of osteoporosis and A-fib
- Labs—mildly depressed TSH, normal fT4 (free T4)
- Management—see table

Subacute thyroiditis

- Etiology—unique syndrome due to post-viral inflammation of the thyroid
- Clinical—patients complain initially of neck pain and tenderness, fever, and hyperthyroid symptoms, then of transient hypothyroidism
- Labs—depressed RAIU
- Management—steroids and NSAIDs

Thyroid storm

- Clinical—delerium, psychosis, fever, A-fib or CHF
- Management—steroids, beta-blockers, PTU, iodine

Treatment of Hyperthyroidism

Tip: Beta-blockers (atenolol or propranolol) can be used in all symptomatic patients to control the sympathetic nervous system symptoms.	
Subclinical hyperthyroidism	Methimazole if TSH <0.1 µU/mL
Graves disease	• Methimazole or PTU • **Avoid** radioactive iodine (risk of worsening ophthalmopathy, unless pretreated with CS) • Thyroidectomy for severe cases
Toxic multinodular goiter	Treat like Graves disease
Subacute thyroiditis	NSAIDs or corticosteroids
Thyroid storm	PTU, iodine-potassium solutions, corticosteroids, and beta-blockers
Pregnancy	• PTU is preferred; **avoid** methimazole (known teratogen/category D) • **Avoid** radioactive iodine (also ablates fetal thyroid tissue)

4

Sick Euthyroid Syndrome

- Etiology—medical illness causes dysfunction of the thyroid
- Labs—decreased secretion of TSH, altered metabolism of T4 → T3 (increase reverse T3), low-normal free T4 (can occasionally be lower or higher) and low T3; during the recovery phase, TSH may be mildly elevated
    - **Tip:** Your clue to getting this right on the test is a low serum T3, **increased rT3** (reverse T3); T4 concentrations are variable.
- Diagnosis often confused with hypothyroidism

Management of Thyroid Nodules

- Best initial step is serum TFTs
    - If all are normal—diagnosis is nonfunctioning thyroid nodule → you must exclude malignancy

- ▸ If TSH is low—most likely diagnosis is toxic multinodular goiter → get thyroid scintigraphy
- ▸ If TSH is high—most likely diagnosis is Hashimoto thyroiditis → get serum anti-thyroperoxidase antibodies
- When **TFTs are normal**, the next best step is **fine-needle aspiration (FNA) biopsy**
  - ▸ 10–15% of samples will be inadequate; 85% are benign adenomatoid, cellular, or cystic cells
    - ▹ Follicular carcinoma **cannot** be diagnosed through FNA, but papillary carcinoma can
  - ▸ Malignant cytology—next step is surgical resection
  - ▸ Indeterminate cytology—next step is thyroid scintigraphy
    - ▹ If nodule is cold (i.e., nonfunctioning)—proceed to surgery
    - ▹ If nodule is hot (i.e., functioning)—observe
  - ▸ Benign cytology—next step is clinical observation
  - ▸ **Tips:**
    - ▹ Papillary carcinoma can be diagnosed by FNA; follicular carcinoma cannot.
    - ▹ Serum thyroglobulin is not helpful in distinguishing benign from malignant.
    - ▹ Order serum calcitonin if hypercalcemia, family history of thyroid cancer, or MEN2.
  - ▸ Nondiagnostic—next step is repeat FNA or ultrasound-guided FNA
- Benign and malignant cells are cytologically identical in follicular neoplasms

Thyroid Cancers

Papillary carcinoma

Most common type, usually slow-growing and spreads via the lymphatics. Most important risk factor is **previous radiation exposure**—look for a patient with previous head and neck irradiation for cancer.

Follicular carcinoma

More common in the **elderly**; early hematogenous spread.

Anaplastic carcinoma

Extremely poor prognosis; seen in the **elderly**, and **directly invades head and neck structures**.

ADRENAL GLAND

Normal Adrenal Physiology

Adrenal cortex

3 Zones	Hormone secreted	Control/feedback
Glomerulosa: "Salt"	Aldosterone (mineralocorticoid)	Sympathetic nervous system (stress, baroreceptors, etc.), decreased renal perfusion or hypokalemia → activates renin-angiotensin system → angiotensin II
Fasciculata: "Sugar"	Cortisol (glucocorticoid)	Negative feedback to hypothalamus inhibits CRH secretion Negative feedback to pituitary inhibits ACTH secretion
Reticularis: "Sex"	DHEA and androgens	Negative feedback to hypothalamus inhibits GnRH secretion Negative feedback to pituitary inhibits FSH and LH secretion

Abbreviations: adrenocorticotropic hormone, ACTH; corticotropin-releasing hormone, CRH; dehydroepiandrosterone, DHEA; follicle-stimulating hormone, FSH; gonodotropin-releasing hormone, GnRH; luteinizing hormone, LH

Adrenal medulla

Secretes epinephrine and is under direct sympathetic nervous system control (stress, etc.).

Adrenal Gland Disorders

Cushing syndrome

- Etiology—excess cortisol production or excess exogenous ingestion of glucocorticoids

- Endogenous hypercortisolism is divided into:
  - ACTH-dependent
    - Bilateral adrenal enlargement
    - 80% → ACTH-secreting pituitary adenoma (known as **Cushing disease**)
    - 10% → ectopic production of ACTH by a tumor (including bronchial carcinoid, small-cell lung cancer, pheochromocytoma, and medullary thyroid cancer)
  - ACTH-independent
    - Most common cause is exogenous glucocorticoid ingestion
    - 10% → **cortisol**-secreting tumor
- Adrenal adenoma—usually secretes only cortisol
- Signs and symptoms
  - Excessive cortisol → depression
  - Osteoporosis → fractures
  - Increased catabolism and hypokalemia → muscle weakness and **proximal muscle loss**
  - Abnormal fat deposits cause characteristic **moon facies**, fat pads (cervicodorsal [**buffalo hump**], supraclavicular), and **central obesity** with thin arms and legs
  - **Facial plethora**
  - Loss of adequate connective tissue → ecchymoses, easy bruisability, purple abdominal striae
  - Peripheral insulin resistance and activation of gluconeogenesis → hyperglycemia
  - Increased serum ACTH → hyperpigmentation (not seen with exogenous ingestion)
  - Inhibition of immune function → frequent infections
  - HTN
- Diagnosis
  - Best test initial test is a 1-mg overnight dexamethasone suppression test (has a lower accuracy, since ACTH and cortisol levels fluctuate throughout the day) or a 24-hour urinary free cortisol

- 8-mg dexamethasone suppression test is the best next step to determine the cause of Cushing syndrome (if the previous tests are abnormal)
  - ▷ If ACTH is suppressed—diagnosis is pituitary adenoma
  - ▷ If ACTH is not suppressed—diagnosis is ectopic ACTH-producing tumor or adrenal tumor
    - – Next step is plasma ACTH
      ACTH is high → ectopic ACTH production (adenoma or other source); next step in management is CT chest (to rule out lung cancer) and MRI of brain (to rule out adenoma); if testing fails to reveal source → inferior petrosal sinus biopsy is a last resort (this is also the gold standard)
      ACTH is low → adrenal gland is the source; next step in management is abdominal CT scan
      - Adrenal hyperplasia
      - Adrenal tumor

- Management—surgical resection if the cause is due to tumor (pituitary, adrenal, extra-adrenal)
  - If not surgically resectable—oral ketoconazole, metyrapone, etomidate, or mitodrine

Adrenal insufficiency

- Etiology—low serum cortisol
  - Most common cause is sudden withdrawal of exogenous glucocorticoids (if given >2 weeks)
  - Primary adrenal insufficiency due to disease of adrenal glands
    - ▷ Results in loss of all three layers of cortex (glomerulosa, fasciculata, reticularis)
    - ▷ Due to autoimmune destruction (MCC: **Addison disease**), surgical removal, trauma, bilateral adrenal hemorrhage (anticoagulant use, Waterhouse-Friderichsen syndrome), infection (**tuberculosis**, fungal)
  - Secondary adrenal insufficiency due to insufficient ACTH
    - ▷ Zona glomerulosa remains intact, so aldosterone is **unaffected → volume and potassium are normal**
    - ▷ Due to pituitary disease (see Hypopituitarism, page 69)

- Signs/symptoms—weakness/fatigue, anorexia, nausea, diarrhea, abdominal pain, fever, **sparse body hair**, orthostatic hypotension, hypoglycemia, weight loss, hyperkalemia, hyponatremia
  - ▸ Hyperpigmentation seen in **primary disease** → due to increased circulating ACTH precursor POMC (proopiomelanocortin) which contains melanocyte-stimulating hormone (MSH) → affects the palmar creases, sun-exposed skin, nipples, scars, buccal mucosa, gingiva, and lips

- Diagnosis
  - ▸ Best initial test is early morning plasma cortisol and ACTH levels before and after ACTH (cosyntropin) stimulation
    - ▹ Normal response is cortisol level >18 µg/dL
    - ▹ Low cortisol + high ACTH = primary adrenal insufficiency → order CT scan of adrenal gland
    - ▹ Low cortisol + normal to low ACTH = secondary (pituitary) or tertiary (hypothalamic) insufficiency → order MRI of brain

- Management
  - ▸ Acute crisis
    - ▹ Suspected adrenal crisis—draw blood cortisol, ACTH, and renin first; then give aggressive IV fluid hydration (corrects volume and hyponatremia) → high-dose IV dexamethasone → remeasure serum cortisol to establish a diagnosis after ACTH suppression
    - ▹ Suspected adrenal crisis in known patients with adrenal insufficiency—above **plus** IV hydrocortisone (takes several days for effect and alters future serum testing); remeasurement is not needed
    - ▹ **Warning:** If the patient has both adrenal and thyroid insufficiency (Schmidt syndrome), management **must** be glucocorticoid replacement, before starting oral levothyroxine, or you **will precipitate adrenal crisis**

► Chronic management

  ▷ Instruct patient on need for stress-dose steroids during infections, surgery, or other stressors

  ▷ Oral replacement with glucocorticoid (hydrocortisone, dexamethasone, or prednisone) for both primary and secondary adrenal insufficiency; plus mineralocorticoid replacement (fludrocortisones) for primary disease **only**

Hypoaldosteronism

- Etiology
  ► Primary causes
    ▷ Hyperreninemic hypoaldosteronism due to loss of adrenal gland function in Addison disease, severe infection, trauma, hemorrhage, surgical resection

    ▷ Inhibition of aldosterone release by ACE inhibitors (due to a decrease in angiotensin [AT]-II)

  ► Secondary causes
    ▷ Hyporeninemic hypoaldosteronism due to loss of renin secretion, seen in type IV renal tubular acidosis (RTA), loss of kidneys, NSAIDs, beta-blockers

- Clinical—hyperkalemia, metabolic acidosis, and hypotension

- Management—oral fludrocortisone (mineralocorticoid)

Hyperaldosteronism

- Clinical—hypokalemia, metabolic alkalosis, and HTN

- **Primary** disorder—adrenal gland is producing **excess aldosterone**

  ► *Hypo*reninemic hyperaldosteronism due to **Conn syndrome** (adrenal adenoma/aldosteronoma), adrenocortical carcinoma, or bilateral hyperplasia (rare)

- **Secondary** disorder—excess **renin** causing excess secretion of aldosterone

  ► *Hyper*reninemic hyperaldosteronism due to renin-secreting tumor or renal artery stenosis

- Diagnosis—diastolic HTN without edema
  - ▶ Best initial test is plasma renin
    - ▷ Primary → **low renin** that fails to increase with volume depletion and high aldosterone
    - ▷ Secondary → high aldosterone that **fails to suppress with saline load** and **high renin**
  - ▶ Best next test is plasma aldosterone-to-renin ratio while patient is supine and hydrated
    - ▷ Plasma ratio >30 is diagnostic of primary disorders
    - ▷ Plasma ratio <10 is diagnostic of secondary disorders
- Management
  - ▶ Primary—surgery for aldosteronoma is first-line treatment; oral spironolactone or eplerenone is first-line therapy for bilateral hyperplasia or surgically nonresectable adenomas
  - ▶ Secondary—angioplasty/stent for renal artery stenosis; surgical resection is first-line for adrenal carcinoma; use oral mitotane if not resectable

Apparent mineralocorticoid excess

- Clinical—hypokalemia, metabolic alkalosis, HTN, and **low renin**
- Similar to primary hyperaldosteronism but will also have **low serum aldosterone**
- Diagnosis—high levels of deoxycorticosterone due to deficiency of 11-B-hydroxysteroid dehydrogenase

Pheochromocytoma

- Mnemonic—remember the 10's: 10% are bilateral, 10% are extra-adrenal, and 10% are malignant
- Familial type—seen in multiple endocrine neoplasia (MEN) type 2, von Hippel-Lindau disease, neurofibromatosis type II, familial carotid body tumors
- Symptoms and signs—due to **excess catecholamines;**
  - ▶ Mnemonic— remember the P's: Pallor, Palpitations, Panic, Pounding headache, Perspiration, abdominal Pain, high blood Pressure

- Diagnosis
  - ► Best initial test—random **plasma free metanephrine and normetanephrine** (simpler with better sensitivity and specificity) or 24-hour urine collection for catecholamines, vanillylmandelic acid (VMA), and metanephrines
    - ▷ If either of these is equivocal and your suspicion is high, perform a clonidine suppression test (serum epinephrine should decrease; if not, you have your diagnosis)
  - ► Best next step—localize tumor with CT or MRI of abdomen → metaiodobenzylguanidine (MIGB); ^{123}I-MIGB or ^{131}I-scan if CT or MRI fails to localize the tumor (helpful in extra-adrenal tumors)
- Management—**you must control the blood pressure**
  - ► Definitive management is surgery to remove tumor; is curable in up to 90% of patients; initiate alpha-, then beta-blockade at least **10–14 days** before surgery
  - ► First, **alpha-blockade** (phenoxybenzamine or phentolamine) and IV fluids (majority of patients are volume-depleted); may also use doxazosin or nicardipine
  - ► After euvolemic—add a **beta-blocker** to control HTN and reflex tachycardia
  - ► Intraoperative control of BP is best accomplished with nitroprusside or phentolamine

Multiple endocrine neoplasia (MEN)

- MEN syndromes are due to autosomal dominant inheritance
- MEN type 1
  - ► Adenomas of at least two of the following (two of the three P's):
    - ▷ **P**ituitary—any secretory pituitary tumor
    - ▷ **P**arathyroid—primary hyperparathyroidism
    - ▷ **P**ancreatic or gastric tumors (often malignant)—gastrinoma, insulinoma, glucagonoma, serotonin, VIPoma

- MEN type 2
  - ► Medullary thyroid cancer
  - ► Pheochromocytoma
    - ▷ Plus parathyroid disease → MEN-2A is your diagnosis
    - ▷ Plus ganglioneuroma → MEN-2B is your diagnosis
  - ► Hyperparathyroidism
  - ► Always check RET-oncogene

Hypogonadism

- Symptoms—fatigue, poor libido, hot flushes, erectile depfunction, gynecomastia

Primary male hypogonadism

- Diagnosis—low serum testosterone (<200 mg/dL), high LH/FSH
- Etiology—trauma, infection (bilateral orchitis, as seen in mumps), radiation, chemotherapy, autoimmune disease of the testes, cryptorchidism, Klinefelter syndrome

Secondary male hypogonadism

- Diagnosis—low serum testosterone, low to normal LH/FSH
- Etiology—Kallmann syndrome and other pituitary/ hypothalamic disorders, uremia, granulomatous disease, hemochromatosis
- Management
  - ► ≤60 years—transdermal, buccal, or IM testosterone replacement (periodically screen for erythrocytosis and prostate cancer)
  - ► >60 years—treatment of patients with no clear, identifiable hypopituitary/thalamic disease is still controversial

Disorders of Glucose Metabolism

Metabolic syndrome

- Etiology—insulin resistance
- Diagnosis—need at least three of the following (ATP III criteria)
  - ► Fasting blood sugar (FBS) between 100 and 125 mg/dL (intermediate DM)

- ▸ Blood pressure greater than either 135 mm Hg systolic or 85 mm Hg diastolic
- ▸ HDL <40 mg/dL for males or <50 mg/dL for females
- ▸ Triglyceride >150 mg/dL
- ▸ Obesity measured by waist >40 inches for males, >35 inches for females
- Acanthosis nigricans is a sign of insulin resistance
- Management—best initial step is therapeutic lifestyle changes (TLCs) and modify risk factors if they persist (e.g., add a statin if LDL remains high)

Diabetes mellitus (DM)

Diagnosis and etiology of DM

- May be diagnosed four ways (any of these may be used):
  1. A random glucose >200 mg/dL
  2. A 2-hour 75-g oral glucose tolerance test >200 mg/dL
  3. An FBS >126 mg/dL, which must be confirmed on a subsequent day
  4. HgA1c ≥ 6.5%

Types of DM

	Type 1 DM	Type 2 DM	Gestational DM	MODY
Prevalence	10%	90%	7% of pregnancies	1–2%
Onset	Sudden	Gradual	Gradual	Gradual
Age at onset	Usually children	Usually adults	Reproductive years	Adults
Usual presentation	DKA	Polyuria, polydipsia	At first obstetric visit or screening at 24–28 weeks	Typically asymptomatic, some forms are symptomatic
Autoantibodies	Anti-GAD	Absent	Absent	• Absent • Diagnose by **specific gene testing**
Treatment	Insulin	TLCs, oral agents, or insulin	TLCs alone or insulin (preferred)	TLCs, oral agents, or insulin

Abbreviations: anti-glutamic acid decarboxylase antibodies, anti-GAD; diabetic ketoacidosis, DKA; maturity onset diabetes of the young, MODY; therapeutic lifestyle changes, TLCs (e.g., diet, exercise, weight loss)

4

Complications of DM

- Microvascular—retinopathy (aneurysms, dot hemorrhages, retinal detachments, macular edema), peripheral neuropathy, symmetric polyneuropathy, mononeuropathy, autonomic dysfunction (impotence, tachycardia, gastroparesis), glomerulopathy → proteinuria

- Macrovascular—coronary artery disease, cerebrovascular disease, peripheral vascular disease

- Acute metabolic complications → diabetic ketoacidosis and hyperosmolar nonketotic coma (HONC)

4

Important phenomena of DM

- Honeymoon effect—initial glucotoxicity on beta cells inhibits insulin secretion; aggressive glucose control with insulin may restore some remaining beta-cell function → patient may develop hypoglycemia from increased endogenous insulin, so strict glucose monitoring and decreased insulin dose are mandatory

- Dawn phenomenon—hyperglycemia prior to awakening due to early morning rise in cortisol

- Somogyi effect—early morning rise in glucose due to nocturnal hypoglycemia; look for signs of nocturnal hypoglycemia: night sweats, nightmares, restless sleep, nonrestorative sleep; manage by decreasing evening insulin

Monitoring DM

- Glycosylated hemoglobin (Hgb) reflects the past 3–4 months of glucose control; this is the preferred method of monitoring glucose control
- Fructosamine (glycosylated albumin) shows the past 3 weeks of glucose control

Treatment of DM

- Outpatient treatment of type I DM—insulin

Insulin

Type	Onset	Peak	Duration
Rapid-acting insulin (lispro, aspart, glulisine)	5–15 min	45–90 min	2–4 hr
Short-acting insulin (regular)	30–60 min	2–4 hr	4–8 hr
Intermediate insulin (NPH)	1–3 hr	4–10 hr	10–18 hr
Basal insulin (glargine, detemir)	1–3 hr	NONE	20–24 hr

Abbreviations: neutral protamine Hagedorn, NPH

Management of diabetic ketoacidosis (DKA) and hyperosmolar nonketotic coma (HONC)

- Diagnosis of DKA—symptoms of nausea and vomiting, **abdominal pain**, hyperglycemia >**250 mg/dL, increased anion gap metabolic acidosis** (serum bicarbonate <18 and arterial pH <7.30); increased serum **beta-hydroxybutyrate, acetoacetate**, and **acetone**; and increased amylase/lipase (unknown causes)

- Underlying infections, acute MI, and non-adherence are the most common precipitator of attacks

- Diagnosis of HONC—**neurologic abnormalities** may progress to coma, profound dehydration, hyperglycemia usually >**600–1,000 mg/dL,** plasma osmolality >330 mOsmol/kg, **pH >7.30**, serum bicarbonate >20 mEq/L, profound dehydration, **minimal to no** ketoacidosis

- Management of volume status
  - ▸ Patients are extremely dehydrated (most are behind 3–6 L in DKA and 8–10 L of fluids in HONC) and volume restoration is the initial step in management → start IV normal saline bolus of 1–2 L, then maintenance fluids

- Management of hyperglycemia
  - ▸ Bolus 0.1 units/kg of regular insulin IV push, then an insulin drip at a rate of 0.1 units/kg/hour
  - ▸ Finger sticks are mandatory every hour

- When the blood glucose is ≤**250 mg/dL,** change IV to a **D5-containing** (D5W or D5 1\2 normal saline) solution
- Continue the insulin drip until the anion gap is closed (ketoacids can be converted to bicarbonate only in the presence of insulin); then overlap with subcutaneous insulin by at least 1 hour

- Management of hypokalemia
  - Although potassium on chem 7 may be high, total body potassium (K) is depleted
  - If K is <3.3 mEq/dL, hold insulin (worsens hypokalemia) and replace K until reaches >3.3 mEq/dL
  - **KCl** must be added to **½ normal saline** (creating an isotonic solution) running at a rate of 20–30 mEq of KCl/hour if the serum K is ≤**5.3 mEq/dL**

- Management of acidosis—bicarbonate should be added to IV fluids only if the pH is <7.10 (applies to DKA patients only)

Outpatient treatment of type 2 diabetics

- Best initial step in management of the newly diagnosed type 2 diabetic is to start TLCs (i.e., weight loss and exercise) and metformin
  - If metformin + TLCs fail—add either insulin or a second oral agent, or switch to insulin therapy alone
    - Insulin therapy alone is preferred in end-stage renal disease (ESRD)
    - If adding a second oral agent, choose a GLP-1 agonist or a DPP-4 inhibitor
      - If dual therapy does not achieve the HgA1C goal, add either a TZD or sulfonylurea as a third agent
    - If adding insulin to oral therapy, choose a long-acting insulin at bedtime

- Mechanism of oral agents
  - Biguanides (metformin)—reduces hepatic gluconeogenesis, stimulates peripheral glucose utilization, reduces intestinal glucose absorption

▷ Beware of **lactic acidosis** (especially if serum creatinine >1.4 in females or >1.5 in males)

▷ Avoid in—chronic renal failure (CRF), hepatic disease, CHF, COPD, and alcohol abuse

▶ Sulfonylureas (glipizide, glyburide, glimepiride)—stimulates insulin secretion from beta cells in pancreas; expect a 2% drop in HgbA1C

▷ Most frequently associated with **hypoglycemia**

▶ Thiazolidinediones "-glitazones" (rosiglitazone, pioglitazone)—improve insulin resistance and pancreatic beta-cell function

▷ May precipitate **acute CHF exacerbations**, especially in those with underlying CHF and **bone loss**

▶ Rapid-acting secretagogues (nateglinide)—very short half-life, cause immediate release of insulin

▶ Incretins (exenatide)

▷ GLP-1—SQ administration BID; reduces gastric emptying, causing early satiety; stimulates insulin secretion; and inhibits glucagon secretion

▷ Causes **nausea** in 30% of patients

▶ Dipeptidyl peptidase-4 inhibitors (sitagliptin)—inhibits the enzyme that metabolizes GLP-1; oral administration

▶ Alpha-glucosidase inhibitors (acarbose, miglitol)—inhibit the enzyme that digests complex carbohydrates

▷ Most common side effect—abdominal cramping

DISORDERS OF CALCIUM

Hypercalcemia

- Serum calcium = bound (chiefly to albumin) and free fractions 50/50

- Corrected serum calcium = add 0.8 mg to serum calcium for every 1 g of albumin <4 mg

- Urine calcium-to-creatinine ratio (more precise method to assess urinary calcium excretion)

- Diagnosed from a urine spot sample
  - ‣ <0.01 = familial benign hypocalciuric hypercalcemia (FHH)
  - ‣ >0.02 = primary hyperparathyroidism

Urinary calcium excretion

- Primary hyperparathyroidism → >4 mg/kg
- Signs and symptoms—osteopenia, resorption of distal phalanges, bone cysts, tapering of distal clavicle, nephrolithiasis, nephrocalcinosis

Primary hyperparathyroidism

- Most common cause is a single adenoma; multiple adenomas cause 10%; hyperplasia in MEN syndrome and rarely parathyroid cancer
- Diagnosis—high serum calcium, low serum phosphate, and **elevated intact parathyroid hormone (PTH) (seen only in FHH and primary hyperparathyroidism**; in all other cases it will be low)
- Management
  - ‣ Surgical exploration and resection indicated if: serum calcium >12 mg/dL, urine calcium excretion >400 mg/day, nephrolithiasis, osteitis fibrosa cystica, low bone density (T score lower than –2), or age <50 years
  - ‣ Medical management indicated if: surgery is contraindicated, serum calcium <12, and patient is asymptomatic
    - ▹ First-line therapy is **bisphosphates**; also recommend decreasing dietary calcium to <400 mg/day, drinking 2–3 L of water per day (if possible), and administering phosphate replacement

Familial benign hypocalciuric hypercalcemia (FHH)

- Rare autosomal dominant disorder
- Partial inactivating mutation of calcium-sensing receptor → resets PTH release leading to ↑ PTH when calcium levels are normal

- Has exactly the same presentation as primary hyperparathyroidism **except urinary calcium excretion is <200 mg/day** with normal serum creatinine
- Look for a family history of "failed" parathyroid surgery or asymptomatic, mild hypercalcemia
- Usually doesn't require treatment, but should recognize syndrome to avoid unnecessary surgery

Other Hypercalcemia Disorders

- Hypercalcemia of malignancy is due to secretion of PTH-related protein seen especially in squamous cell carcinomas; diagnosis with history of malignancy and high serum calcium
  - ▸ Bisphosphonates are the mainstay of therapy

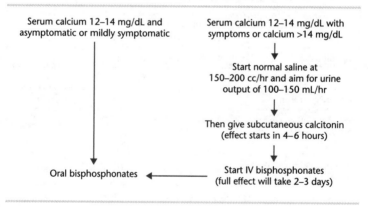

Management of Hypercalcemia

- Hypercalcemia in granulomatous disease due to macrophages containing 1-alpha-hydroxylase and seen in tuberculosis, sarcoidosis, histoplasmosis, berylliosis, and silicone breast implants
- Thiazides, vitamin D intoxication, vitamin A intoxication, immobilization, and lithium all cause hypercalcemia

Milk alkali syndrome

- Symptoms—hypercalcemia, metabolic alkalosis, and renal failure
- Most common cause is calcium carbonate; this combination decreases renal excretion of calcium and HCO_3
- Pathogenesis—PTH is suppressed → decreased phosphate clearance → hyperphosphatemia → nephrocalcinosis → renal failure
- Management—stop the offending drug

Secondary Hyperparathyroidism

High PTH with low or low-normal serum calcium

Hypercalcemia (>10 mg/dL)

	Serum PTH	Serum P	Serum 25 VitD	Serum 1,25 VitD
Primary hyperparathyroidism	N or ⇑	N or ⇓	N	N or ⇑
Malignancy secreting PTHrP	⇓	N or ⇓	N	N or ⇓
Multiple myeloma	⇓	N or ⇑	N	N or ⇓
Sarcoidosis	⇓	N or ⇑	N	⇑
Vitamin D intoxication	⇓	N or ⇑	⇑⇑⇑	N or ⇑
Hyperthyroidism	⇓	N	N	N
Familial hypocalciuric hypercalcemia (FHH)— very rare	N or ⇑	⇓	N	N
Immobilization or Paget disease of the bone	⇓	N or ⇑	N	N or ⇓

Abbreviations: 1,25 dihydroxycholecalciferol, 1,25 VitD; 25 hydroxycholecalciferol, 25 VitD; parathyroid hormone-related peptide, PTHrP

Hypocalcemia

- Signs and symptoms—neuromuscular irritability, **prolonged QT** interval, **numbness**, cramps, fatigue, anxiety, depression
- Etiology—primary hypoparathyroidism, accidental surgical removal of **all parathyroid glands**, autoimmune destruction of parathyroids, magnesium deficiency (required for PTH release and action), hungry bone syndrome, and vitamin D deficiency

- ▶ **Tip:** Prolonged primary hyperparathyroidism → very calcium-depleted bones will take up calcium when parathyroid(s) resected.
  - ▷ Look for a patient who is immediately post-op after parathyroid or thyroid resection and has the above symptoms
- Pseudohypoparathyroidism—defect in PTH receptor → low calcium, high phosphate, high PTH
- Pseudohypocalcemia—low calcium but normal ionized calcium, due to low albumin levels
  - ▶ Calcium will be normal when corrected for the low albumin (add 0.8 mg to serum calcium for each 1 g of albumin below 4 g)

Paget Disease

- Clinical—bony deformities cause **bowing of legs**, and **increased skull growth** compresses cranial nerve (CN) VIII → **deafness**
  - ▶ Erythema, pain, and warmth over affected sites
- Labs—elevated **alkaline phosphatase**
  - ▶ **Tip:** Look for an older patient with **normal calcium**, no history of liver disease, and an isolated increase in serum alkaline phosphatase.
  - ▶ X-ray evidence does not reflect metabolic activity, but the classic test question mentions a skull x-ray with a **"hair-on-end"** or **"cotton wool"** appearance
  - ▶ Most sensitive test—bone scan; will detect more lesions than x-rays, and shows multiple "hot spots"
- Diagnosis—positive bone scan plus high alkaline phosphatase confirms the diagnosis
- Indications for treatment—pain, deformity, fracture, skull or weight-bearing joint involvement, neurologic complications (CN palsies, etc.)
- Management—bisphosphonates are first-line; if not tolerated → calcitonin

4

III. GASTROENTEROLOGY

ESOPHAGEAL DISORDERS

- General approach to GI symptoms—**any patient with alarm symptoms** should **always** have upper **endoscopy as the first step in management**

- Alarm symptoms—age >45 years, progressive weight loss, anemia, melena, hematemesis, strong family history of malignancy, or **progressive** dysphagia

Symptoms Suggestive of Oropharyngeal/Gastrointestinal Disorders

	Common Etiologies	Keys to Diagnosis
Dysphagia: "difficulty swallowing"	• Oropharyngeal • Esophageal (see below)	**Solids** only? → think **structural** **Liquids first?** → think **motility** Weight loss? → think **cancer**
Odynophagia: "painful swallowing"	• Infectious esophagitis (*Candida albicans*, CMV, HSV, HPV, TB) • GERD • Pill-induced • Exposure to radiation	Oral thrush (present in >50% candidal esophagitis) Immunosuppressed? e.g., corticosteroids (inhaled or systemic), TNF inhibitors, chemotherapy, AIDS Pill-induced (tetracycline, iron sulfate, bisphosphonates, potassium, NSAIDs, quinidine)
Chest pain, noncardiac	• Esophageal spasm • GERD	Persists >1 hr Typically postprandial Usually lacks radiation
Globus sensation: "feeling a lump or tightness in the throat"	• Psychological factors • GERD (rare)	Emotional problems Unrelated to meals Transient
Pyrosis: "heartburn"	GERD	Improves with antacids

Abbreviations: cytomegalovirus, CMV; herpes simplex virus, HSV; human papillomavirus, HPV; gastroesophageal reflux disease, GERD; non-steroidal anti-inflammatory drugs, NSAIDs; tuberculosis, TB; tumor necrosis factor inhibitor, TNF inhibitor

Achalasia

- Clinical—dysphagia for **liquids and solids**, nocturnal cough from aspiration, chest pain infrequent

- Diagnosis—best initial test is barium swallow (shows "bird's-beak" appearance of distal esophagus); gold standard is esophageal manometry (shows elevated resting lower esophageal sphincter [LES] pressure, incomplete relaxation of LES and aperistalsis); esophagogastroduodenoscopy (EGD) if alarm symptoms

- Management
  - ▸ Poor operative risk—calcium-channel blocker (CCB) or nitroglycerin is first-line; botulinum toxin injection into LES if medical therapy fails (relief >1 year for some)
  - ▸ Good operative risk—laparoscopic myotomy first-line

Diffuse Esophageal Spasm

- Clinical—**intermittent** dysphagia for **solids and liquids** (especially **cold**); chest pain may radiate to neck and arm like acute MI, but not to jaw and teeth

- Diagnosis—barium swallow is first-line (shows "corkscrew" esophagus); gold standard is esophageal manometry (shows high-amplitude, repetitive contractions)

- Management—trial of proton pump inhibitor (PPI) is first line, CCB, TCA, or antispasmodic agents (e.g., nitric oxide) may be helpful

Gastroesophageal Reflux Disease (GERD)

- Complications—ulcerative esophagitis, bleeding, stricture, Barrett esophagitis, and esophageal cancer

- Clinical—**metallic taste, nocturnal cough**; substernal, burning chest pain; **asthma** or recurrent pneumonia

- Diagnosis—clinical if typical symptoms (go straight to treatment); gold standard is 24-hour esophageal pH monitoring

4

- Management—daily PPI (e.g., omeprazole) is first-line, if no response, you can add an H$_2$ blocker at night; consider surgical management with Nissen fundoplication if the patient cannot be tapered off PPIs

Barrett Esophagus

- Pathophysiology
  - ► Intestinal columnar metaplasia of the distal esophagus secondary to chronic GERD
  - ► 0.5% yearly risk of adenocarcinoma (30- to 50-fold increased risk)
- Management—endoscopic surveillance for cancer
  - ► No dysplasia: 3 years
  - ► Low-grade dysplasia: 6 months, then yearly if no change
  - ► High-grade dysplasia: endoscopic ablation, repeat in 3 months
    - ▷ Esophagectomy is optional
  - ► Tip: PPIs **do not** result in regression of abnormal histology.

Eosinophilic Esophagitis

- A common cause of **chronic solid-food dysphagia** and **food impaction** due to narrow and stiffened esophagus
- Etiology—probably allergic response to food or airborne allergen; male predominance
- Diagnosis—EGD shows mucosal rings, linear furrows, strictures, papules or exudates; **biopsy is key to diagnosis**
  - ► >15 **eosinophils/hpf** in the **upper esophagus** (high eosinophil counts can be seen in lower esophagus of GERD patients, but not in the upper esophagus)
- Management
  - ► **6-food elimination diet** (milk protein, eggs, nuts, seafood, soy, and wheat)

- ▸ Immune modulation: swallow 4 puffs of fluticasone (rinse and spit to prevent thrush, do not eat or drink for 30 minutes)
  - ▸ Duration of treatment: 6 weeks–indefinitely; systemic steroids and taper for refractory disease
- **Esophageal dilation** for severe strictures

Esophageal Cancer

- Clinical—dysphagia to **solids first, liquids later**; odynophagia, weight loss, choking, cervical lymphadenopathy
- Risk factors—smoking, ethanol (ETOH), lye stricture, Plummer-Vinson syndrome, head and neck cancer
- Two clinical types: squamous cell carcinoma and adenocarcinoma; equal in frequency
  - ▸ Squamous cell carcinoma—affects the esophagus, men three times more common, African American, smoking, ETOH abuse
  - ▸ Adenocarcinoma—affects **lower two-thirds** (most commonly at the **gastroesophageal junction**) of the esophagus, men seven times more common, usually with history of chronic GERD (i.e., progression of **Barrett esophagus**)
- Diagnosis—barium swallow is first-line (may show stricture or mass effects; gold standard is EGD with biopsy)
- Management—surgery if localized; neoadjuvant treatment with radiation therapy and combination cis-platin plus 5-FU

Esophageal Varices

- Clinical—**sudden** onset of **painless upper GI bleeding** → hematemesis or melena
- Typically associated with signs of **cirrhosis**—spider angiomata, splenomegaly, hepatomegaly, ascites, palmar erythema
- Acute management
  - ▸ **Start** IV octreotide (somatostatin analogue) **plus** IV ciprofloxacin or ceftriaxone (decreases mortality)

4

> ► **Then** upper endoscopy with sclerotherapy (preferred) or band ligation as soon as possible
>   > ▷ **Note:** If endoscopy is delayed, balloon tamponade may be used temporarily to control bleeding
> ► Transjugular intrahepatic portosystemic shunting (TIPS) only if the above fail

- Long-term management
  - ► Endoscopic band ligation—superior to sclerotherapy for long-term management of varices
  - ► Nonselective beta-blockers decrease portal pressure and prevent variceal bleeding
  - ► TIPS—indicated when the above fail; lowers portal pressure (can cause encephalopathy and liver failure)
  - ► Only cure is liver transplant—to qualify, candidates must have end-stage liver disease, be abstinent from drugs and alcohol for at least 6 months, and have no severe cardiopulmonary disease or extensive malignancy

Mallory-Weiss Syndrome

- Clinical—**continuous retching**, usually after binge-drinking, causes longitudinal tears in the esophageal mucosa → bright-red hematemesis
  - ► **Tip:** Most have concomitant hiatal hernia.
- Diagnosis and management—clinical history is most important → hemodynamically stabilize → upper endoscopy (both diagnostic and therapeutic)

Plummer-Vinson Syndrome

Web located in the **upper esophagus** due to esophagitis, iron deficiency, bullous skin disorders, and pemphigus vulgaris.

Schatzki Ring or "Steakhouse Syndrome"

- Web located at the **gastroesophageal junction**
- Clinical presentation—history of **intermittent dysphagia to solids, especially meat and bread**
- Diagnosis—barium swallow
- Management—endoscopy with balloon dilation

Zenker Diverticulum

- Clinical—**foul-smelling breath** with **oral regurgitation** and **coughing** during meals, and aspiration pneumonia
- Diagnosis—barium swallow is first-line; **avoid** blind endoscopy (may perforate diverticulum)
- Management—surgical repair with resection of the diverticulum, myotomy

Gastric Volvulus

- Paraesophageal and large sliding hiatal hernias
- Occasionally occurs with large hiatal hernias
- Tortuous esophagus and stomach

Acute Gastric Volvulus	Chronic Gastric Volvulus
Sudden, severe pain in upper abdomen	Intermittent epigastric discomfort
Dysphagia (solids only)	Dysphagia (solids only)
Persistent retching	Fullness after eating

4

ACUTE GI BLEEDING

- Upper GI bleeding originates above the ligament of Treitz →
  usually presents as hematemesis (blood or "coffee grounds") or
  melena (black, tarry stool)
  - ▸ Most common causes—peptic ulcers, gastric erosions,
    esophageal varices
  - ▸ Other causes—esophagitis, erosive duodenitis, Mallory-Weiss
    tear, neoplasm, esophageal ulcer, stomal ulcer, Osler-Weber-
    Rendu syndrome (hereditary telangiectasias)
  - ▸ Most bleeding stops spontaneously; exception: acute variceal
    bleeding, which has 30–50% mortality
  - ▸ Syncope and presyncope may occur in severe upper GI bleeding
- Lower GI bleeding originates below the ligament of Treitz
  → usually presents with wine-colored or bright-red blood
  per rectum
  - ▸ Most common cause is diverticulosis, followed by arterio-
    venous malformations (think of Meckel diverticulum in
    young patients)
- Diagnosis—endoscopy should be done within 24 hours or
  immediately if rapid blood loss or variceal bleeding is suspected
- Treatment
  - ▸ Fluid resuscitation with IV crystalloid solution and/or blood
    products
    - ▹ Caution: Hgb and Hct are not reliable indicators of volume
      status
  - ▸ FFP, vitamin K if INR >2; platelet infusion if <40,000/mL
- Discharge—stable Hgb/Hct with a low risk for rebleeding (e.g.,
  clean-based ulcers or Mallory-Weiss tears) can be discharged
  after 12 hours

Management of Acute GI Bleeding

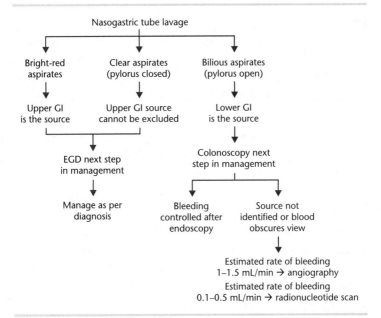

Abbreviations: esophagogastroduodenoscopy, EGD; gastrointestinal, GI

Recurrent GI Bleeding

- When EGD and colonoscopy do not identify a cause → repeat both endoscopies → diagnostic in 40% of cases
- If negative again → suspect **small bowel bleeding**

Small bowel evaluation

- **Wireless capsule endoscopy** can evaluate the entire small bowel, *but only the mucosa is viewed*
- **CT enterography**—evaluates the bowel wall (e.g., vascular tumors)
- Other studies—RBC scanning, angiography, push enteroscopy

STOMACH DISEASE

Dyspepsia

- Clinical—epigastric pain, epigastric burning, postprandial fullness, and early satiety; 75% of cases have no clear underlying cause (termed a functional dyspepsia)

- Diagnosis—above clinical history for 3 months with symptom onset at least 6 months prior to diagnosis

- Management— <50 years without alarm signs → test for *Helicobacter pylori*. If negative, PPI trial for 4–6 weeks.

- If **alarm signs/symptoms** → upper endoscopy

Peptic Ulcer Disease (PUD)

- Includes both gastric and duodenal ulcers

- Risk factors and etiology—***H. pylori* infection** and **NSAIDs are the most common**; also smoking, alcohol, and stress (e.g., emotional, surgery, trauma, burns, mechanical ventilation)

  - ▶ **ICU and trauma** patients should be on **prophylactic PPI** therapy to prevent development of stress ulcers; **proven to decrease mortality** related to GI bleeding

- Clinical—typically **gnawing or burning** epigastric pain, with or without nausea and vomiting

  - ▶ Early satiety

  - ▶ **Gastric ulcer** pain is typically **worse with meals**

  - ▶ Duodenal ulcer pain **improves** with meals and antacids, and increases an hour later (due to rebound hypersecretion of acid)

  - ▶ May have weight loss

- Complications of PUD

  - ▶ **Bleeding**—hematemesis, melena, or hematochezia

  - ▶ **Obstruction**—nausea, vomiting, early satiety, and a succussion splash

  - ▶ **Perforation**—sudden, severe abdominal pain, later peritoneal signs and shock

- Diagnosis
  - If >**50 years** or with **alarm signs/symptoms** → upper endoscopy
  - If <50 years and no alarm signs/symptoms → ***H. pylori* test** and a trial of PPIs or H$_2$ antagonists
- Treatment
  - PPI for 2–4 weeks for duodenal ulcers, 4–8 weeks for gastric ulcers
  - Eradicate *H. pylori* if testing is positive
  - Long-term PPI use if chronic NSAID use is required

4

H. pylori Testing

- Gold standard—gastric mucosal biopsy with rapid urease testing
- Noninvasive tests
  - Best initial tests
    - **Fecal antigen testing**—test of choice for initial testing and eradication (fast, accurate, and cost-effective)
    - IgG serology—serum antibody test for *H. pylori* **remains positive for life**. Do not repeat if there is a need to prove eradication.
  - Best test to **confirm eradication** = stool antigen
    - Urease breath test (less cost-effective)
- **Tip:** *H. pylori* infection is strongly associated with the development of MALT (mucosal associated lymphoid tissue) lymphoma. Treatment of *H. pylori* can cure disease in some!

Dumping Syndrome

- Clinical—symptoms of **bloating**, cramping, abdominal discomfort, and/or **diarrhea** after **gastrectomy**; due to overdistention of the jejunum from excess carbohydrates (early dumping) or hypoglycemia (late dumping)
- Diagnosis—clinical history is sufficient
- Management—encourage well-balanced diet, limit liquids with meals, and **avoid** simple carbohydrates

4

Gastritis

- Clinical—**burning epigastric pain** (with tenderness or discomfort), nausea, and/or anorexia

- Pathophysiology—**NSAIDs, steroids**, viral infection, alcohol, *H. pylori*

- Diagnosis—epigastric tenderness, possible serum test for *H. pylori*

- Management—discontinue offending drugs; try antacids, H_2 blockers or PPI; eradicate *H. pylori* if test is positive

- Refer for EGD if >45 years old or alarm symptoms

Gastroparesis

- Clinical/Pathophysiology—autonomic dysfunction from long-standing DM; symptoms of **early satiety, abdominal bloating**, and **nausea/vomiting**

- Diagnosis—clinical history; gold standard is gastric emptying studies (rarely done)

- Management—small, frequent low-fat meals; avoidance of carbonated beverages and indigestible fiber. May add oral metoclopramide (preferred) or erythromycin (beware of tachyphylaxis).

Management of Helicobacter pylori *Infection*

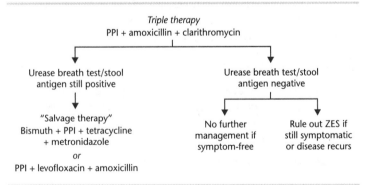

Abbreviations: proton pump inhibitor, PPI; Zollinger-Ellison syndrome, ZES

Zollinger-Ellison Syndrome (ZES)

- Clinical—**recurrent peptic and duodenal ulcers**, but simple duodenal ulcer is most common, diarrhea (30%), family history of MEN syndrome

- EGD—postbulbar (duodenal) and peptic ulcers → seen in ZES (common test question)

- Pathophysiology—**gastrinoma** (65% are malignant)

- Diagnosis
  - ▶ Best initial test—fasting serum gastrin; if >1,000 pg/mL, do gastric pH study; pH <4.0 is diagnostic of ZES
  - ▶ If fasting serum gastrin is not diagnostic (i.e., <1,000 pg/mL)—secretin stimulation test is the best next step; positive test is diagnostic
  - ▶ Once ZES is confirmed—do somatostatin-receptor scan and endoscopic ultrasound (EUS) to localize tumor

- Management—high-dose PPIs is first-line; then surgical resection, if possible
  - ▶ Octreotide is effective in slowing tumor growth

4

COLONIC DISEASE

Colon Polyps

- Hyperplastic polyps—no risk for cancer

- Sessile serrated adenomas— >1 cm, pale, nearly flat, usually right colon
  - ▶ Histologically more similar to hyperplastic polyps than to tubular or villous adenomas, but have *malignant potential* like the adenomas
  - ▶ >50% of patients with multiple large sessile serrated adenomas will have synchronous cancers

Management of Colon Polyps

Condition	Repeat colonoscopy
No dysplasia, completely removed, 1 or 2, and ≤1 cm	5 years
No dysplasia, completely removed, *3 or more or >1 cm*	3 years
Dysplasia or not completely removed	Shorter interval
Villous adenoma	3 years
Colon cancer (resected)	3 years

Colon Cancer

Guidelines for Colon Cancer Surveillance
(from the American Gastroenterological Association)

Risk Stratification	Starting Age	Screening Options
Average risk *No family history or predisposing factors; or family history and relative was >60 years of age at time of diagnosis*	50 years	Either: • Yearly FOBT, **or** • Flexible sigmoidoscopy or double-contrast barium enema every 5 years, **or** • Colonoscopy every 10 years No single test listed above has yet been shown to be superior to the others, but **colonoscopy** is presumed to be the single best test.
Intermediate risk *First-degree relative <60 years of age with colorectal cancer; or two first-degree relatives of any age*	40 years **or** 10 years prior to the age at which the relative was diagnosed	Colonoscopy every 5 years
High risk *Known predisposing factors for colorectal cancer*	*See Screening Options, right*	• Advanced histology or multiple polyps on previous exam—colonoscopy every 3 years • Small or benign polyps on previous exam—colonoscopy every 5 years • History of IBD—colonoscopy every 1–2 years, 8 years after initial diagnosis if pancolitis **or** 15 years after diagnosis with left-sided colitis

Abbreviations: fecal occult blood test, FOBT; inflammatory bowel disease, IBD
Source: *www.gastro.org*

Familial Colon Cancer Syndromes

Diagnosis	Clinical Presentation	Management
Familial adenomatous polyposis	• Mutated **APC gene** • **Hundreds to thousands of colonic adenomas** with malignant transformation by age 45	• Annual sigmoidoscopy starting at age 10–12 years • Colectomy
Gardner syndrome	**FAP plus extraintestinal tumors;** may include nasopharyngeal fibroma, osteoma, lipoma, etc.	Same as FAP
Turcot syndrome	**FAP plus brain tumors** (medulloblastoma most common); also have café-au-lait spots, multiple lipomas/fibromas and basal cell carcinomas	Same as FAP
Peutz-Jeghers syndrome	• Multiple **hyperpigmented spots on lips and buccal mucosa** • Multiple **hamartomous polyps** in stomach, small intestine, and colon • Increased risk of childhood **intussusception**	• Start EGD + colonoscopy at age 8 years • Remove all polyps >1 cm in diameter
Lynch syndrome (hereditary nonpolyposis colorectal cancer)	• Defective **mismatch-repair gene** • Markedly increased risk of **non-colonic tumors,** especially **endometrial cancer**	Colonoscopy every 1–2 years starting either at age 20–25 years or at 10 years earlier than the youngest age of colon cancer diagnosis in the family

Abbreviations: adenomatous polyposis coli, APC; esophagogastroduodenoscopy, EGD; familial adenomatous polyposis, FAP

Note: All hereditary cancer syndromes are transmitted in an autosomal dominant pattern and all patients will have a strong history of premature or multiple malignancies.

Management of colon cancer

- First, determine the extent of spread
  - ▸ If localized to the colon—surgical resection is first-line; then perform colonoscopy in 6 months to confirm eradication

- ▸ If there is a **single metastatic lesion to the liver**—surgical resection is first-line
- ▸ If multiple liver metastases or widely metastasized—chemotherapy is first-line

DIVERTICULAR DISEASE

Diverticulosis and Diverticular Bleeding

- Pathophysiology—increased intraluminal pressure causes sac-like protrusion of the colonic wall at areas of greatest weakness, i.e., the vasa recta → erosion into the vasa recta

- Clinical—sudden onset of bright-red blood per rectum ranging from minimal to massive in volume

- Diagnosis—colonoscopy is the best initial step; may require angiography if massive bleeding

- Management—for further acute management, see Acute GI Bleeding (page 100); for long-term outpatient management, recommend high-fiber diet

Diverticulitis

- Pathophysiology—increased intraluminal pressure or inspissated food particles → microscopic to macroscopic perforation of colonic diverticula → focal necrosis and inflammatory process

- Clinical—classic presentation is an **older patient with left lower quadrant (LLQ) colicky pain and tenderness** for **several days**; labs show leukocytosis
  - ▸ If palpable LLQ mass—think of abscess formation
  - ▸ If generalized abdominal pain and guarding—worry about large perforation → stat upright chest x-ray (to rule out free air)

- Diagnosis—best initial test is abdominal and pelvic CT scan with oral and IV contrast; reveals bowel-wall thickening, fat stranding, and/or abscess formation

- Management
  - ► Complicated diverticulitis
    - ▷ Evidence of perforation or obstruction—broad-spectrum antibiotics, then surgical intervention
    - ▷ Evidence of abscess formation—CT-guided percutaneous drainage is the best initial step; if it fails, then proceed to surgery
  - ► Uncomplicated diverticulitis
    - ▷ NPO with IV fluid hydration and either a (1) a fluoro-quinolone plus metronidazole or (2) a third-generation cephalosporin plus metronidazole
    - ▷ Start a clear liquid diet when abdominal pain and leuko-cytosis improve

LIVER DISEASE

Gilbert Syndrome

- 5–7% of the population
- Indirect hyperbilirubinemia, increases with illness
- Not caused by hemolysis or resolving blood from a hematoma
- Normal Hgb/Hct and reticulocyte count (unlike hemolysis)

Dubin-Johnson Syndrome

- Highest incidence in Iranian Jews
- Jaundiced entire life, but feel perfectly well
- More than half the bilirubin is conjugated

Alpha-1-Antitrypsin Deficiency

- Pathophysiology—severe deficiency results in pulmonary, liver, and skin disease
- Clinical—**panacinar emphysema** in **young** nonsmokers to minimal smokers, **strong family history** of COPD/emphysema, necrotizing **panniculitis** (hot, painful skin nodules), and unexplained **chronic liver disease**

- Diagnosis—clinical history and serum alpha-1-antitrypsin levels
- Management—if severe deficiency plus evidence of COPD, may use pooled human alpha-1-antitrypsin; lung/liver transplant for end-stage disease
- At high risk of developing hepatocellular carcinoma

Cirrhosis and End-Stage Liver Disease

- Pathophysiology—chronic hepatitis from any cause can progress to cirrhosis, i.e., fibrotic liver
- Clinical
  - ▶ Gynecomastia, spider angiomata, and palmar erythema caused by **high circulating estrogens**
  - ▶ Muehrcke nails, peripheral edema, and prolonged bleeding times due to **hypoalbuminemia/hypoproteinemia**
  - ▶ Thrombocytopenia, anemia, and leukopenia due to hypersplenism
- Complications
  - ▶ Variceal hemorrhage—portal hypertension causes esophageal varix formation (see Management of Acute GI Bleeding, page 101)
  - ▶ Ascites
    - ▷ Calculate the serum ascites albumin gradient (SAAG)
      - If >1.1, etiology is **portal hypertension** from liver or cardiac disease (constrictive pericarditis, tricuspid regurgitation, severe heart failure)
      - If <1.1, etiology is **malignancy** or **infection** (e.g., tuberculosis)
  - ▶ Spontaneous bacterial peritonitis (SBP)—idiopathic infection of ascitic fluid; diagnostic criteria are ascitic fluid white blood cells (WBCs) >500/dL or polymorphonuclear cells (PMNs) >250/dL
    - ▷ Treatment of choice is IV cefotaxime or other third-generation cephalosporin plus IV albumin infusion

- ► Hepatic encephalopathy—asterixis (hand-flapping tremor), confusion, stupor, and coma
  - ▷ Management—lactulose, protein restriction (i.e., meat; legumes are OK), neomycin, or metronidazole
- ► Hepatorenal syndrome—often iatrogenic, poor survival rate, urinary Na is <10; only treatment is midodrine and octreotide until liver transplant, but usually by time hepatorenal syndrome develops, it is too late for liver transplant
- ► Hepatocellular carcinoma—screen cirrhotics with alpha-fetoprotein and liver ultrasound every 6 months

Hemochromatosis

- Pathophysiology—autosomal recessive defect causing abnormal intestinal iron absorption → massive iron deposition in the liver (**cirrhosis**), heart (CHF), pancreas (DM), pituitary gland (**hypogonadism**), skin (characteristic **bronze discoloration**), and joints (arthropathy of second and third metacarpophalangeal joints)
  - ► High risk of infection with *Yersinia enterocolitica, Listeria monocytogenes,* and *Vibrio vulnificus*
- Highest risk for liver cancer of all the cirrhotic diseases
- Diagnosis
  - ► Best initial test is serum iron studies → increased serum iron and ferritin with decreased total iron-binding capacity (TIBC)
  - ► Definitive test → C282Y and H63D gene testing for HFE; screen family members
- Management—weekly phlebotomy is first-line; defuroxime if this is not possible

Primary Biliary Cirrhosis

- Pathophysiology—autoimmune disorder causing chronic progressive cholestasis; affects **women age 40–60 years** who usually have history of other **autoimmune diseases**

- Clinical—persistent **fatigue; intense pruritus** typically begins in perineum or palmar/plantar areas and becomes generalized, causing thickened skin; jaundice, abdominal pain, xanthomas, xanthelasma, hepatomegaly
  - ▸ Many are asymptomatic and present with **very elevated alkaline phosphatase and gamma-glutamyl transferase (GGT)**
- Diagnosis—**antimitochondrial antibody** is the best initial test → high sensitivity and specificity; gold standard is liver biopsy showing nonsuppurative cholangitis
- Management—**ursodeoxycholic acid** → reduces pruritus, delays cirrhosis and need for liver transplantation; ultraviolet (UV) light also shown to help decrease pruritus

Primary Sclerosing Cholangitis (PSC)

- Pathophysiology—idiopathic disease occurring in **males <45 years of age** with a history of **inflammatory bowel disease (IBD)** (especially ulcerative colitis)
- Clinical—right upper quadrant (RUQ) pain, fever, chills, jaundice, and **pruritus**; will have **high alkaline phosphatase and GGT** with **negative** antimitochondrial antibody; high risk of progression to **cholangiocarcinoma**
- Diagnosis—best test is magnetic resonance cholangiopancreatography (MRCP) → dilatations/constrictions of the bile ducts with **"beaded-string"** appearance
- Management—**ursodeoxycholic acid** is first-line; antibiotics for acute attacks and endoscopic retrograde cholangiopancreatography (ERCP) with stenting for duct constrictions

Wilson Disease

- Pathophysiology—autosomal recessive defect causing increased copper absorption with excessive copper buildup in tissues
- Clinical—several characteristic clinical findings
  - ▸ Copper deposition in eye → **Kayser-Fleischer ring** (brown to grey-green) on slit-lamp examination (if present, **always** indicates underlying neurologic involvement)

- ► Basal ganglia → tremors
- ► Liver → **cirrhosis**, elevated transaminases
- ► Kidneys → **RTA type II**
- ► Blood → toxic effect causes **hemolytic anemia**

- Diagnosis—best initial test → low serum ceruloplasmin (also high urinary copper concentration); gold standard is liver biopsy

- Management
  - ► Asymptomatic or symptomatic patients—**trientine** (now favored as first-line therapy), or penicillamine; high-dose zinc used for maintenance therapy
  - ► Fulminant hepatic failure—transplant

4

PANCREATIC DISEASE

Acute Pancreatitis

- Etiology—alcohol is by far the most common cause in the United States (alcohol abusers); other causes include gallstones, hypertriglyceridemia, some medications (e.g., azathioprine)

- Clinical—**severe continuous epigastric**, RUQ, or LUQ **pain** that radiates commonly to **back** but also to shoulder; nausea, vomiting, anorexia, and low-grade fever

- Best test of severity is abdominal/pelvic CT scan with IV contrast followed by **Ranson criteria** (see table)

Ranson Criteria

At Presentation	At 48 Hours
Age >55 years	Hct fall by ≥10%
WBCs >16,000 mm³	BUN ≥5 mg/dL, even with IV hydration
Glucose > 200 mg/dL	Serum calcium <8 mg/dL
LDH >350 U/L	pO$_2$ <60 mm Hg
AST >250 U/L	Base deficit > 4 mEq/L
	Fluid sequestration >6L

Abbreviations: aspartate aminotransferase, AST; hematocrit, Hct; white blood cells, WBCs
Note: Mortality <3% with a score <3, 11–15% with a score ≥3, and 40% with a score ≥6.

- Diagnosis—best initial test is increased serum amylase and lipase (most specific); serum amylase assay is suppressed by hypertriglyceridemia
  - ▶ Abdominal x-ray—may show ileus or "sentinel loop" pattern (dilated bowel adjacent to pancreas)
  - ▶ CT scan—also helps show pseudocyst or abscess formation
  - ▶ MRCP or ERCP indicated to evaluate possible blockage if jaundice is present

Stepwise Management of Acute Pancreatitis

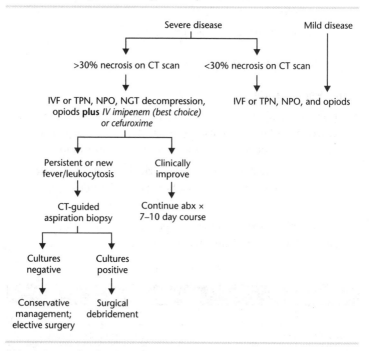

Abbreviations: antibiotics, abx; IV fluids, IVF; nasogastric tube, NGT; nothing by mouth, NPO; total parenteral nutrition, TPN

- Surgical consult for biliary pancreatitis, pseudocyst, or abscess
  - ▸ Pseudocyst—occurs **2–4 weeks after** a bout of pancreatitis; CT-guided drainage warranted if abdominal pain, increasing size or size >5 cm; if loculated or signs of infected pseudocyst, surgical removal required
  - ▸ Pancreatic abscess formation is a poor prognostic indicator; urgent surgical intervention is warranted
  - ▸ Biliary pancreatitis—look for symptoms of pancreatitis plus evidence of obstruction from gallstones within the pancreatic duct or ampulla of Vater

Chronic Pancreatitis

- Pathophysiology—alcohol abuse; never due to repeated attacks of biliary pancreatitis
- Clinical—**abdominal pain plus pancreatic insufficiency**
- Diagnosis—triad of **pancreatic calcifications** on CT, severe **steatorrhea**, and **DM**
- Management—small, low-fat meals and pancreatic enzyme replacement

Autoimmune Pancreatitis

- An IgG4-related sclerosing disease
- A chronic pancreatitis, usually with normal amylase and lipase levels
- Diagnosis
  - ▸ **CT scan**—diffusely enlarged pancreas (**"sausage-shaped"**), often with an enhanced peripheral rim of hypoattenuation ("halo")
  - ▸ **IgG4** levels elevated
  - ▸ Look for *other autoimmune diseases* (e.g., RA, IBD, Sjögren syndrome)
- Management—very good response to steroids

INFLAMMATORY BOWEL DISEASE (IBD)

Distinguishing Features of Crohn Disease and Ulcerative Colitis

Crohn Disease	Ulcerative Colitis
Bimodal; patients age 20s and 50–70s	Most common in 20–30s or the elderly
Mouth to anus; terminal ileum most commonly involved	• **Colon only**; starts distally in rectum, terminal ileum ("backwash ileitis") 10% • Only 10% have pan-colitis
Nonbloody diarrhea, RLQ pain, low-grade fever	**Bloody** diarrhea, cramping, pain, low-grade fever
Pyoderma gangrenosum, erythema nodosum iritis, episcleritis, gallstones, **kidney stones**, arthritis	**Primary sclerosing cholangitis**, pyoderma gangrenosum, erythema nodosum, iritis, arthritis, **ankylosing spondylitis**
• **Transmural** involvement, focal and **skip lesions** • Fissures and fistula formation • **Cobblestoning** of mucosa seen on colonoscopy	• **Mucosal** only, **continuous** • Ulcers and erosions, **lead-pipe colon/ loss of haustra** • Biopsy shows **crypt abscesses**
ASCA	p-ANCA
Therapy: Oral 5-ASA (balsalazide disodium) ↓ Trial of ciprofloxacin plus metronidazole ↓ Add or switch to oral budesonide ↓ Azathioprine, 6-MP, or methotrexate with or without systemic steroids (may also use this regimen initially if disease is severe or of recent onset) ↓ Anti-TNF-alpha	Therapy: Oral 5-ASA (mesalamine or balsalazide disodium) *or* 5-ASA or steroid suppository with or without steroid enemas ↓ Oral prednisone ↓ Azathioprine, 6-MP, or methotrexate

Abbreviations: 5-aminosalicylic acid, 5-ASA; anti-Saccharomyces cerevisiae antibodies, ASCA; mercaptopurine, MP; perinuclear antineutrophil cytoplasmic autoantibodies, p-ANCA; right lower quadrant, RLQ; tumor necrosis factor, TNF

CARCINOID SYNDROME

- Pathophysiology—tumor produces serotonin and kallikreins resulting in **sudden skin flushing** and **wheezing/bronchospasm** lasting up to **30 minutes**; secretory **diarrhea**, and pathognomic **plaque-like fibrinous** deposits on the **heart**

- Clinical—clinical syndrome occurs only in metastatic small- or large-bowel tumors or primary ovarian or bronchial/lung carcinoid tumors (bypasses liver metabolism)

- Diagnosis—best initial test is **24-hour urinary 5-HIAA** → if not diagnostic, next step is whole blood serotonin concentration; use CT scan or octreotide-scan to localize tumor location

- Management—control symptoms with **octreotide or lanreotide**; surgical resection for localized disease

4

CLOSTRIDIUM DIFFICILE COLITIS (ANTIBIOTIC-ASSOCIATED DIARRHEA)

- Pathophysiology—pseudomembranous colitis associated with recent antibiotic use (e.g., **clindamycin, amoxicillin**), but may be without recent antibiotic or hospitalization
  - ▸ Toxin A—enterotoxin, causes inflammation and mucosal damage
  - ▸ Toxin B—cytotoxin 10 times more potent in causing mucosal damage
  - ▸ Binary toxin produced by a hypervirulent toxic strain (NAP1/B1/027)

- Clinical—**abdominal pain**, fever, moderate to very **high WBC, diarrhea** may or may not have blood; toxic megacolon is possible

- Diagnosis—*C. diff* **PCR test** is 95% sensitive
  - ▸ ELISA for stool toxins A and B: NPV 73%, PPV 96%
  - ▸ If negative, repeat testing is not recommended

- Management
  - ▸ Discontinue the causative antibiotic
  - ▸ Discontinue PPI use if possible
  - ▸ Mild colitis → PO metronidazole for 10–14 days
  - ▸ Severe colitis or pregnant
    - ▹ PO vancomycin is probably the best initial therapy
    - ▹ Add IV metronidazole if ileus or megacolon
  - ▸ Relapse treatment (outpatient)
    - ▹ First recurrence → second course of same antibiotic if disease severity is unchanged (metronidazole 500 mg q8h × 14 days)
    - ▹ Second recurrence → vancomycin tapering course over 8 weeks
  - ▸ Fulminant colitis with perforation or toxic megacolon → total colectomy
- Prevention—**hand-washing** with water and soap for spore eradication

INFECTIOUS DIARRHEA

Osmotic Gap = 290 − 2 ([stool Na+] + [stool K+])

- Stool osmolality (OSM) should be close to that of plasma (290)
- **High** stool OSM due to osmotic causes
- **Very high** stool OSM can be accounted for only by:
  - ▸ Addition of solutes to stool after collection but before measurement (i.e., urine contamination, accidentally or purposefully) or
  - ▸ Bacterial fermentation of unabsorbed nutrients (most likely source)
- **Low** osmotic gap (<50) = secretory diarrhea (e.g., hyperthyroidism or VIPoma)

Infectious Diarrhea

INVASIVE Inflammatory Diarrhea	
Watery, **bloody**, mucoid diarrhea with increased **stool WBCs**, fever, fatigue	
Shigella	• Fecal contamination of food products, easily spread in day care centers (low inoculum) • Can result in HUS
Salmonella	• Undercooked **eggs and poultry** • At particular risk: sickle cell disease and achlorhydria
Campylobacter jejuni	• MCC bacterial colitis • Undercooked **poultry** (or other food contaminated by the chef's hands) • Mucosal ulcerations and erosions • Associated with the Miller Fischer variant of Guillain-Barré syndrome
Yersinia enterocolitica	• Undercooked **pork** • RLQ pain (mimics appendicitis) • Reactive arthritis, rash
Hemorrhagic *E. coli* (O157:H7)	• Undercooked **beef** • Shiga-like toxin associated with HUS and TTP in children (especially after antibiotic use)
ENTEROTOXIGENIC Noninflammatory Diarrhea	
Watery, large-volume stools, nonbloody, no stool WBCs, no systemic symptoms	
Enterotoxigenic *E. coli* (ETEC)	• "Traveler's diarrhea," "turista," "Montezuma's revenge" • 3–5 days duration
Viruses	• **Norovirus:** common in **nursing home and cruise ship** outbreaks • **Rotavirus:** children in **day care centers**
Bacillus cereus	• Within hours of eating **reheated rice** • **Vomiting** predominates
Staphylococcus aureus	• Severe **nausea/vomiting** within 1–8 hours of ingesting unrefrigerated **mayonnaise and eggs** (e.g., **picnics**) • May not have diarrhea
Giardia lamblia	• **Stream water, camping trips** (MCC parasitic cause of diarrhea) • Bloating, cramps, **foul-smelling** diarrhea, weight loss • Stool antigen test • Treatment: metronidazole

4

(continued)

Infectious Diarrhea (continued)

Cryptosporidium	• Usually **immunosuppressed** patients (e.g., AIDS), **stream water** • Diagnosis: acid-fast stain of stool: **oocysts**
Vibrio vulnificus	Usually chronic **liver disease patients, raw seafood** may cause **skin bullae**, rapid **septicemia**, and death
Scombroid poisoning	• **Reef fish** (grouper, parrot fish, snapper) • Within **minutes to hours** → **wheezing, flushing,** and diarrhea • Treatment: antihistamines

Abbreviations: hemolytic-uremic syndrome, HUS; most common cause, MCC; right lower quadrant, RLQ; thrombotic thrombocytopenic purpura, TTP; white blood cells, WBCs

IRRITABLE BOWEL SYNDROME (IBS)

- Diagnosis—Rome III criteria
  - ▶ Recurrent, **crampy** abdominal *pain/discomfort* at least **3 days/ month** in the **last 3 months** associated with 2 or more of the following:
    - ▷ **Improvement with defecation**
    - ▷ Onset associated with a **change in frequency of stool**
    - ▷ Onset associated with a **change in form of stool**
  - ▶ **Postprandial fecal urgency** is also a key feature
  - ▶ Should rule out celiac disease (20–30% of IBS cases): IgA transglutaminase antibody
- Management
  - ▶ Mild symptoms—avoid foods that increase flatulence; increase dietary fiber or take bulking agents; stress management
  - ▶ Pharmacotherapy
    - ▷ Antispasmodics—initial agents of choice by most physicians; include hyoscine, cimetropium, pinaverium, peppermint
    - ▷ TCAs—useful if history of neuropathic pain
    - ▷ Rifaximin—improves abdominal bloating and flatulence
    - ▷ Tegaserod—constipation-predominant and mixed-type IBS
    - ▷ Lubiprostone—constipation-predominant IBS

LACTOSE INTOLERANCE (LACTASE DEFICIENCY)

- Pathophysiology—loss of lactase brush border enzyme with aging; more common in African Americans and Asian Americans; may be transient after infection

- Clinical—gaseous distention, flatulence, and diarrhea after consuming dairy products

- Diagnosis—lactose tolerance test

- Management—avoid dairy products and/or take lactase enzyme supplements

MALABSORPTION SYNDROMES

Celiac Disease

- See also page 362

- Pathophysiology—immune-mediated gluten sensitivity to wheat, barley, and rye results in small-bowel villous atrophy and malabsorption syndrome

- Classic GI presentation—triad of **chronic diarrhea, weight loss**, and **abdominal distention**
  - ▸ Can present as **iron deficiency anemia**, osteoporosis, peripheral neuropathy, ataxia, **dermatitis herpetiformis**
  - ▸ High association with other autoimmune diseases (e.g., DM type 1, Hashimoto thyroiditis)

- Diagnosis—best initial test is **anti-endomysial** or **anti-transglutaminase antibodies** (skin biopsy of dermatitis herpetiformis lesions also diagnostic, if present); gold standard and confirmatory test is small-intestinal biopsy showing **blunted intestinal villi/villous atrophy**

- Increased risk of developing **gastrointestinal lymphoma**

- Management—strict gluten-free diet

4

Whipple Disease

- Pathophysiology—infection with *Tropheryma whippelii* results in **malabsorption syndrome**

- Clinical—pentad of **weight loss**, migratory **arthralgias, abdominal pain, foul-smelling diarrhea**; may also have adenopathy

- At risk for central nervous system (CNS) infection (cognitive dysfunction) and lesions of cardiac valves

- Diagnosis—upper endoscopy with small-bowel biopsy → **strongly periodic acid-Schiff (PAS)–positive foamy macrophages** in the lamina propria and **blunted intestinal villi**

- Management—IV ceftriaxone or penicillin/streptomycin for 2–4 weeks, then trimethoprim-sulfamethoxazole (TMP-SMZ) orally for 1 year

Tropical Sprue

- Pathophysiology—endemic to tropical regions of 30 degrees latitude; thought to be infectious, but no agent has been identified to date

- Clinical—**chronic, malabsorptive diarrhea** with **vitamin B-12 and folate deficiency** in a person from an endemic area

- Diagnosis—intestinal biopsy reveals flattening of duodenal folds and **"scalloping"**

- Management—oral tetracycline and folate for 3–6 months

IV. GERIATRIC MEDICINE

GERIATRIC WELLNESS VISIT

Assessment of the following should be addressed in the geriatric population (i.e., age >60 years):

- Ability to perform activities of daily living (ADLs), and at what level
  - ▸ Basic ADLs—bathing, dressing, using the toilet, continence, self-feeding
  - ▸ Intermediate ADLs—grocery shopping, cleaning, driving, cooking, laundry
  - ▸ Advanced ADLs—exercise regimens, caring for grand-children, etc.

- Social support system, if any (family, friends, daily activities like chess or bingo)

- History of falls and assessment of fall risk
  - ▸ The most common cause of falls in the elderly is mechanical
  - ▸ Assess speed of gait, ability to arise from a chair; if these are impaired, fall risk is increased
  - ▸ More than half of those age >80 have at least one fall per year

- Symptoms of depression
  - ▸ Very common in the elderly; more likely with increased comorbidity and frequent hospitalization rates
    - ▹ MDD rate among elderly in the community: around 2%
    - ▹ MDD rate in frequently hospitalized geriatric patients: >40%
  - ▸ Best depression screening questions:
    - ▹ "Are you feeling down?"
    - ▹ "Have you lost interest or pleasure in doing things?"

- Visual or hearing difficulties
  - ▸ All should have routine hearing and visual testing
  - ▸ Visual difficulties can go unrecognized and contribute to mechanical falls

- ▸ Hearing difficulties may lead to isolation from family/friends due to embarrassment

- Documentation of a health-care proxy and advance directives

- Elimination of polypharmacy
  - ▸ Have geriatric patients bring all medicine to the outpatient appointment, including herbal remedies
  - ▸ More meds = more drug interactions = increased likelihood of adverse effects

ACUTE DELIRIUM

- Acute altered mental status in the elderly (delirium)—common during inpatient hospitalization of the elderly with underlying dementia; also referred to as "sundowning"
  - ▸ Acute confusion, more common at night with delirium—treatment of choice is PRN (as needed) **haloperidol** or other antipsychotic; **avoid benzodiazepines**, which worsen confusion and increase fall risk

DEMENTIA

Distinguishing Dementia Syndromes

Syndrome	Clinical Course	Characteristics	Diagnosis
Alzheimer dementia	• Chronic over years • Spares motor, sensory, and visual areas	• Memory loss and either: aphasia, agnosia, apraxia, or loss of executive function* • Paranoia	• Clinical • Definitive at autopsy: shows plaques, neurofibrillary tangles, amyloid
Multi-infarct dementia	**Stepwise decline**	Progressive, stepwise loss of function after each stroke	MRI shows multiple infarcts

(continued)

Distinguishing Dementia Syndromes (continued)

Syndrome	Clinical Course	Characteristics	Diagnosis
Dementia with Lewy bodies	Waxing/waning course	**Vivid hallucinations and parkinsonian symptoms**	• Clinical • Definitive diagnosis at autopsy
Frontotemporal dementia (Pick disease)	Ability to perform executive function worse than memory	• **Personality changes:** disinhibited or very quiet • Abulia, lost initiative • Better memory than with AD	MRI shows disproportionate **atrophy of anterior frontal and temporal lobes**
Vitamin B-12 deficiency	Dementia can be severe	• **Loss of vibratory sense in legs** • **No DTRs** • Babinski is positive	Decreased serum B-12 level
Creutzfeldt-Jakob	Dementia over weeks to months due to infection with prion disease	Also have **tremors** and **myoclonic jerks** of extremities	CSF shows 14-3-3 protein

Abbreviations: Alzheimer disease, AD; cerebrospinal fluid, CSF; deep tendon reflexes, DTRs
* Note: Executive function *involves initiating behavior, planning, shifting between activities flexibly, and the ability to inhibit or delay responding.*

Treatment of Alzheimer Dementia

Acetylcholinesterase inhibitors are first-line therapy (include donepezil, rivastigmine, galantamine) for mild to moderate dementia. Add memantine if this fails to control symptoms or in those with severe dementia.

SLEEP

Both REM (rapid eye movement) sleep and total length of sleep decrease with age. Sleeping aids should be avoided if sleep loss is due to natural aging (ask if patient feels tired, fatigued, or groggy, which points toward sleep deprivation) and because the elderly are particularly at risk for adverse effects from drug therapy (e.g., increased fall risk).

- **Tip:** Remember to *eliminate drugs of questionable benefit* in those with advanced end-stage dementia or other diseases (e.g., simvastatin in a patient with a terminal illness) in order to decrease the pill burden and preserve quality of life.

DECUBITUS ULCERS

See page 250.

END-OF-LIFE CARE

- Advance directives should be discussed with all patients, but particularly with older patients in order to avoid confusion if/when they are admitted to the hospital

- Elderly patients should be encouraged to have a living will and/or a health-care proxy in the event they cannot make medical decisions for themselves

- The primary physician should clearly document the patient's wishes in the record (either outpatient or inpatient) while the patient is still lucid. This will avoid unnecessary confusion if a life-altering event occurs and the patient is no longer able to speak for himself or herself.

V. HEMATOLOGY AND ONCOLOGY

MACROCYTIC ANEMIA (MEAN CORPUSCULAR VOLUME [MCV] >100)

B-12 Deficiency

- Etiology—vegan diet or small-bowel disease

- Pernicious anemia—autoimmune variety associated with achlorhydria → antiparietal and intrinsic factor antibody-positive; can be associated with other autoimmune disorders

- Clinical—**neurologic deficits** affecting dorsal columns may precede the anemia (peripheral neuropathy, foot drop, vibratory/position sense loss)

- Diagnosis
  - ► Best initial test—peripheral smear shows **hypersegmented** neutrophils (≥5 lobes)
  - ► Most specific test—low serum B-12
    - ▷ May be normal in 30%; best next step is serum methylmalonic acid (MMA) → if MMA is high, get serum antiparietal and anti-intrinsic factor antibodies
  - ► Schilling test—use when serum B-12 and MMA are nondiagnostic

- Management—IM replacement with 1,000 mcg/day for 1 week, then once a month
  - ► Watch for **hypokalemia** after starting treatment

Folate Deficiency

- Etiology—dietary deficiency common in **alcoholics**, drug addicts, and the **elderly**; malabsorption, chronic hemolytic states, folate antagonists, and pregnancy

- Diagnosis
  - ► Best initial test—peripheral smear shows **hypersegmented neutrophils** (≥5 lobes)
  - ► Most specific test—low serum folate

4

▸ Assays for vitamin B-12 are not accurate, especially in the elderly. Best tests for vitamin B-12 and folate deficiency are **methylmalonic acid** and **homocysteine** (see table below)

- Management—folate 1 mg PO daily

B-12 Deficiency versus Folate Deficiency

	Methylmalonic acid <0.4 µmol/L	Homocysteine 4–12 µmol/L
Vitamin B-12 deficiency	Elevated	Elevated
Folate deficiency	Normal	Elevated

MICROCYTIC ANEMIA (MCV <80)

Iron Deficiency

- Most common anemia
  - ▸ In an elderly patient with iron-deficiency anemia—you must rule out colon cancer *but* anemia of chronic disease is the most common cause. Your key to getting this right is the TIBC.
  - ▸ In a young female—think of menstrual blood loss
  - ▸ In an adult patient with symptoms of diarrhea—think of celiac disease

- Diagnosis
  - ▸ Best initial test—serum ferritin
  - ▸ Other iron studies—low serum iron, high TIBC, low transferrin saturation, increased red-cell distribution width, high soluble transferrin receptor assay
  - ▸ Gold standard—bone marrow biopsy → lack of stainable iron with Prussian blue in erythrocyte precursors

- Management—oral ferrous sulfate or ferrous citrate; IV therapy if severe malabsorption

Thalassemia

Alpha-thalassemia

- Etiology—decreased alpha-chain production
- Diagnosis—**profoundly low MCV** (<70), normal iron studies, elevated reticulocytes, **target cells** in peripheral smear
- Four alpha alleles
  - ▸ One deficit = alpha-thalassemia trait → **asymptomatic**
  - ▸ Two deficits = alpha-thalassemia minor → no anemia to mild anemia, **normal** Hgb electrophoresis, so diagnosis is presumptive after excluding Fe deficiency and beta-thalassemia
    - ▹ Molecular DNA studies for definitive diagnosis, but not widely available
  - ▸ Three deficits = Hgb H (four beta chains) → severe anemia (Hgb 7–9 g/dL), jaundice, splenomegaly, Hgb electrophoresis shows 5–30% Hgb H
    - ▹ Management—transfusion every 3–4 months, rigorous hydration, and treat iron overload (common)
  - ▸ Four deficits = Hgb Barts (hydrops fetalis due to **gamma tetramers**) → stillborn

Beta-thalassemia

- Etiology—decreased beta-chain production
- Diagnosis—as above, plus **elevated Hgb A2** on electrophoresis
- Beta-thalassemia minor—mild anemia with marked microcytosis
- Beta-thalassemia intermedia—some beta-globulin produced
- Beta-thalassemia major (Cooley anemia)—no production of Hgb → transfusion-dependent

Anemia of Chronic Disease

- Etiology—elevated hepcidin (protein made by liver inhibits iron transfer from macrophages to bone marrow and inhibits absorption of iron from the intestine)

4

- Diagnosis—normal to **elevated serum ferritin, low** serum iron and TIBC; gold standard is bone marrow biopsy showing **macrophages that stain densely with Prussian blue** (due to sequestered stores)

- Management—treat underlying disease; transfuse only if symptomatic or severe

	Iron Deficiency Anemia	Anemia of Chronic Disease
MCC of	Anemia in adults, especially women	Anemia in elderly
Iron	Low	Low
TIBC	High Low if ACD is also present	Low
Ferritin	Low	High (>100 ng/mL)
EPO	High	Low

Abbreviations: anemia of chronic disease, ACD; erythropoeitin, EPO; total iron-binding capacity, TIBC

Sideroblastic Anemia

- Etiology—hereditary (deficiency of **ALA synthetase**) or acquired (drugs, lead poisoning, alcohol abuse)

- Diagnosis—**elevated serum ferritin and low TIBC**; gold standard is bone marrow biopsy showing **ringed sideroblasts** with Prussian blue staining

- Management—treat underlying disease or give oral B-6 if hereditary

Lead Poisoning

See page 370.

NORMOCYTIC ANEMIA (NORMAL MCV)

Best initial test—reticulocyte count

- Increased reticulocyte count: think hemolytic causes or acute bleeding

- Decreased reticulocyte count: think of hypoproliferative states

Hemolytic Anemia

- Etiology—intravascular (destruction within vasculature) or extravascular (destruction within spleen); may be chronic (like sickle-cell disease) or acute (usually drug-induced)

  ▸ See also Chapter 8: Pediatrics for discussion of sickle-cell disease, spherocytosis, and glucose-6-phosphate dehydrogenase (G6PD) deficiency

- Diagnosis—normal to slightly increased MCV, **increased indirect bilirubin, increased lactate dehydrogenase (LDH)** and **schistocytes** on peripheral smear

  ▸ Paroxysmal nocturnal hemoglobinuria (PNH)—defect in red-cell membrane phosphatidylinositol glycan A → increased complement binding resulting in hemolysis especially during acidosis (infection, acute CO_2 retention, and during sleep)

    ▹ Clinically present with darkened urine upon awakening

    ▹ Increased risk of acute thrombosis → Budd-Chiari syndrome from circulating thrombogenic particles

    ▹ Diagnosis—best initial test is flow cytometry for **CD55** (decay-accelerating factor) and **CD59**

    ▹ Management—steroids if severe disease; anticoagulate if history of thrombosis

      – Immune suppression therapy may also be appropriate

      – Bone marrow transplant (BMT) is curative

APLASTIC ANEMIA

- Etiology—**pancytopenia** due to bone marrow failure (stem cell disorder)

  ▸ In 50%, most common causes are: idiopathic, drugs (benzene, gold, sulfa, chloramphenicol, insecticides), radiation, PNH, viruses

- Clinical—symptoms due to cytopenias (infections, bleeding, anemia)

- Diagnosis—bone marrow is **fatty and hypocellular** (5% cellularity)

- Management
  - ► Age <45 and healthy with donor available—BMT is first-line. Best survival rates; up to 90% of young patients with a suitable donor will survive.
  - ► Age >45 or high operative risk—immunosuppression with antithymocyte globulin, cyclosporine, and prednisone is first-line

COAGULOPATHIES

Etiology—factor-type bleeding and platelet-type bleeding, hemophilias, vitamin deficiency, disseminated intravascular coagulation (DIC), and effect of hepatic or renal disease on platelet function.

Disorders of Primary Hemostasis

Includes thrombocytopenia or dysfunctional platelets.

Thrombocytopenia

- Etiology
  - ► Decreased production—primary marrow failure, marrow replacement, viral, drug-induced
  - ► Sequestration—hypersplenism, liver disease
  - ► Increased destruction—idiopathic thrombocytopenic purpura (ITP), TTP/HUS, DIC, heparin-induced thrombocytopenia (HIT)

Dysfunctional platelets

Most often seen in chronic renal failure.

Idiopathic Thrombocytopenic Purpura (ITP)

- Etiology—IgG autoantibodies directed against GP (glycoprotein) Ib-IX or IIb-IIIa; cause may be idiopathic (30%), drug-induced (30%), lymphoma, leukemia, collagen vascular diseases (SLE, scleroderma) or viral (HCV, HIV)

- Diagnosis of exclusion; best initial test is an adequate history, physical exam, and **peripheral smear**; confirmatory test is **antiplatelet antibodies**
  - ▸ Absence of antiplatelet antibodies does not exclude disease, especially when clinical picture is suggestive of ITP

- Management—some cases resolve spontaneously
  - ▸ If platelet count >50,000—watchful waiting
  - ▸ If platelet count <50,000—steroids are best initial therapy, IV immunoglobulin (IVIG) is first-line in children
    - ▹ Transfusion indicated if any acute bleeding

- Indications for splenectomy—if platelet count remains low after 4–6 weeks of therapy

- Chronic refractory ITP—ITP for >3 months, platelet count <50,000, and failure to respond to splenectomy; treatment with immunosuppression, steroids, or observation (no one therapy has been shown to be superior to the next); other options are rituximab and Rho(D) immunoglobulin
  - ▸ **Tip:** Remember that ITP patients usually do not bleed; therefore, continued treatment may not be indicated.

Thrombotic Thrombocytopenic Purpura and Hemolytic Uremic Syndrome (TTP-HUS)

- Etiology—defect in **ADAMTS13 gene** (codes for a protease which cleaves very large von Willebrand multimers → accumulation of these multimers leads to thrombotic phenomenon); idiopathic or due to *E. coli* 0157:H7

- Clinical presentation/diagnosis—triad of fever, microangiopathic hemolytic anemia (schistocytes, reticulocytosis, elevated bilirubin, decreased haptoglobin), and thrombocytopenia **plus** renal dysfunction and neurologic deficits
  - ▸ → Predominantly renal dysfunction = HUS
  - ▸ → Predominantly neurologic dysfunction = TTP

- Management—daily plasma exchange is first-line until symptoms improve; add steroids if etiology is known to **not** be drug-induced and/or if thrombocytopenia recurs despite plasma exchange
  - ▸ **Avoid** platelet transfusions—makes the disease worse
  - ▸ Recurrent or refractory TTP-HUS—increase plasma exchange to twice daily and add cyclosporine or rituximab

Disseminated Intravascular Coagulation (DIC)

- Etiology—due to tissue factor release or damaged endothelium → clotting (small thrombi) and continued consumption of procoagulants
  - ▸ Secondary to retained product(s) of conception, postpartum hemorrhage, any cause of prolonged hemorrhage, malignancy, trauma, or sepsis
- Clinical—case scenario will describe a patient with bleeding and/or oozing from **multiple body sites** including **IV lines, small cuts, mucosal surfaces**
- Diagnosis—schistocytes, thrombocytopenia, reticulocytosis, **decreased fibrinogen, elevated prothrombin time (PT)/partial thromboplastin time (PTT)/INR, and increased d-dimer/ fibrin-split products levels**
- Management—treat the underlying disorder, and provide supportive therapy with transfusions of packed red blood cells (RBCs), platelets, fresh frozen plasma (FFP), cryoprecipitate
  - ▸ If DIC develops intraoperatively—immediately stop surgery, treat the DIC, and return to the operating room (OR) when bleeding stops
- Heparin still controversial—may be used in cases of acute thrombosis

DISORDERS OF PLATELET FUNCTION

von Willebrand Disease

- Most common inherited bleeding disorder; autosomal dominant, with affected patients being heterozygous

- Etiology—deficiency of one or more multimers of the proteins which compose von Willebrand factor (vWF)

- Clinical—bleeding ranging from mild to severe; common case scenario is young female with **menorrhagia** or young child/ adult with **recurrent nosebleeds**

- Diagnosis—normal platelet count and morphology with **increased bleeding time**; gold standard is the **ristocetin cofactor test**

- Management
  - ► Desmopressin (DDAVP®) is first-line for mild bleeding—raises plasma vWF and factor VIII levels by releasing them from endothelium
    - ▷ IV during and after minor surgery
    - ▷ Intranasally prior to surgery, during active nosebleed, or just before menses
  - ► Factor VIII concentrate with high vWF content—use in emergencies, major surgery, or bleeding refractory to desmopressin
  - ► Cryoprecipitate—has large amounts of vWF and factor VIII; use only in emergencies with severe bleeding

Bernard-Soulier Syndrome (Giant Platelet Syndrome)

- Etiology—defect in GPIb prevents platelet binding to vWF, preventing adhesion and platelet activation

- Diagnosis—giant platelets on peripheral smear, mild thrombocytopenia, abnormal ristocetin aggregation in a patient with bleeding that is out of proportion to severity of platelet count

Glanzmann Thromboasthenia

- Etiology—autosomal recessive defect in GPIIb-IIIa; cannot bind to fibrinogen, causing abnormal aggregation

- Diagnosis—childhood mucosal bleeding with normal platelet counts but single, isolated platelets and lack of clumping on peripheral smear

4

Drug-Induced Coagulopathy

- Aspirin—binds **irreversibly** to cyclooxygenase, preventing platelet activation
- NSAIDs—bind **reversibly** to cyclooxygenase

MYELODYSPLASTIC SYNDROMES

- Etiology—clonal disorder of hematopoietic stem cells associated with deletions of chromosomes 3, 5, 7, 8, and 17 → ineffective hematopoesis with **crowded, hypercellular marrow** and **cytopenia** in ≥2 cell lines
- Clinical—usually >50 years of age with pancytopenia and **<20% blasts** → respective signs and symptoms
- Diagnosis—peripheral smear may show **macroovalocytes** and/or **bilobed neutrophil** (called the Pelger-Huët anomaly), which are the most specific findings; bone marrow biopsy is the gold-standard test
- Can progress to acute leukemia (**>30% blasts**)
- Management—if patient is <60 years of age and has a matched donor → SCT is first-line; otherwise, management is individualized but should include erythropoietin (EPO) injections and transfusions as needed if symptomatic. Drug therapy with lenalidomide and azacitidine if indicated in 5q syndrome.

MYELOPROLIFERATIVE SYNDROMES

- Definition—clonal stem cell disorders of chronic unregulated proliferation with differentiation into mature blood elements; always rule out secondary causes of elevated cell counts

POLYCYTHEMIA VERA

- Diagnosis—Hct >60% in males or Hct >56% in females, thrombocytosis (platelet count >400,000), WBC count >12,000, plus signs and symptoms

- **Secondary polycythemia due to identifiable causative factor— e.g., smoking is a common cause of secondary polycythemia**

- Symptoms—headache, aquagenic pruritus (**intense itching after hot showers**), dyspnea, blurred vision, night sweats, **facial plethora, transient ischemic attack (TIA)/stroke**
  - ▸ **Tip:** Any patient diagnosed with portal vein thrombosis has PV until proven otherwise.

- Signs—splenomegaly, bleeding, thrombotic events (mesenteric)

- Prognosis—median survival ~15 years

- Diagnosis
  - ▸ Best initial test is serum EPO
    - ▹ Serum EPO increased—secondary polycythemia
    - ▹ Serum EPO normal—get bone marrow biopsy → panmyelosis
    - ▹ Serum EPO decreased—primary polycythemia
  - ▸ 97% of primary cases are **JAK2**-positive

- Management—phlebotomy is first-line → to keep hematocrit (Hct) < 45% in men and <42% in women
  - ▸ Add hydroxyurea if age >50, history of thrombotic event, platelet count >1,500,000/uL, or cardiovascular risk factors
  - ▸ Aspirin—for all patients without contraindications (81 mg)
  - ▸ Elective surgical procedures—lower the Hct several months before the surgery

ESSENTIAL THROMBOCYTOSIS

- Diagnostic criteria—platelet count persistently >450,000, megakaryocyte hyperplasia on bone marrow biopsy, absent Philadelphia chromosome or evidence of another myelodysplastic syndrome, absence of secondary causes of thrombocytosis (bleeding, etc.), and normal iron stores and studies
  - ▸ JAK2—seen in 50% of cases

- Clinical—middle-aged and older with evidence of splenomegaly, erythromelalgia (**burning pain in hands/feet with erythema/warmth**), livedo reticularis, acral dysesthesia, headache, and visual disturbances

- Complications—thrombotic (arterial or venous) and hemorrhagic complications (platelet dysfunction when >1,500,000/uL) most common

- Management—see table below

  ▸ **Tip: Must** correct platelet count before elective surgery to reduce perioperative bleeding and thrombosis.

- Prognosis—near normal life

- Rarely—converts to myelofibrosis or leukemia

Management of Myeloproliferative Syndromes

Asymptomatic, age <60 years	Erythromelalgia	Mildly urgent symptoms	Life-threatening symptoms*
Observation or aspirin (81 mg)	Aspirin	Hydroxyurea plus aspirin	Platelet apheresis with hydroxyurea

*e.g., TIA, stroke, MI, GI bleeding

PRIMARY MYELOFIBROSIS

- Etiology—clonal proliferation of abnormal hematopoietic stem cells, which release fibroblast growth factors stimulating collagen production, impaired marrow function, and extra medullary hematopoesis

- Clinical—splenomegaly and hepatomegaly from extramedullary hematopoiesis, normocytic anemia, teardrop cells from circulating erythroblasts and myeloid precursors, giant platelets, and portal hypertension

- Diagnosis—gold standard is bone marrow biopsy showing extensive fibrosis, also called a **"dry tap"**; JAK-2 positive in 50%

- Prognosis—3 to 5 years median survival

- Management
  - ▸ If few to no symptoms—supportive therapy/palliation
  - ▸ If age <60 years with symptoms—allogeneic SCT is first-line
  - ▸ If age >60 years with symptoms—palliation with chemotherapy, ruxolitinib (a JAK inhibitor) improves symptoms in some
  - ▸ Splenectomy is contraindicated due to high perioperative morbidity and mortality

LEUKEMIA

- Children—think acute lymphocytic leukemia (ALL)
- Adults—think acute myelocytic leukemia (AML) or chronic myeloid leukemia (CML)
- Elderly—think chronic leukocytic leukemia (CLL) or hairy cell leukemia

Acute Myelocytic Leukemia (AML)

- Peripheral smear likely to show **blasts** with **Auer rods** and/or **myeloperoxidase** granules
- Bone marrow biopsy must demonstrate **>20% blast forms on biopsy**
- Eight FAB (French-American-British) categories
  - ▸ M0—undifferentiated
  - ▸ M1—without maturation
  - ▸ M2—with maturation → t(8;21); good prognosis
  - ▸ M3—promyelocytic → t(15;17); involves retinoic acid receptor gene on chromosome 17
    - ▹ Associated with **DIC**, although heparin usually not needed
    - ▹ Uses **all-trans-retinoic acid (ATRA)** as a maturational agent for induction therapy and follow with a full course of chemotherapy
    - ▹ Good prognosis

4

- ▸ M4—myelomonocytic → inverted chromosome 16; associated with **peripheral eosinophilia**, leukemia cutis and CNS disease
- ▸ M5—monocytic → rearrangement of chromosome 11q; associated with skin and soft-tissue disease, **gingival hyperplasia** and CNS disease/hemorrhage
- ▸ M6—erythroid
- ▸ M7—megakaryotic
- Prognosis—cytogenetics is the best factor; t(8;21), t(15;17), inv 16 have a good prognosis; age adversely affects prognosis. Secondary AML has a poorer prognosis.
- Management
  - ▸ First, perform induction chemotherapy with daunorubicin or idarubicin plus cytarabine
    - ▷ If M3 subtype → **add ATRA** followed by chemotherapy
    - ▷ **Tip:** To prevent tumor lysis syndrome, all should receive aggressive pretreatment IV fluids with allopurinol or rasburicase.
    - ▷ Leukapheresis if blast count >100,000 or symptoms of leukostasis syndrome (TIA, hypoxia, diffuse pulmonary infiltrates, other CNS symptoms)
  - ▸ Allogenic or autologous stem cell transplant after first relapse or second complete remission

Acute Lymphocytic Leukemia (ALL)

- >20% blasts on bone marrow biopsy; **CALLA antigen**-positive
- Three FAB categories, but it is not necessary to know them
- Clinical—typically a young child with fatigue, pallor, and new-onset epistaxis/bleeding gums; lymphadenopathy and splenomegaly in 50%; an anterior mediastinal mass is common in T-cell subtypes, and CNS involvement common

- Prognosis—children do better, with majority being cured; adults have 30–40% survival rate
  - ▸ If blasts >30,000—tend to do poorly
  - ▸ Cytogenetics—if Philadelphia chromosome t(9,22) positive, poor prognosis (unlike CML, which has a good prognosis)
- Management
  - ▸ First, induction chemotherapy with vincristine + asparaginase + daunorubicin + steroids
  - ▸ Second, consolidation therapy—must add intrathecal methotrexate to prevent CNS disease
  - ▸ Third, maintenance therapy
  - ▸ **Leukaphoresis**—not usually needed, cells are smaller

Chronic Lymphocytic Leukemia (CLL)

- Clinical—older adults present with lymphadenopathy, splenomegaly, and asymptomatic lymphocytosis; may present with infection, anemia, or thrombocytopenia
  - ▸ Transformation of disease (Richter syndrome)—rapid growth of nodes or increase in extranodal disease
- Diagnosis—peripheral blood smear with **lymphocytosis** and **smudge** cells; flow cytometry is **CD5-positive** (which is a T-cell marker) with CD19+, CD20+ and **CD23+**. Bone marrow biopsy not typically needed for diagnosis.
- Quantitative immunoglobulins since diffuse hypogammaglobulinemia is common
- Associated with warm autoimmune hemolytic anemia
- Management
  - ▸ Treat only if symptomatic, rapid doubling of WBC count in 1 year, anemia, thrombocytopenia, B symptoms, or recurrent infections
    - ▹ If age <70 and good performance status—fludarabine plus cyclophosphamide and rituximab is first-line
    - ▹ If age >70 and/or poor performance status—chlorambucil is first-line

Chronic Myeloid Leukemia (CML)

- Etiology—a myeloproliferative disease with myeloid proliferation and differentiation into mature neutrophils caused by a translocation **(t9,22)**, the **Philadelphia chromosome**, forming a novel **bcr-abl gene**, which produces the **bcr-abl tyrosine kinase** (responsible for the myeloid proliferation)

- Clinical—asymptomatic for years with high WBC counts or fatigue

- Diagnosis—best initial test is **leukocyte alkaline phosphatase:** will be decreased in CML, and increased in leukemoid reactions. Bone marrow biopsy will demonstrate t(9:22)

4

CML Disease Course

Chronic phase	Accelerated phase	Blast crisis
Years of asymptomatic elevated WBC	Increasing WBC count, fatigue becomes more prominent	Transformation to acute leukemia (67% myeloid, 33% lymphoid)
• PE shows splenomegaly • Peripheral smear shows 1–5% blasts	Peripheral smear with 10–20% blasts	Smear now with >20% blasts
Treatment: hydroxyurea and bcr-abl tyrosine kinase inhibitors (includes imatinib, dasatinib, and nilotinib) will control most disease	Treatment: allogenic stem cell transplantation (best hope for cure)	Treatment: allogenic stem cell transplantation

Hairy Cell Leukemia

- Rare leukemia of B-cell origin predominantly affecting older males

- Usually presents with triad of **pancytopenia, massive splenomegaly**, and **dry tap** on bone marrow biopsy

- Diagnosis—several unique markers
  - ▸ Bone marrow biopsy or peripheral smear shows cells with **"fried-egg" appearance** that stain positive for tartrate resistant acid-phosphatase, specific to hairy cell (**TRAP, tartrate resistant acid phosphatase**) and express B-cell–positive flow cytometry (CD19+, CD20+, **CD11c+**, **CD103+**)

- Prognosis—usually indolent course

- Management—development of symptoms is an indication for treatment (infectious complications, anemia, thrombocytopenia) → **cladribine** is first-line; splenectomy for abdominal pain or refractory disease

4

LYMPHOMA

- Clinical—painless lymphadenopathy with or without B symptoms (fever, night sweats, pruritus)

- Diagnosis—best step is **excisional biopsy** of the entire lymph node or mass
  - ▸ Flow cytometry—helps with specific subtypes, clonality, and lineage (B or T)
  - ▸ Staging—CT chest, abdomen, and pelvis; gallium or PET scan

Ann Arbor Staging and Management of Hodgkin Lymphoma

Stage	Extent of Disease	Management
Stage I	Unilateral node or group of nodes or single extranodal site	Short course ABVD + irradiation
Stage II	Two or more nodes/groups on same side of diaphragm	Full course ABVD + irradiation
Stage III	Nodes on both sides of diaphragms involved	ABVD
Stage IV	Disseminated	ABVD

Abbreviations: Adriamycin® (Doxorubicin), bleomycin, vinblastine, dacarbazine, ABVD

Note: In those age <70 who relapse after initial *therapy*, bone marrow transplant is the best next step.

Hodgkin Lymphoma

- Biopsy shows characteristic **Reed-Sternberg cells**
- Classification includes
  - ▸ **Lymphocyte-predominant**—has the **best prognosis**; CD 57+
  - ▸ Mixed cellularity
  - ▸ Nodular sclerosing
  - ▸ Lymphocyte-depleted—has the worst prognosis
- Bimodal age distribution, pruritus common, pain with alcohol ingestion

Non-Hodgkin Lymphoma

- Most are B-cell type; **LDH** and **beta-2 microglobulin** are markers; flow cytometry and cytogenetics (CD20) helpful in classification
- Classification
  - ▸ Low grade—indolent course, older patients, fewer B symptoms, mostly B cells, and have 7-to-10-year survival (e.g., follicular type lymphoma, CLL/small lymphocytic type)
  - ▸ Intermediate grade—younger, more B symptoms, 1-to-2-year survival
  - ▸ High grade—younger patients, B symptoms, lower stage at time of diagnosis, B or T cells. May be cured even if advanced (e.g., diffuse large B cell lymphoma, Burkitt lymphoma, lymphoblastic lymphoma)
- Management—cyclophosphamide, hydroxy-doxorubicin (Adriamycin®), Vincristine (Oncovin®), and prednisone (CHOP); add rituximab if CD20+

MONOCLONAL GAMMOPATHY OF UNKNOWN SIGNIFICANCE (MGUS)

- Increased total protein with monoclonal spike, **absence** of clinical features of multiple myeloma (MM)

- Present in up to 5% of those >80 years of age, increasing to 12% by age 90 years → may progress to MM, macroglobulinemia, other lymphoproliferative disorders, or amyloidosis
- Diagnosis—**<10% plasma cells** on bone marrow biopsy
- Management—follow-up in 6–12 months; no treatment

MULTIPLE MYELOMA (MM)

- Etiology—clonal proliferation of malignant plasma cells in bones and bone marrow leads to bone marrow failure, renal dysfunction, spinal cord or cranial nerve compression, polyneuropathy, hyperviscosity syndrome

4

Diagnosis of Multiple Myeloma

Major Criteria	Minor Criteria
Plasmacytoma on biopsy	Bone marrow 10–30% plasma cells
Bone marrow >**30% plasma cells**	**Lytic bone lesions**
High M-protein IgG >3.5g/dL or IgA >2.0g/dL	M-protein IgG <3.5 g/dL, IgA <2.0 g/dL
Bence-Jones proteinuria >1.0 g/24 hours	Diminished levels of nonmonoclonal Igs IgM <50 mg/dL, IgA <100 mg/dL, or IgG <600 mg/dL

- Management
  - ▸ Candidate for stem cell transplantation (< 75 years)—may use either thalidomide or lenalidomide plus dexamethasone or bortezomib alone or combined prior to SCT
  - ▸ Not a candidate for SCT—melphalan, prednisone, and bortezomib
- Smoldering myeloma—meets criteria for MM but is **asymptomatic**

[1]

BREAST CANCER

- MC malignancy in women; second leading cause of death in women
- Risk factors—age is the most important (1 in 8 by 85 years old)
  - ► Genetic syndromes account for 10% of breast cancers
    - ▷ BRCA1 and BRCA2 account for 30–50% of all inherited cancers
    - ▷ BRCA1 has a 50–85% lifetime risk of breast cancer; 33% lifetime risk for ovarian cancer; men have an increased risk for breast and prostate cancer
    - ▷ BRCA2—similar risk for breast cancer, less for ovarian cancer
  - ► Malignant proliferation of the cells lining the ducts
- Physical findings—breast mass, asymmetry, nipple inversion, edema and thickening of the skin (peau d'orange), and/or lymph nodes in the axilla or supraclavicular fossa
- Diagnosis
  - ► Premenopausal women should be followed through one menstrual cycle; fibroadenomas are benign and extremely common
  - ► **Biopsy all suspicious lesions** (found by breast exam or mammography)
  - ► **Nipple discharge** must be sent for cytology
    - ▷ **Tip:** The most common cause of bloody or abnormal discharge in a woman who is *not* lactating is ductal papilloma. These are usually benign, but always excise to exclude malignancy.
  - ► If the tumor is invasive, **receptor status** must be determined (i.e., ER, PR, HER2/neu)
  - ► Normal mammograms or ultrasounds **do not rule out** breast cancer
  - ► Breast lumps should always be biopsied
  - ► Sentinel node biopsy is as reliable as full-node dissection
- Prognosis
  - ► Tumor size and axillary nodes are the most important
  - ► Oncotype diagnosis: 21 genes tested → recurrence score for the next 10 years

Types of Breast Cancer

Ductal carcinoma (originating from the lining cells of the milk ducts) is the most common histological type	**Lobular carcinoma** (originating from the lobules where milk is produced) is less likely to form a breast lump and is the 2nd most common type
Ductal carcinoma in situ (DCIS) (good prognosis) dose not invade the stoma	Lobular carcinoma in situ (not really a cancer but considered a risk factor)
Invasive carcinoma	**Invasive carcinoma**

Breast Cancer Survival Rates

Staging	Size of Tumor	10-Year Survival
Stage I	<2 cm	75%
Stage II	2–5 cm	50%
Stage III	>5 cm or fixed nodes, chest wall involvement	27%
Stage IV	Metastatic	<10%

4

- Treatment options
    - Lumpectomy followed by radiation therapy ("conservation surgery")—tumor <5 cm; ductal carcinoma in situ
    - Mastectomy—for large tumors or if radiation therapy is contraindicated
    - Chemotherapy—receptor-positive tumors are generally **more responsive** to therapy than receptor negative breast cancer. Use the following drugs unless contraindications or intolerance
        - ER/PR receptor-positive tumors
            - Tamoxifen (watch out for thrombosis) is preferred in **pre**menopausal women
            - Aromatase inhibitors (e.g., anastrazole) are preferred for **post**menopausal women, but watch out for osteoporosis. Monitor with routine DEXA scans.

▷ HER2-positive tumors
  – Trastuzumab (cardiotoxic, check LV function before starting therapy) should be part of the regimen
  – In invasive breast cancer: adjuvant chemotherapy with anthracyclines, taxanes, cyclophosphamide, methotrexate, and 5-FU
  – With lytic bone lesions: include a bisphosphonate (typically IV zoledronic acid) in the regimen with or without radiation therapy

4

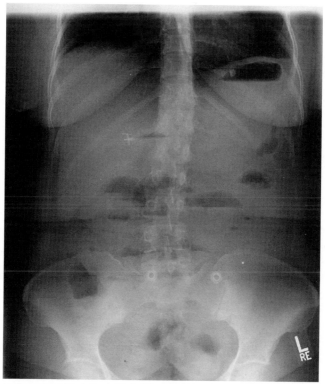

Upright abdominal x-ray showing multiple air-fluid levels in the small bowel

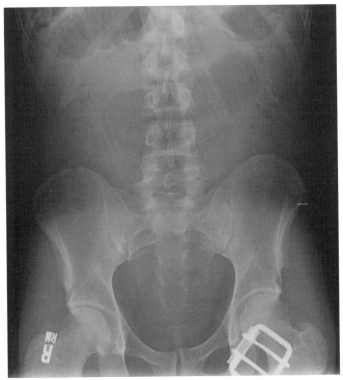

Image courtesy of the Lutheran Medical Center Radiology Department

Upright abdominal x-ray showing multiple dilated loops of small bowel

When you see multiple air-fluid levels and dilated loops of small bowel, keep the following in mind:

- If the patient is in the immediate post-laparotomy period (several days) → think of paralytic ileus
- If the patient has a history of multiple abdominal surgeries months-years prior to presentation → think of small-bowel obstruction secondary to intraperitoneal adhesions
- Always look for and correct hypokalemia → worsens ileus

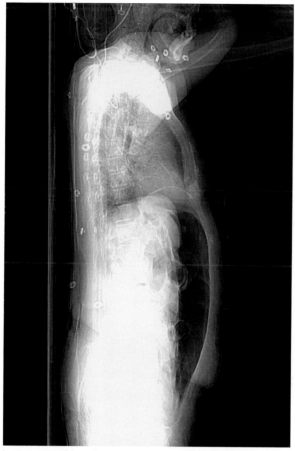

CT scan showing massive pneumoperitoneum (known as "football sign"); only one thing can cause this: acute bowel perforation; look for a diffusely tympanitic abdomen with peritoneal signs with or without sepsis

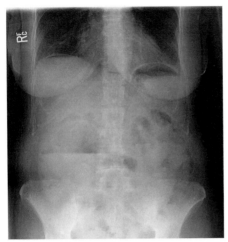

Upright chest x-ray showing free air under the diaphragm (note the sharply demarcated hemidiaphragm) → due to bowel perforation; peritoneal signs with or without sepsis should be present

Image courtesy of the Lutheran Medical Center Radiology Department

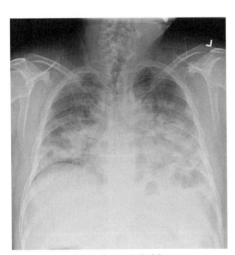

Chest x-ray revealing bilateral ground-glass infiltrates

- When you see this picture plus a PaO$_2$/FiO$_2$ ratio <200 → think of ARDS

Image courtesy of the Lutheran Medical Center Radiology Department

CT scan of the head showing a large, lentiform-shaped hemorrhage due to epidural hematoma; look for a patient with a history of head trauma, and/or initial loss of consciousness followed by a **lucid interval**, who becomes acutely confused or loses consciousness again (the re-losing of consciousness is a bad sign and means the patient has probably herniated)

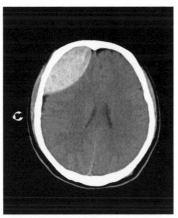

Image courtesy of the Lutheran Medical Center Radiology Department

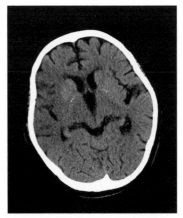

Image courtesy of the Lutheran Medical Center Radiology Department

Head CT scan without contrast showing a large area of hypoattenuation (notice the darkened area) in the distribution of the middle cerebral artery due to acute ischemic CVA

Middle cerebral artery strokes present with:

- Contralateral hemiparesis
- Contralateral sensory denervation
- Homonymous hemianopsia with deviation **toward** the lesion
- If **dominant** hemisphere → **aphasia**
- If **nondominant** hemisphere → confusion and **apraxia**

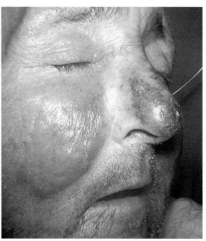

Notice the sharply demarcated, erythematous borders and superficial edema consistent with acute facial erysipelas (MCC is beta-hemolytic streptococci); the disease can be rapidly fulminant in the elderly, so hospitalize the elderly patient and treat with IV ceftriaxone or cefazolin

Image courtesy of Dr. Thomas F. Sellers of Emory University and the Public Health Image Library (*http://phil.cdc.gov*)

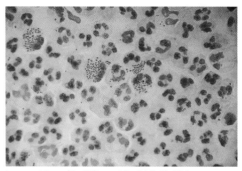

Image courtesy of Joe Millar and the Public Health Image Library (*http://phil.cdc.gov*)

Urethral swab showing multiple PMNs with Gram-negative intracellular diplococci due to *Neisseria gonorrhea* infection; look for a history of purulent penile discharge, dysuria, and recent unprotected sexual intercourse

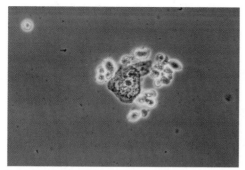

Image courtesy of the Public Health Image Library
(*http://phil.cdc.gov*)

Note the flagella of trichomonads in the upper left-hand
corner of this epithelial cell. Look for a history of increased,
non-odorous, frothy, purulent vaginal discharge in a young
female who has had recent unprotected intercourse.
A friable, erythematous (so-called "strawberry") cervix is
also characteristic of this infection.

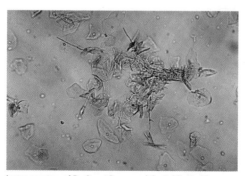

Image courtesy of Dr. Stuart Brown and the Public Health
Image Library (*http://phil.cdc.gov*)

Note the hyphae in this wet mount from the cervix indicating
vaginal candidiasis. History usually includes increased white
cottage cheese–like vaginal discharge with external pruritus.
Frequent sexual intercourse and recent antibiotic usage are the
most common precipitators of infection.

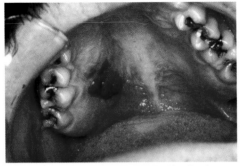

Note the distinctly purple, sharply demarcated lesion consistent with mucocutaneous Kaposi sarcoma (due to HHV-8) in AIDS and immunosuppressed patients

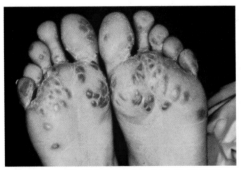

Note the hyperkeratotic appearance of these lesions on the soles consistent with the extra-articular manifestations of reactive arthritis (Reiter syndrome), which is an immune complex–mediated disease more common in those with the HLA-B27 haplotype

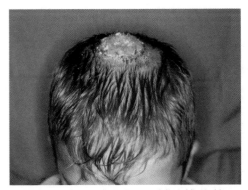

Image courtesy of Dr. Lucille K. Georg and the Public Health Image Library (*http://phil.cdc.gov*)

A tender, boggy scalp lesion with central loss of hair is consistent with a kerion in this patient (due to dermatophyte infection) and must be treated with systemic antifungal therapy. Griseofulvin is still the drug of choice for these infections.

Note the asymmetry and difference in color of this skin lesion, which was diagnosed as malignant melanoma. Remember the ABCDEs, especially in a patient with extensive history of sun exposure or sunburn.

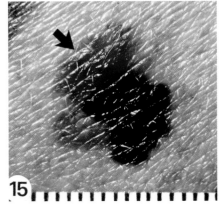

Image courtesy of the National Cancer Institute (*http://visualsonline.cancer.gov*)

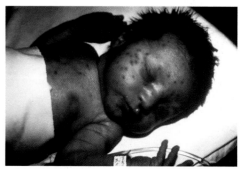

Image courtesy of the Public Health Image Library
(*http://phil.cdc.gov*)

A newborn infant with diffuse, hyperpigmented macular
lesions ("blueberry-muffin" spots) consistent with congenital
rubella syndrome

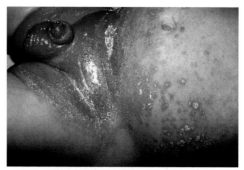

Image courtesy of the Public Health Image Library
(*http://phil.cdc.gov*)

In this infant, note the involvement of the **groin creases** from
superficial candidiasis of the skin; diaper rash **does not** involve
the skin creases. (Very important!)

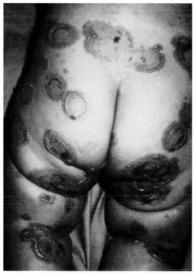

Note the target-like appearance of these diffuse skin lesions due to erythema multiforme. The most common causes are viral infection and drug hypersensitivity.

Image courtesy of Arthur E. Kaye and the Public Health Image Library (*http://phil.cdc.gov*)

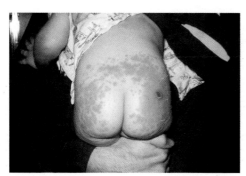

Image courtesy of Allen W. Mathies, MD, and the Public Health Image Library (*http://phil.cdc.gov*)

Note the sloughing and superficial necrosis of the epidermis in this infant due to Stevens-Johnson syndrome with <10% of BSA involved. Toxic epidermal necrolysis has the same presentation except that it involves >10% of the BSA. The most common cause is idiosyncratic drug reactions.

This is a classic targetoid lesion of Lyme disease. Note the central erythema (erythema migrans) with clearing and erythematous borders. The lesions must be >5 cm in diameter.

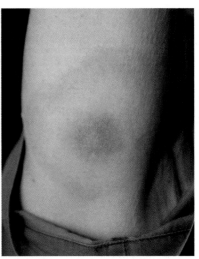

Courtesy of James Gathany and the Public Health Image Library (*http://phil.cdc.gov*)

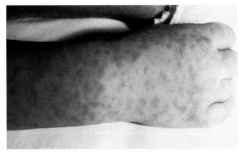

Image courtesy of the Public Health Image Library (*http://phil.cdc.gov*)

This maculopapular rash is due to Rocky Mountain spotted fever. It starts on the wrists and ankles, then spreads centrally and turns into a petechial (non-blanching) rash. Look for a recent history of outdoor activities or camping in the Southeastern or South Central United States. There may or may not be a history of a tick bite. Most patients will have constitutional, nonspecific symptoms.

VI. INFECTIOUS DISEASES

TOXIC SHOCK SYNDROME (TSS)

- Erythematous, **sunburn-like** rash involving the palms and soles with systemic hypotension; **very sick patients**; precipitated by **foreign bodies** including tampons, surgical wounds, and cutaneous and subcutaneous infections with toxin-producing strains of *Staph. aureus* and *Strep. pyogenes*
  - ▶ **Remove** all foreign bodies → aggressive fluid hydration and intravenous clindamycin plus nafcillin → pressors if required
  - ▶ IVIG has been shown to decrease sepsis-related organ failure
- Bacterial exotoxin (TSS-toxin-1, enterotoxin A and B) are superantigens—widespread T-cell activation → massive cytokine activation → fever, rash, and muscle proteolysis and increased sensitivity to endotoxin from GI tract → septic shock

4

BACTEREMIA

Best time to draw blood cultures is 1 hour **prior to** anticipated fever (phagocytes remove bacteria quickly during fever)

MANAGEMENT OF HIV AND AIDS

Principles of HIV Management

- Check viral load and CD4 count every 3–4 months
- When to start HAART (see page 151)
  - ▶ AIDS defining illness
  - ▶ Asymptomatic with CD4 count <500; discuss risk and benefits when CD4 count is >500
  - ▶ Rapidly declining CD4 count of >100/year

Management of Dysphagia in HIV

Dysphagia and/or odynophagia in HIV: assume infection with *Candida albicans* and start empiric course of oral fluconazole	No improvement → perform EGD with biopsy Better → continue fluconazole until T-cells >200 cells/mm³	>1-cm-deep, large ulcer → CMV esophagitis → ganciclovir Multiple, small, shallow ulcers → herpes esophagitis → acyclovir or famciclovir

Abbreviations: cytomegalovirus, CMV; esophagogastroduodenoscopy, EGD

Prophylaxis in HIV

Disease	Start	Drug of Choice	Alternative
PCP*	<200 cells/μL	TMP-SMZ	Dapsone, atovaquone, aerosolized pentamidine
Toxoplasmosis*	<100 cells/μL and IgG seropositive	TMP-SMZ	Dapsone plus leucovorin, pyrimethamine, or atovaquone
MAC	<50 cells/μL	Azithromycin	Clarithromycin, rifabutin
CMV	<50 cells/μL	Ganciclovir	Not routinely recommended

Abbreviations: cytomegalovirus, CMV; Mycobacterium avium *complex*, MAC; Pneumocystis jiroveci *pneumonia*, PCP; trimethoprim-sulfamethoxazole, TMP-SMZ

* May discontinue therapy if CD4 count >**200 cells/μL for >3 months**

Highly Active Antiretroviral Therapy (HAART)

- An adequate antiretroviral regimen consists of **a base and a backbone: ideally, a non-nucleoside (and -nucleotide) reverse transcriptase inhibitor (NNRTI) or protease inhibitor (PI) or integrase inhibitor plus two nucleoside (and nucleotide) reverse transcriptase inhibitors (NRTIs)**
  - NRTIs include abacavir (ABC), didanosine (ddI), emtricitabine (FTC), lamivudine (3TC), stavudine (d4T), tenofovir (TDF), zalcitabine (ddC), zidovudine (ZDV, AZT)
    - ▷ **Tip:** If a patient also has chronic hepatitis B, use two drugs with activity against hepatitis B (lamivudine/emtricitabine/tenofovir are preferred).
  - NNRTIs include delavirdine (DLV), efavirenz (EFV), nevirapine (NVP)
    - ▷ EFV is absolutely contraindicated in pregnancy
  - PIs include saquinavir, ritonavir, indinavir, nelfinavir, atazanavir, darunavir
    - ▷ Most common side effects are **insulin resistance**, hyperglycemia, diabetes, **hyperlipidemia, lipodystrophy**, hepatotoxicity, bleeding
    - ▷ **Tip:** Beware of **crystal-induced nephropathy with indinavir.**
  - Integrase inhibitors include raltegravir and elvitegravir

Cutaneous Cryptococcosis

- Suspect in any HIV-positive patient presenting with **molluscum-like** lesions; papules with central umbilication covered by hemorrhagic crust, oral ulcers, and/or tumors
- Diagnosis through biopsy with culture
  - **Note: Warn lab**, because it is **very contagious**

Pneumocystis jiroveci Pneumonia (PCP) (Formerly *P. carinii* Pneumonia)

- When CD4 count <200 cells/mm^3, should receive prophylaxis with TMP-SMZ

- Symptoms include nonproductive cough, fever, malaise, progressive dyspnea, tachypnea, and **diffuse bilateral "ground-glass"** infiltrates on chest x-ray. Best next actions:

    1. Perform bronchoalveolar lavage (BAL) for specific diagnosis (stain with methamine silver)

    2. Treatment with intravenous TMP-SMZ
        ▷ IV pentamidine is second-line

    3. Add corticosteroids (decreases mortality) when A-A gradient is ≥35 mm Hg and/or PaO$_2$ ≤70 mm Hg on room air

Progressive Multifocal Leukoencephalopathy

- Suspect in any HIV (CD4 count usually <200) or immunocompromised patient with focal findings

- Due to infection with the JC virus

- Most common presentation is hemiparesis and disturbances in speech, vision, and gait

- Best test is **MRI** of the brain, revealing multiple demyelinating lesions

- No treatment available and death usually in <6 months, but should attempt to optimize HAART therapy. Reversal of immunosuppression is key.

Cryptococcal Meningitis

- Suspect in HIV patients with a CD4 cell count <100

- Best initial step is lumbar puncture (LP)—cerebrospinal fluid (CSF) findings include increased opening pressure, leukocytosis with predominant lymphocytes, decreased glucose, increased protein, and positive **India ink** stain; should send for cryptococcal antigen and culture of CSF

- Management—induction treatment with intravenous **amphotericin B and flucytosine for 14 days** → consolidation treatment with fluconazole for 10 weeks → then fluconazole daily for maintenance therapy
  - ▸ Daily LPs are indicated in those with signs of increased pressure (nausea and vomiting, altered mental status [AMS]) to maintain CSF pressure <200 mm H_2O
  - ▸ If no response to initial pharmacotherapy → switch to fluconazole and continue indefinitely

MENINGITIS AND ENCEPHALITIS

Definitions and Initial Management

- Meningitis—infection of the meninges → fever, nuchal rigidity, systemic signs of illness
- Encephalitis—infection of the meninges **plus** brain parenchyma → signs of meningitis **plus** altered mental status

In **any patient with suspected meningitis or encephalitis**, follow these rules for initial management:

- Most sensitive test is CSF protein; most accurate test is CSF culture
- Worrisome findings (focal deficits/seizure/AMS/papilledema)— CT scan first; follow with LP
- No worrisome findings—LP **first**; do not do CT scan
- **Always** start antibiotics **before** sending patient for CT **or** if there is a delay in getting the LP (best next step)
- Predominant PMNs on LP—bacterial meningitis
- Predominant lymphocytes on LP—numerous (see discussion of lymphocyte-predominant LP, following the next tables)

Results of the Lumbar Puncture

CSF Glucose	CSF Protein	CSF WBC Count	Diagnosis
50–75 mg/dL	15–45 mg/dL	0–5 cells/µL	Normal LP
0–45 mg/dL	>250 mg/dL	100–1,000 cells/µL	Bacterial
<10 mg/dL	>250 mg/dL	5–100 cells/µL	Tuberculosis
10–45 mg/dL	50–250 mg/dL	5–1,000 cells/µL	Viral

Abbreviations: cerebrospinal fluid, CSF; lumbar puncture, LP; white blood cell, WBC

Epidemiology of Bacterial Meningitis

Age	MCC	Empiric Coverage
Neonate	Group B Beta-hemolytic streptococci	• 0–7 days: ampicillin plus gentamicin • >7 days: Gram-negative coverage is required: add cefotaxime
Adolescent with a purpuric rash (beware of sudden decompensation due to bilateral adrenal hemorrhage; Dx: Waterhouse-Friderichsen syndrome)	Neisseria meningitides	IV ceftriaxone plus vancomycin
Adult	Streptococcus pneumoniae	As for Adolescent, plus: give IV steroids just prior to or with the first dose of antibiotics (decreases mortality)
Immunocompromised (i.e., with leukemia, lymphoma, or HIV; or age >50 years)	Streptococcus pneumoniae except increased risk of Listeria	Add ampicillin to empiric coverage

Abbreviations: diagnosis, Dx; most common cause, MCC

Lymphocyte-predominant LP: history and physical examination will provide the biggest clue to care of the patient and suspected pathogens.

• Lyme disease (*Borrelia burgdorferi*)—history of recent tick bite or camping in woods; **"bull's-eye" rash**, peripheral rash moving to trunk; do serology; first-line is ceftriaxone

- Rocky Mountain spotted fever (RMSF)—history of recent tick bite or camping in woods; do serology; first-line is doxycycline

- Tuberculosis (TB)—may have history of pulmonary TB, **high CSF protein**; first-line is same as for pulmonary TB **plus steroids**

- Cryptococcal infection—history of AIDS with <100 CD4+ cells; get cryptococcal antigen testing; amphotericin B is first-line, fluconazole second-line acutely; lifelong fluconazole prophylaxis unless CD4 count rises after primary infection resolved

- Viral—nonspecific; supportive care only

Herpes Encephalitis

- Clinical—fever and **confusion** (altered mental status)

- Best initial test is CT scan of brain, may show **temporal** lobe lesions; second-line (if CT or MRI is negative) and most accurate test is CSF PCR-DNA for herpes simplex virus (HSV); IV acyclovir

BRAIN ABSCESS

- Brain abscess—fever and **focal** findings

- Etiology—local spread from ear, nose, and throat infections or embolization from endocarditis **or** severe immunodeficiency (AIDS)-related opportunistic infections

  ▸ Best initial test is CT or MRI scan (but MRI is the most sensitive test) showing **ring-enhancing lesion**

    ▹ If HIV-positive—empiric treatment of toxoplasmosis with pyrimethamine plus sulfadiazine for 7–10 days → repeat CT scan → if better, continue therapy; if not, probably CNS lymphoma; next step in management is brain biopsy

    ▹ If HIV-negative—stereotactic aspiration of abscess **required** for identification of organisms; until cultures positive, **must** initiate broad-spectrum therapy (third-generation cephalosporin plus metronidazole is preferred)

4

OTITIS MEDIA, OTITIS EXTERNA, SINUSITIS, AND PHARYNGITIS

- The organisms associated with both otitis and sinusitis are the **same**: most common cause *Strep. pneumoniae* → *H. influenzae* → *Moraxella*

- Vast majority of acute sinusitis, however, is due to **viral infections**, with bacterial causes accounting for secondary infections

Otitis Media

- Clinical—unilateral ear pain, decreased hearing, bulging tympanic membrane

- Most sensitive finding—immobile membrane with air insufflation

- Best initial treatment is oral amoxicillin

- If treatment fails or otitis recurs—tympanocentesis (most accurate) for culture → amoxicillin/clavulanate (first-line), first- or second-generation cephalosporin, or azithromycin/clarithromycin

Bacterial or Fungal Sinusitis

- Clinical—**purulent** nasal discharge, pain, headache, **point tenderness** on sinuses, lasting >7–10 days (viral etiology less likely)

- If diagnosis is clear—empiric therapy

- If diagnosis is not clear—CT scan of sinuses

- Most accurate test—sinus needle aspiration biopsy for culture

- Criteria to treat as acute bacterial rhinosinusitis are as follows:

  ► Symptoms >10 days with *no* improvement

  ► Severe symptoms (fever >102°F, purulent discharge/facial pain ≥3 days)

  ► Sudden worsening of symptoms after a recent clinical viral infection

- Beware of **mucormycosis in diabetic patients** → fever, sinus pain, thin and **bloody** nasal discharge, diplopia, **dusky-red nasal turbinates** (necrosis) → get endoscopic evaluation with biopsy → broad septated hyphae → sinus CT (or MRI) to assess involvement → surgical debridement and amphotericin B intravenously as soon as possible; **do not delay treatment**, otherwise fulminant, rapid clinical deterioration

Streptococcal Pharyngitis

- For managing possible streptococcal pharyngitis patients, use the Centor criteria:
  - ▸ Fever
  - ▸ Tonsillar exudates
  - ▸ Tender adenopathy
  - ▸ No cough

- Routine testing for GAS pharyngitis is **not necessary** when clear signs/symptoms of upper respiratory infection are present (rhinorrhea, cough, hoarseness, oral ulcers)

- If one criterion, no further study or treatment indicated; if 2 criteria, do rapid strep test; if 3 or more criteria, empiric treatment for Group A *Streptococcus*
  - ▸ Negative rapid strep test in adults = streptococcal pharyngitis unlikely—routine culture not recommended
  - ▸ Negative rapid strep test in children = possible strep pharyngitis → do culture and treat empirically

- Group A *Streptococcus* in 90% of cases causes streptococcal pharyngitis; skin infections cause only renal sequelae, and throat infections cause **both** cardiac and renal sequelae

Diphtheria (*Corynebacterium diphtheriae*)

- Infectious droplet spread more likely in developing countries or immigrants (disease rare in U.S. due to vaccination)

- Clinical—sore throat, **hoarseness**, dry cough, fever, **grayish pseudomembrane**, pharyngeal edema, and tender cervical adenopathy

- Diagnosis with throat cultures

- Management—**diphtheria antitoxin** (from horse serum) can improve course but beware of **serum sickness (10%)** and **anaphylaxis (<1%)**, plus antibiotic therapy (penicillin or erythromycin)

Infectious Mononucleosis

- Etiology—Epstein-Barr virus infection; **"kissing virus,"** salivary transmission

- Clinical—fever, malaise, adenopathy, fatigue

- Diagnosis—heterophil antibody test; EBV serology if negative

- Management

  ▶ Symptomatic treatment and advise to **avoid sports until splenomegaly abates** (due to increased risk of rupture)

  ▶ **Do not give penicillin or amoxicillin;** if you do, the patient will develop a **rash** (mechanism is not known)

  ▶ Give **corticosteroids** if signs of airway compromise or severe infection (aplastic anemia, thrombocytopenia) **only**

- Sequelae—increased risk of nasopharyngeal carcinoma

BRONCHITIS, PNEUMONIA, AND INFLUENZA

Key to differentiating bronchitis from pneumonia is the chest x-ray.

- If no infiltrate—bronchitis

- If positive infiltrate—pneumonia

Use the **CURB-65 criteria** when you must decide on hospital admission: **c**onfusion, **u**remia, **r**espiratory rate (>30), low **b**lood pressure, or age ≥**65** years

- If two or more criteria are present—admit
- If hypotension requiring vasopressors is present—admit to ICU; otherwise, medical floor is adequate

Nursing Home-Acquired or Hospital-Acquired Pneumonia

- No multidrug-resistant (MDR) risk factors/early onset—ceftriaxone **or** a fluoroquinolone **or** ampicillin-sulbactam **or** ertapenem
- MDR risk factors/late onset—an antipseudomonal penicillin or cephalosporin, plus either a fluoroquinolone or aminoglycoside **plus** vancomycin
  - ▶ **Note:** You will essentially need broad-spectrum coverage of atypicals, gram-negatives, and MRSA until cultures and sensitivity are available.

Guidelines for the Treatment of Community-Acquired Pneumonia

Outpatient	Inpatient (Non-ICU)	Inpatient (ICU)
• Healthy adults: macrolide or doxycycline • With comorbidities*: respiratory fluoroquinolone (moxi/levo/gemifloxacin) or a beta-lactam (amoxicillin-clavulanate, cefuroxime) **plus** a macrolide or doxycycline	Respiratory fluoroquinolone **or** Beta-lactam† plus a macrolide or doxycycline	• Beta-lactam† plus azithromycin or a fluoroquinolone (if *Pseudomonas* is suspected‡) • If penicillin-allergic: fluoroquinolone plus aztreonam

Notes:

*Comorbidities include chronic heart/lung/kidney disease, immunosuppression, alcoholism, etc.

†The best beta-lactam antibiotics include cefotaxime, ceftriaxone, and ampicillin-sulbactam.

‡Suspected *Pseudomonas* pneumonia should be treated with an antipseudomonal, antipneumococcal beta-lactam (piperacillin-tazobactam, cefepime, imipenem or meropenem) plus either ciprofloxacin or levofloxacin, or with a beta-lactam plus an aminoglycoside and azithromycin.

4

Influenza Virus

- Type A or B—initially upper respiratory symptoms with prominent **myalgia and arthralgia**; the very old and very young are at highest risk of severe infection, sequelae, and death

- Best test—nasopharyngeal swab for enzyme-linked immunosorbent assay (ELISA) or PCR testing

- Treatment
    - Anti-influenza therapy with a neuramidase inhibitor (oseltamivir, zanamivir) should be offered to those at high risk of sequelae—e.g., those with comorbidities, age <2 years or >65 years, immunosuppressed, pregnant women, residents of chronic care facilities, morbidly obese, Native Americans or Alaskan natives
    - Most effective if given within the first 48 hours of illness; can be considered even after this time has elapsed
    - Can be offered to non-high-risk patients within the first 48 hours of illness to shorten illness duration; otherwise symptomatic therapy is recommended
    - Amantidine and rimantidine are effective only against influenza A. They are not routinely recommended for treatment.

- Vaccination—high yield
    - In 2010, ACIP updated recommendations to vaccinate all individuals six months of age and older
    - If supply is limited, priority is to vaccinate high risk populations first (health-care workers, immunosuppressed, etc.)
    - Inactivated intramuscular vaccine—most commonly used
    - Live intranasal vaccine—avoid in egg allergy, pregnancy, immunocompromised, history of GBS

TUBERCULOSIS (TB)

- Due to *Mycobacterium* tuberculosis infection
- Acute pulmonary TB—key features are copious **blood-tinged** sputum, fever, malaise, cough, **weight loss, night sweats**, lymphadenopathy in a patient with **risk factors** (prisoner, health-care worker, immunosuppressed, or immigrant)
- Latent TB—usually asymptomatic with or without diffuse adenopathy
- Best initial test—chest x-ray revealing apical infiltrates with cavitation with or without mediastinal adenopathy and calcified Ghon complex if active disease

Management of Multidrug-Resistant TB (MDR-TB)

- Treatment for MDR-TB is recommended in those with history of contact with a known MDR patient, with one who has a confirmed case of MDR-TB, or with one from a population of high MDR-TB patterns (China, India, Russia)
- Multiple regimens are available but the best choice without sensitivity results available is a fluoroquinolone plus an aminoglycoside plus ethambutol and pyrazinamide (MDR strains are most commonly resistant to INH and rifampin) until C&S available

4

Management of Suspected Pulmonary TB

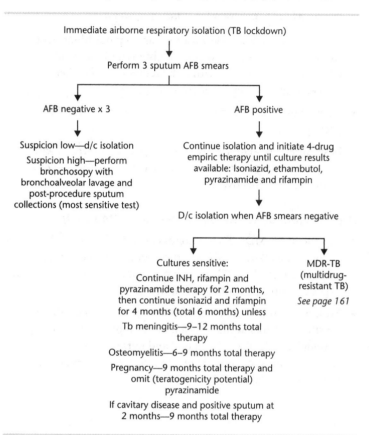

Immediate airborne respiratory isolation (TB lockdown)

↓

Perform 3 sputum AFB smears

AFB negative x 3 | AFB positive

AFB negative x 3

Suspicion low—d/c isolation

Suspicion high—perform bronchosopy with bronchoalveolar lavage and post-procedure sputum collections (most sensitive test)

AFB positive

Continue isolation and initiate 4-drug empiric therapy until culture results available: Isoniazid, ethambutol, pyrazinamide and rifampin

↓

D/c isolation when AFB smears negative

Cultures sensitive:

Continue INH, rifampin and pyrazinamide therapy for 2 months, then continue isoniazid and rifampin for 4 months (total 6 months) unless

Tb meningitis—9–12 months total therapy

Osteomyelitis—6–9 months total therapy

Pregnancy—9 months total therapy and omit (teratogenicity potential) pyrazinamide

If cavitary disease and positive sputum at 2 months—9 months total therapy

MDR-TB (multidrug-resistant TB)

See page 161

Abbreviations: acid-fast bacilli, AFB; discontinue, d/c; isoniazid, INH; tuberculosis, TB

Tip: Addition of dexamethasone in the first month of treatment of TB meningitis has been proven to decrease mortality and morbidity.

Management of Latent TB Infection

Criteria for Positive PPD in Patient Populations

Induration*	Population Considered PPD-Reactive
>5 mm	• HIV-positive, long-term steroid use, or transplant recipients • Chest x-ray consistent with prior infection • Close adult contacts of known TB cases
>10 mm	• Health-care workers • Prisoners • Nursing-home residents • Immunosuppression other than above • Any chronic disease state (cardiac/pulmonary/renal/diabetes) • Close child contacts of known TB cases
>15 mm	Population at low risk of exposure

Abbreviations: purified protein derivative, PPD; tuberculosis, TB
*Must be a localized swelling, not redness at the injection site.

- After positive PPD is confirmed (read within 48 hours) →
  perform chest x-ray
  ► If chest x-ray normal—INH and pyridoxine (vitamin B-6) for
    9 months regardless of age
  ► If chest x-ray abnormal—isolation and three AFBs (acid-fast
    bacilli smears; see Management of Suspected Pulmonary TB,
    preceding page)

- Two-step TST or PPD
  ► If result is indeterminate (e.g., positive PPD but <10 mm
    induration in someone from an area of high prevalence),
    repeat TST within one week
  ► Use the results of the **second TST** to determine management

- Interferon gamma release assay (IGRA)
  ► Specific for M-TB; does not cross-react with most nontuber-
    culous mycobacteria or those who have received the BCG
    vaccine
  ► CDC recommends IGRA over TST for
    ▷ those who have previously received the BCG vaccine
    ▷ those unlikely to return to follow up on the TST reading

Important Side Effects of TB Drugs

- Isoniazid—peripheral neuropathy if not accompanied by vitamin B-6 replacement, drug-induced hepatitis
- Rifampin—orange-red tinge of secretions, drug-induced hepatitis
- Pyrazinamide—hyperuricemia (treat only if symptomatic), drug-induced hepatitis
- Ethambutol—optic neuritis and/or blindness

VIRAL HEPATITIS

Hepatitis A

- Transmitted through feco-oral route
- Clinical—typical hepatitis symptoms in travelers (should be vaccinated if visiting endemic areas) or children who attend **day care**
- Diagnosis—acute disease diagnosed with positive **IgM** anti-hepatitis A virus (HAV)
- Management—treatment is supportive, **no** chronic disease; all household contacts should receive Ig within 2 weeks of last exposure

Hepatitis C

- Epidemiology—most common cause of chronic hepatitis in the United States; seen in IV drug abusers, those who practice unsafe sex, and, rarely, with blood transfusion
- Diagnosis—establish diagnosis with anti-HCV antibody (may take 18 weeks to become positive, in these patients, PCR-RNA viral load is best test)
- Chronic hepatitis C—treatment with pegylated interferon (IFN)-alpha-2b and ribavirin recommended
  - ▸ Genotypes 2 and 3 are most likely to respond to treatment
  - ▸ Genotype 1—must add either telaprevir or boceprevir to treatment regimen

- Side effects of pegylated IFN—depression and suicidality (screen all patients before/during therapy), and flulike symptoms

- Side effect of ribavirin—hemolysis

- Monitor disease activity and effectiveness of treatment with PCR-RNA viral load

Hepatitis B

- Vaccination—three doses of the vaccine administered and test for HbSAb; if negative → administer up to three more doses → test again for HbSAb; if negative, deemed a "nonresponder" (titer < 10 mIU/mL) and must receive hepatitis B Ig whenever exposed to hepatitis B-positive blood (e.g., fingerstick injury)

- Determining hepatitis B status:
  - ▸ HbsAb-positive = previous vaccination and immunity
  - ▸ HbsAg-positive = chronic infection
  - ▸ IgM HbcAb + HbeAg = acute infection and highly infectious (eAg)
  - ▸ IgG HbcAb and HbsAb-positive = recovery from acute infection

- Treatment of hepatitis B infection should be started in those with:
  - ▸ Positive HbeAg with no evidence of cirrhosis, HBV DNA >20,000, and ALT >2 times normal *or* in those with compensated cirrhosis, HBV DNA >2,000, *or* any patient with detectable HBV DNA and decompensated cirrhosis
  - ▸ Negative HbeAg with HBV DNA >2,000 and ALT >2 times normal

- Many options available for treatment (interferon, lamivudine, adefovir, entecavir, telbivudine); details of treatment are beyond the scope of the USMLE exams

4

Cryoglobulinemia

- A small to medium vessel vasculitis caused by immune complex formation

- Seen in HIV, HCV (very high in co-infection), HBV, and connective tissue diseases (e.g., SLE)

- Clinical—history of joint pain, neuropathy, and purpuric skin lesions (usually in lower extremities) in a patient with chronic HIV/hepatitis; may also have glomerulonephritis syndrome

- Diagnosis—best initial test is serum erythrocyte sedimentation rate (ESR) (elevated), also with decreased complement; most accurate test is serum cryoglobulins

- Treatment—treat underlying hepatitis; **steroids** if moderate disease; **plasmapheresis** only if severe (e.g., renal failure, amputation, or advanced neuropathy)

SEXUALLY TRANSMITTED DISEASES (STDs)

See Gynecology, page 291.

CYSTITIS AND PYELONEPHRITIS

Cystitis

- 30% of females will have cystitis in their lifetime, and 30% of those will have recurrent episodes; associated with sexual activity, urinary catheterization, and urinary stasis

- Most common cause is *E. coli* and other gram-negatives (*Proteus, Klebsiella pneumoniae, Enterococci*) and *Staph. saprophyticus*

- Clinical—dysuria, urgency, frequency, suprapubic pain/tenderness, foul-smelling urine with or without fever

- Diagnosis—best initial test is urinalysis: RBCs (>5), WBCs (>5), and bacteria; leukocyte esterase positive on dipstick; nitrite positive if gram-negative organism
  - ▶ Gold standard—culture (>100,000 colonies)

- Treatment—drug of choice is TMP-SMZ, a quinolone, or nitro-furantoin (but extend to 5 days even if uncomplicated)
  - ► Uncomplicated infection—3 days
  - ► Diabetics—7 days

Pyelonephritis

- Etiologies are the same as for cystitis; infection has now ascended into the kidneys/collecting system

- Clinical—same symptoms as cystitis **plus flank tenderness**

- Diagnosis—same as cystitis plus presence of **WBC casts**; more often toxic, febrile with leukocytosis. May or may not have concomitant bacteremia.

- Treatment
  - ► Criteria for hospitalization—toxic-appearing, nausea/vomiting, pregnancy
    - ▷ IV fluoroquinolone, ampicillin plus gentamicin or third-generation cephalosporin until C&S available; treat for 14 days
  - ► Outpatient—adequate if able to tolerate PO meds
    - ▷ Oral fluoroquinolone for 5–7 days
  - ► Failure to respond to therapy after 48–72 hours
    - ▷ Get CT scan of abdomen/pelvis to rule out perinephric abscess; if present, must perform percutaneous drainage
    - ▷ Renal sonogram is also acceptable
    - ▷ In all males, rule out obstructive uropathy or complicated GU pathology

INFECTIOUS DISEASES OF THE SKIN

See Dermatology, Chapter 5.

SEPTIC ARTHRITIS

Divided into gonococcal and nongonococcal arthritis

- Nongonococcal arthritis is by far the most common cause and usually due to *Staph. aureus* **infection followed by streptococcal infection, rare gram-negatives**

- ▶ **Single joint** involvement with erythema, edema, decreased range of motion, pain; knee is the most common site
- ▶ Diagnosis—first step is to perform joint fluid aspiration
  - ▷ Gram stain may or may not be positive
  - ▷ WBC count >50,000 with predominant PMNs and low glucose is diagnostic
- ▶ Treatment—vancomycin plus third-generation cephalosporin until culture results available

- Gonococcal arthritis must be considered in a younger, sexually active patient with risk factors or previous history of gonococcal infection
  - ▶ **Multiple joints** involved, with evidence of **tenosynovitis** (tenderness along tendon insertion); history of **migratory arthralgia, petechiae**, and purpura are common
  - ▶ Diagnosis—first step is to perform joint fluid aspiration, but Gram stain and culture **rarely** positive; must also culture sites of sexual contact, including **urethra, cervix, oropharynx, anus (if MSM)**
  - ▶ Treatment—IV or IM ceftriaxone; if stain reveals Gram-positive cocci in clusters, consider adding IV vancomycin until workup is complete

OSTEOMYELITIS

Spread is either hematogenous or from direct extension of superficial infection.

- Ulcer with necrotic base and foul-smelling discharge (diabetics, decubitus, and peripheral vascular disease) or bone pain and systemic symptoms with no obvious site of superficial infection (intravenous drug abuser, TB, prosthetic joints, or endocarditis)
- Diagnosis
  - ▶ Best initial test—x-ray of affected bones; shows **periosteal elevation** but may take weeks to be abnormal

> ▸ Most accurate test—MRI (next step if x-ray is negative)
>> ▹ If MRI cannot be performed (contraindications), bone scan is next best test
>> ▹ **Tip:** If you can poke a Q-tip into a wound and feel bone, **it is osteomyelitis.**
> ▸ ESR and CRP—elevated during acute infection; both are used to monitor **response to therapy**
> ▸ Bone biopsy—perform blood cultures first; if positive, may sometimes treat based on results; bone biopsy is preferred in all cases of osteomyelitis

- Treatment—requires combined surgical (debridement) and antibiotic treatment for 4–6 weeks
  - ▸ Empiric coverage—vancomycin plus third-generation cephalosporin or an aminoglycoside until cultures available. If a patient is stable, most recommend to start antibiotics empirically after bone biopsy is done (to minimise risk of false negative/low-yield culture).

4

GAS GANGRENE

- Infection of soft tissues with anaerobic organisms (most common cause: *Clostridium perfringens*) leads to rapid spread and myonecrosis, **crepitus**; x-rays reveal feathery gas pattern in tissue; requires **rapid surgical debridement**, IV antibiotics, and hyperbaric oxygen
- Definitive diagnosis made at time of surgery—characteristic pale, dead tissue with sweet-smelling discharge is pathognomonic
- Empiric therapy—high-dose IV penicillin and clindamycin (combined therapy)

LYME DISEASE AND ROCKY MOUNTAIN SPOTTED FEVER

Lyme Disease

- Infection due to *Borrelia burgdorferi*; *Ixodes* tick in Northeastern United States requires **>24 hours** of attachment for transmission

- Presentation—approximately 14–21 days after tick bite, development of **erythema migrans rash** ("bull's-eye" center with >5 cm diameter) and nonspecific illness; 1 week to months later (early disseminated disease), including neurologic symptoms such as Bell palsy, meningitis; or encephalitis; AV node block (most common cardiac manifestation); chronic infection (months to years later) with polyarthritis of large joints, especially the knee

- Treatment—if high suspicion, treat empirically; if not, perform ELISA with Western blot confirmation

- If any sign of neurologic involvement, spinal tap with CSF examination is required; if positive, IV ceftriaxone **must** be used

Management of Lyme Disease

Rash, Bell palsy, joint pain	Cardiac arrhythmia or CNS infection (meningitis, encephalitis)
↓	↓
Doxycyeline preferred; amoxicillin or cefuroxime is also effective	IV ceftriaxone
Length of therapy: Erythema migrans, 10–21 days Bell palsy, 14–28 days Arthritis, 28 days	Length of therapy: CNS disease, 28 days Cardiac disease (symptomatic AV-block or P-R >300 mg), 28 days

Abbreviations: central nervous system, CNS

Rocky Mountain Spotted Fever

- Infection from *Rickettsia rickettsi*; *Dermacentor* tick found in southeastern and south central United States; endemic in **North Carolina**

- Incubation period 5–7 days after exposure in most
- Clinical—fever, headache, and erythematous maculopapular rash starting on the wrists and ankles (involving **palms and soles**) and **spreading centrally,** rash then becomes **petechial**; history of recent camping/outdoor trip
- Labs—look for **thrombocytopenia**, elevated LFTs, azotemia, prolonged PT/PTT. True DIC is rare.
- Diagnosis—best initial test is serology (takes 7 days to become positive); skin biopsy is most sensitive test
- Treatment—doxycycline; second-line chloramphenicol (use in pregnant women)
  - ▸ **Tip:** If you suspect RMSF, start therapy immediately based on your clinical suspicion alone.

4

SYSTEMIC FUNGAL INFECTIONS

Blastomycosis

- Due to infection with *Blastomyces dermatitidis;* results in **pulmonary infection** and frequent dissemination
  - ▸ Usually seen in farmers and outdoor enthusiasts exposed to contaminated soil; multiple clinical presentations, but look for **erythema nodosum** verrucous skin lesions (mimics squamous cell carcinoma), osteomyelitis, and/or prostatitis/epididymo-orchitis
  - ▸ Endemic in North America in the Southeastern and South-central United States; especially the **Mississippi and Ohio river basins**
- Diagnosis—best initial test is sputum, tissue, or purulent fluid culture with wet mount using calcofluor white stain—reveals **broad-based buds**
  - ▸ **Tip:** Remember the B's in blastomycosis—Bone involvement and Broad-Based Buds.

- Treatment
  - ▸ For mild disease, itraconazole is first-line
  - ▸ For severe or CNS disease, amphotericin B is first-line

Aspergillosis

- Due to *Aspergillus fumigatus* (ubiquitous); usually causing pulmonary infection (rarely disseminates) or allergic bronchopulmonary asthma
  - ▸ History will include a patient with neutropenia, chronic steroid use, or chronic immunosuppression, because it is an opportunistic pathogen
  - ▸ Clinical—varies upon disease
  - ▸ Bronchopulmonary asthma—asthma-like symptoms with **high serum IgE and peripheral eosinophilia**
  - ▸ *Mycetoma*—fungal ball on chest x-ray; hemoptysis is often the only presenting symptom
  - ▸ Invasive pulmonary disease—biopsy required for diagnosis; CT scan may show "halo" sign (low attenuation surrounding a nodular pulmonary lesion)
  - ▸ Treatment
    - ▹ Allergic bronchopulmonary disease—steroid taper and bronchodilator
    - ▹ *Mycetoma* (fungal ball)—surgical resection if symptomatically bothersome
    - ▹ Invasive *Aspergillosis*—drug of choice is voriconazole; amphotericin B and caspofungin are alternatives

Histoplasmosis

- Due to infection with *Histoplasma capsulatum;* seen in **cave explorers** and **farmers** exposed to bird droppings (especially chicken coops)
  - ▸ Endemic in the **midwestern United States**, Central America, and South America

- Clinical—suspect in a patient with **hilar adenopathy, cavitary lung lesions, erythema nodosum,** polyarticular symmetric arthritis with or without pericarditis
- Diagnosis—urine and/or serum antigen is best initial test; gold standard is cultures from blood, sputum, or BAL or biopsy of affected sites
- Treatment
  - ▸ Mild disease—oral itraconazole
  - ▸ Moderate to severe—IV amphotericin; add IV methylprednisolone if hypoxemic

4

VII. NEPHROLOGY

ELECTROLYTE DISORDERS

Hyponatremia

- Most common cause is fluid overload (CHF, ARF), syndrome of inappropriate antidiuretic secretion (SIADH), psychogenic polydipsia, or excessive sodium losses

- Important points on hyponatremia

  ▸ Always correct for hyperglycemia (falsely lowers sodium), BUN, and hyperlipidemia

  ▸ Serum osmolarity = $(2 \times$ serum sodium$)$ + (BUN/2.8) + (glucose/18)

  ▸ Hyperglycemia—for every 100 mg/dL of glucose over normal, sodium decreases by 1.6 mg/dL

  ▸ BUN—correct with formula

  ▸ Hyperlipidemia—lab testing equipment causes false hyponatremia

Hyponatremia

Hypotonic	Isotonic	Hypertonic
• Water shifts into the cells (cells swell)	• No change in water shifting	• Water shifts out of the cells (cells shrink)
• **Subdivided into 3 categories** (see table on page 175)	• Plasma volume expanded by lipids or proteins	• Hyperglycemia* or mannitol

Correction for hyperglycemia: For every 100 mg/dL of glucose add 1.6 mEq/L.

- Clinical—the more rapid the drop, the more likely there will be symptoms; symptoms are **neurologic** and range from altered mental status to coma

- Treatment

  ▸ No change in mental status—restrict fluids and correct underlying cause

- ▸ Altered mental status—IV normal saline plus loop diuretic (furosemide or acetazolamide)
- ▸ Stupor or coma—IV hypertonic saline
  - ▹ Correct at rate of 0.5 mEq /hour to prevent **central pontine myelinolysis**

Hypotonic Hyponatremia

Hypovolemic	Euvolemic	Hypervolemic
Salt loss, RENAL (urine Na >20 mEq/L) Diuretics Salt-losing nephropathy RTA Bicarbonaturia Ketonuria	SIADH** Hypothyroid (↑ ADH) Hypopituitarism (↑ ADH) Addison's (↑ ADH) Primary polydipsia	Urine Na <10 mEq/L CHF** Cirrhosis (ascites) Nephrotic syndrome Third spacing (e.g., ileus) Pancreatitis Traumatized muscle
Salt loss, NON-renal (urine Na <10 mEq/L) Diarrhea** Sweating Vomiting		Urine Na >20 mEq/L AKI and CKD

Abbreviations: acute kidney injury, AKI; antidiuretic hormone, ADH; chronic kidney disease, CKD; congestive heart failure, CHF; renal tubular acidosis, RTA; syndrome of inappropriate antidiuretic hormone, SIADH

**CHF, diarrhea, and SIADH together account for 95% of hyponatremia cases.

Hypernatremia

- Most common cause is excessive fluid loss (diarrhea, vomiting, sweat), cellular shift, or diabetes insipidus

Causes of Hypernatremia (>145 mEq/L)

Hypotonic Fluid Loss	Pure Water Loss	Hypertonic Fluid Gain
• GI: vomiting, diarrhea • Diuretics, osmotic diuresis • Relief of urinary obstruction • Recovery from ATN	• Insensible water losses • Central DI • Nephrogenic DI (hereditary, X-linked) • Drugs: lithium, demeclocycline, amphotericin • Hypercalcemia • Hypokalemia • Sjögren syndrome	• Salt ingestion • Sodium bicarbonate or hypertonic saline administration

Abbreviations: acute tubular necrosis, ATN; diabetes insipidus, DI; gastrointestinal, GI

- Clinical—neurologic changes just like hyponatremia
- Treatment
  - No change in mental status—free water replacement (orally or via nasogastric tube)
  - Altered mental status—IV D5W or ½-normal saline with maximum correction of 12 mEq/day
  - Seizures, stupor, or coma—IV D5W or ½-normal saline with maximum correction rate of 1 mEq/hour
  - **Tip:** If circulatory collapse is present, always use **isotonic saline** to correct organ hypoperfusion **first**.

Hypokalemia

- Most common cause is insensible loss (mainly GI; vomiting and diarrhea), transcellular shift, hypomagnesemia, hyperaldosteronemia, and loop or thiazide diuretics
- Clinical—skeletal muscle weakness may progress to paralysis, **ileus**, cardiac **arrhythmias** (**ECG** may show flat T waves or U waves)
- Treatment
  - First, always **check magnesium levels**; if low, supplement either IV (magnesium sulfate) or orally (magnesium oxide; decrease dose if diarrhea occurs)
  - Asymptomatic—oral potassium replacement is adequate; if diuretic-induced, switch to potassium sparing (spironolactone) or add supplemental potassium to daily meds (usually 10–40 mEq/day)
  - Symptomatic (ileus, arrhythmia, etc.)—IV potassium chloride or potassium phosphate in normal or 50%-normal saline at maximum rate of 20 mEq/hour; avoid any dextrose-containing IV fluids (causes transcellular shift and worsens hypokalemia)

Hyperkalemia

- Clinical—most feared complication is fatal arrhythmia; first **check ECG**

- ▶ **ECG changes (in order of progression)**—prolonged PR interval → short QT interval → diffuse peaked T waves → wide QRS complex → torsade de pointes → ventricular tachycardia → ventricular fibrillation → death
- Treatment
  - ▶ Potassium <5.8 mEq/dL and asymptomatic—review medications (especially ACE or ARB) and discontinue; limit oral potassium intake
  - ▶ Potassium >5.8 mEq/dL or symptomatic (muscular weakness)—sodium polystyrene sulfonate (Kayexalate®), either orally (first-line) or as retention enema (second-line)
  - ▶ ECG changes present—first-line treatment is IV calcium chloride (stabilizes myocardial membranes), follow with IV sodium bicarbonate drip, IV dextrose (50 g, prevents hypoglycemia) followed by IV insulin (10 U) to drive potassium intracellularly
    - ▷ Arrange hemodialysis emergently after above measures, if needed

ACID-BASE DISORDERS

- The basics:
  - ▶ Metabolic alkalosis: increased serum HCO_3
    - ▷ Excessive oral or IV bicarbonate, milk-alkali syndrome, transcellular shift, diuretics, vomiting, Conn and/or Cushing syndromes
  - ▶ Respiratory alkalosis: decreased PCO_2
    - ▷ Hyperventilation from any cause: acute anxiety, increased progesterone (pregnancy and chronic liver disease), pain
  - ▶ Metabolic acidosis: decreased serum HCO_3
    - ▷ Increased anion gap: DKA, ethylene glycol poisoning, lactic acidosis, methanol ingestion, uremia
    - ▷ Normal anion gap: diarrhea, RTA
    - ▷ Decreased anion gap: multiple myeloma, hypoalbuminemia, lithium

- ► Respiratory acidosis: increased PCO_2
  - ▷ Hypoventilation from any cause: COPD, asthma exacerbation, chest wall disorders, opiate overdose
- Anion gap = serum sodium – (chloride + serum bicarbonate)
- Primary disorder with compensation: arrows move in the **same** direction (e.g., respiratory acidosis ↑ PCO_2 compensates with metabolic alkalosis ↑ serum HCO_3)
- Mixed disorder: arrows move in **opposite** direction (e.g., respiratory acidosis ↑ PCO_2 with metabolic acidosis ↓ serum HCO_3)
- Practice arterial blood gases (ABGs):
  1. pH 7.35, PCO_2 45, PO_2 80, HCO_3 28 = _____
  2. pH 7.10, PCO_2 40, PO_2 80, HCO_3 7 = _____
  3. pH 7.49, PCO_2 30, PO_2 80, HCO_3 28 = _____
  4. pH 7.38, PCO_2 60, PO_2 70, HCO_3 30 = _____
  - ► Answers
    1. Metabolic alkalosis with respiratory acidosis (compensated)
    2. Metabolic acidosis with no respiratory compensation
    3. Metabolic alkalosis with some respiratory acidosis
    4. Respiratory acidosis with metabolic alkalosis (compensated)

ACUTE RENAL FAILURE—PRERENAL, INTRARENAL, AND POSTRENAL CAUSES

- Pathophysiology—elevation of blood urea nitrogen (BUN) over several hours to days with or without uremia
  - ► Uremia indicates a need for urgent dialysis—includes metabolic acidosis, hyperkalemia, hyperphosphatemia, hypocalcemia, pleuritis or pericarditis, pleural effusions, and/or mental status changes
- Best measure of renal function is creatinine clearance—if age >65 years and creatinine <1.0 mg/dL, you must round creatinine up to 1.0 mg/dL

Prerenal

- Most common cause is dehydration and shock; due to decreased renal perfusion from any cause: CHF, diuretics, vomiting, diarrhea, etc.

- Diagnosis: BUN/Cr ratio of ≥**20:1**, decreased **FeNa (<1%), high** urine **osmolality** (high specific gravity; >1.030 on urine dipstick)

Prerenal Syndromes

Diagnosis	Clinical Findings	Diagnosis	Treatment/ Complications
Bilateral renal artery stenosis	**Multidrug-resistant HTN** and signs of **prerenal azotemia**	1. Rapid rise in BUN/Cr after starting therapy 2. Suspect in **young** patient with **fibromuscular dysplasia** 3. Suspect in **elderly** with history of **atherosclerotic disease**	First-line: stenting
Hepatorenal syndrome	**Prerenal azotemia** and history of **liver disease**	Failure of BUN/Cr ratio to improve after ≥**1.5 L** of IV normal saline	• Treat liver disease • Dialysis if evidence of uremia
ACE inhibitor-induced renal insufficiency or failure	**Rise in BUN/Cr** after initiating therapy; seen in those with **baseline** renal insufficiency or bilateral RAS	Monitor BUN/Cr weekly after starting therapy	**Continue** if rise is ≤**30% increase from pretreatment creatinine** (benefit outweighs the risk); discontinue if greater

Abbreviations: angiotensin-converting enzyme, ACE; blood urine nitrogen, BUN; hypertension, HTN; renal artery stenosis, RAS

Intrarenal

- Most common cause based upon age and risk factors; due to intrinsic renal defects, including glomerulonephritis and acute tubular necrosis

- Diagnosis—look for BUN/Cr ratio of 10:1; other findings dependent on cause

Intrarenal Causes of Renal Failure

Diagnosis	Important History	Studies	Treatment
Acute papillary necrosis	Use of **NSAIDs** in **elderly or baseline renal disease; sickle-cell crisis; sudden fever and flank pain**	• Best initial test: UA with microscopy and culture shows: **WBCs; negative urine cultures; and granular, necrotic sediment** • Most accurate test: abdominal/pelvic CT scan shows **irregular renal contours**	Stop NSAIDs; treat underlying cause
Cholesterol embolization syndrome	**Recent catheterization** (causes embolization from vessel walls) **followed by ARF and bluish discoloration of fingers/toes** (vascular occlusion from emboli)	• Best initial test: UA with microscopy shows **increased eosinophils on Wright-Hansel stain** • Most accurate test: skin biopsy shows cholesterol crystals	Supportive
Allergic interstitial nephritis	**New medication** causing **allergic drug reaction** or **infection; fever**	Best initial test: UA with microscopy shows **increased eosinophils on Wright-Hansel stain**	• First-line: stop drug or treat infection • Second-line: if failure to improve, start steroids

(continued)

Intrarenal Causes of Renal Failure (continued)

Diagnosis	Important History	Studies	Treatment
Contrast-induced renal failure	History of **recent IV contrast**, usually in a person with **baseline renal disease** or diabetes on **oral hypoglycemics**	Best initial test: UA; disease usually causes acute tubular necrosis; look for **muddy brown casts on UA**	• First-line: vigorous IV hydration • Prevention: stop all oral hypoglycemics at least 48 hours before contrast and provide IV hydration with or without N-acetylcysteine
Ethylene glycol poisoning	**Antifreeze** ingestion with **suicidal** ideations; look for **drunk** person with **increased anion gap metabolic acidosis**	Best initial test: UA with microscopy shows **oxalate crystals**	First-line: IV fomepizole followed by dialysis
Rhabdomyolysis	**Severe trauma** (crushing injuries), recent **strenuous physical exertion, hypokalemia*** or **ABO incompatibility** with ARF	• Best initial test: UA shows **positive urine dipstick for hemoglobin**, and microscopy reveals **absence of red blood cells** • Also check serum CPK if muscular damage suspected	• First-line: check ECG to rule out hyperkalemic changes, and treat if needed • Then: **IV normal saline plus sodium bicarbonate**; add mannitol if severe
Tumor lysis syndrome	**Recent chemotherapy with ARF shortly thereafter**	Best initial test: UA with microscopy shows **urate crystals**	• First-line: **vigorous IV hydration with sodium bicarbonate** • Prevent with prechemotherapy IV hydration plus allopurinol

Abbreviations: A,B,O blood groups, ABO; acute renal failure, ARF; creatinine phosphokinase, CPK; nonsteroidal anti-inflammatory drugs, NSAIDs; urinalysis, UA

*Hypokalemia may cause rhabdomyolysis, but hyperkalemia is the result of rapid muscular breakdown.

Postrenal

- Most common cause depends on age group; due to **bilateral** obstruction of urine outflow such as obstructing calculi or pelvic tumors; look for **oliguria** in history
  - ▶ In the young—obstructing calculi at level of bladder neck
  - ▶ In the elderly—benign prostatic hyperplasia (BPH)
- Diagnosis: BUN/Cr ratio of ≥20:1, decreased **FeNa (<1%)**, **distended bladder** on examination **or** bilateral hydronephrosis on renal sonogram or CT scan or postvoid **residual volume of >50 mL** (use Foley catheter to measure)
- Treatment—relieve obstruction; start prazosin or terazosin if elderly male with newly diagnosed BPH

CHRONIC RENAL FAILURE AND END-STAGE RENAL DISEASE (ESRD)

- Indications for dialysis—fluid overload with oliguria or anuria; "-itis" including pericarditis, pleuritis; uremia, significant platelet dysfunction, significant electrolyte abnormalities, and/or altered mental status
- Two methods available: hemodialysis (through Tesio® catheter, AV fistula, or AV graft), and peritoneal dialysis (can be done at home)
  - ▶ Peritoneal dialysis should be used only with a **reliable** patient; carries increased incidence of infection—i.e., peritonitis
- Place on transplant list as long as criteria are met (less mortality compared to long-term hemodialysis)
- Almost all dialysis patients require EPO injections to prevent normocytic anemia (kidneys no longer produce EPO)
- Hypocalcemia and hyperphosphatemia—secondary to inability to produce 1,25-dihydroxy vitamin D; need vitamin D replacement and calcium acetate or calcium carbonate (phosphate binders)

- Coronary artery disease (CAD)—ESRD is an **equivalent** of **CAD**; all hemodialysis patients should be on a beta-blocker, a statin, and an ACE inhibitor (monitor potassium levels); keep blood pressure <130/80 mm Hg
- Diet—all hemodialysis patients should be on a protein- and element-restricted diet (sodium, potassium, magnesium, and phosphate)

Glomerulonephritis

- Multiple types, but all have at least one specific feature you can identify; the most accurate (gold-standard test) for all forms is renal biopsy
- May cause nephrotic or nephritic syndrome

VASCULITIC DISORDERS

See Rheumatology, page 224.

GOODPASTURE SYNDROME

- Clinical—lung and renal involvement causes **hemoptysis, cough**, dyspnea, and **hematuria**
- Diagnosis—best initial test is anti–basement membrane antibody; confirm with lung (hemosiderin-laden macrophages) or renal biopsy
- Treatment—plasmapheresis and IV methylprednisolone

IgA NEPHROPATHY (BERGER DISEASE)

- Pathophysiology/clinical—deposition of IgA after recent viral infection; most common in **young Asian American** patients
- Clinical—hematuria and hypertension 1–2 days after a sore throat/URI syndrome causing acute or chronic renal failure
- Diagnosis—best initial test is serum IgA, but is not always elevated; gold standard is renal biopsy
- Treatment—fish oil may improve symptoms; otherwise treatment is symptomatic

AUTOSOMAL DOMINANT POLYCYSTIC KIDNEY DISEASE

- Clinical—hypertension, renal cysts (may become infected or hemorrhage, causing pain), CKD, nephrolithiasis, hepatic cysts, cerebral aneurysms, MVP, aortic root dilation, and/or colonic diverticula

- Diagnosis—renal ultrasound; positive family history

- Treatment—control hypertension; infected or bleeding cysts may require drainage or nephrectomy if severe. May progress to requiring dialysis until renal transplant can be done.

HEMOLYTIC UREMIC SYNDROME AND THROMBOTIC THROMBOCYTOPENIC PURPURA

Hemolytic Uremic Syndrome (HUS)

- **Triad** of **microangiopathic hemolytic anemia** (shistocytes on peripheral smear and increased serum LDH with normal GGT, indicating hemolysis), **thrombocytopenia, and renal insufficiency**

- Usually in **children** (see Nephritic and Nephrotic Syndromes, page 391) and associated with *E. coli* **0157:H7**; common scenario is a child eating undercooked hamburger

Thrombotic Thrombocytopenic Purpura (TTP)

- **Pentad** of (1) **microangiopathic hemolytic anemia,** (2) **thrombocytopenia,** (3) **fever,** (4) **neurologic findings** (which may include headache, neurologic deficit, and others), **and** (5) **renal insufficiency**

- The first 2 criteria *must* be present to make a diagnosis. Urinalysis typically shows several schistocytes in every high-power field

- More common in **adults** and associated with **HIV/AIDS** or **ticlopidine** (antiplatelet)
- Treatment—try to avoid platelet transfusions unless life-threatening bleeding (causes worsening of thrombosis); dipyrimidole to inhibit platelet aggregation if needed; **plasmapheresis** if disease is severe

RAPIDLY PROGRESSIVE GLOMERULONEPHRITIS (RPGN)

- Idiopathic glomerulonephritis associated with **HIV and AIDS**
- Clinical—rapid onset of ARF; look for **crescent formation** on renal biopsy
- Treatment—steroids plus cyclophosphamide, but will usually progress to ESRD requiring hemodialysis

4

NEPHROTIC SYNDROMES (NS)

- Diagnosis—**proteinuria > 3.5 g** in 24 hours, **hypoalbuminemia, edema** (from reduced oncotic pressure), **hyperlipidemia** (loss of chylomicron substrate), and **hyperlipiduria** ("cross" formations on urine microscopy)
  - ▸ **Tip:** All have fusion of the foot processes on electron microscopy.
- Treatment—remove or treat the underlying cause

Nephrotic Syndromes

Diagnosis	Etiologies	Presentation	Treatment
Minimal change	NSAIDs, leukemia, lymphoma, allergy	MCC of NS in **children**	Steroids: • 90% go into remission • 25% are long-term
Focal segmental GN (30–35% of adult NS)	HIV, obesity, heroin use, ureterovescical reflux	Segments of some glomeruli are diseased	• ACE-I or ARB + corticosteroids: 50–70% remission • In those that fail: cyclosporine, tacrolimus → despite this, will likely progress to ESRD in 5 years
Membranous	• HBV, HCV, syphilis • Cancer: breast, lung, colon • Hydralazine • NSAIDs	• MCC of NS in **adults** • All and entire glomeruli diseased • Light microscopy shows thick capillary walls • **Subepithelial spikes on EM**	As above
Membrano-proliferative	Same causes as Membranous	• Light microscopy shows mesangial proliferation • Electron microscopy shows either subendothelial (type I) or dense (type II) deposits • **C3 nephritic factor** is specific to diagnosis but not widely available	As above

Abbreviations: angiotensin-converting enzyme inhibitor, ACE-I; angiotensin receptor blocker, ARB; electron microscopy, EM; end-stage renal disease, ESRD; glomuleronephritis, GN; hepatitis B virus, HBV; hepatitis C virus, HCV; most common cause, MCC; nephrotic syndromes, NS; non-steroidal anti-inflammatory drugs, NSAIDs

RENAL TUBULAR ACIDOSIS (RTA)

Type 1 (Distal)	Type 2 (Proximal)	Type 4
Cannot excrete H^+ ions	Cannot reabsorb HCO_3^-	Deficiency of aldosterone or resistance to its effects
Primary RTA Secondary • Sjögren syndrome • SLE • RA • Familial • Hyperparathyroidism	Primary RTA Secondary • Sjögren syndrome • Heavy metals • Ifosfamide • Myeloma • VitD deficiency • Amyloidosis	Aldosterone Deficiency • Addison • Hyporeninemic hypoaldosteronism • MCC DM (50% of cases) • Interstitial nephritis (50% of cases) • Idiopathic • HTN • Gout Aldosterone Resistance NSAIDs, ACE-I, ARB, amiloride, trimethoprim, pentmidine
Urine pH >5.5	Urine pH <5.5	Urine pH <5.5
Hypokalemia	Hypokalemia	Hyperkalemia
Normal gap metabolic acidosis	Normal gap metabolic acidosis	Normal gap hyperchloremic metabolic acidosis
Calcium phosphate stones, **nephrocalcinosis**	**Osteomalacia, rickets**	Renal insufficiency
• Dx with acid load test (oral ammonium chloride fails to decrease urine pH) • Increased urine anion gap ([urine $Na^+ + K^+$] – urine Cl^-)	• Dx with IV sodium bicarbonate load test • Urine remains acidic (pH <5.0)	Dx with oral sodium restriction test: will show high urinary sodium
Treatment: **oral sodium bicarbonate and potassium replacement**	Treatment: oral sodium bicarbonate, potassium replacement and thiazide	Treatment: oral **fludrocortisone**

Abbreviations: angiotensin-converting enzyme inhibitor, ACE-I; angiotensin receptor blocker, ARB; diabetes mellitus, DM; diagnosis, Dx; electron microscopy, EM; end-stage renal disease, ESRD; glomerulonephritis, GN; hepatitis B virus, HBV; hepatitis C virus, HCV; most common cause, MCC; non-steroidal anti-inflammatory drugs, NSAIDs; rheumatoid arthritis, RA; renal tubular acidosis, RTA; systemic lupus erythematosus, SLE

Nephrolithiasis

Type	Causes	Appearance
Calcium oxalate	**Hereditary,** malabsorption syndromes, vitamin D deficiency, metastatic disease or multiple myeloma	O⊠ALATE
Cysteine	**Hereditary**	⬡YSTINE
Indinavir and acyclovir	Antiretroviral and antiviral drugs	✗ NEEDLE SHAPED
Struvite	Urease producing bacteria-causing cystitis and pyelonephritis (*Proteus, Klebsiella, and Pseudomonas*)	Coffin Lids / AMMONIUM MAGNESIUM TRIPHOSPHATE OR "STRUVITE"
Uric acid	Gout, malignancy, Chron disease	☐RIC ACID

MANAGEMENT OF RENAL STONES

- Same for all types of stone
  - ▸ If <4 mm in diameter—will likely pass spontaneously; aggressive hydration and adequate pain control are the best next steps
  - ▸ If 5–10 mm in diameter—may or may not pass spontaneously; shock-wave lithotripsy is the best initial management
  - ▸ If >10 mm—flexible ureteroscopy combined with laser lithotripsy is probably the best management

VIII. NEUROLOGY

TRANSIENT ISCHEMIC ATTACK (TIA) AND STROKE

- Both TIA and stroke are due to embolic phenomena
  - ► TIA—transient focal neurologic deficit **resolving** within <24 hours of onset (usually resolves within **minutes**); patient usually presents to the clinic after event has resolved
  - ► Stroke—permanent, irreversible focal neurologic deficit; patients usually present to emergency department hours after event occurred
  - ► **Tip:** TIA is considered a neurologic emergency because there is a significant risk of stroke within 48 hours.
- Source—carotid stenosis or cardiac thrombi

Management of Acute Cerebrovascular Accident (CVA)

- Initial test of choice is noncontrast CT (may be normal for 24 hours after event); if negative, next best test is noncontrast MRI of brain (gold standard; may be normal in initial 6 hours after event)
- First 4.5 hours from symptom onset—tPA is the drug of choice if no contraindications exist
  - ► Contraindications to use of tPA:
    - ▷ Seizure with stroke onset
    - ▷ Previous CVA or trauma in <3 months
    - ▷ Hemorrhage within 21 days
    - ▷ Surgery within 14 days
    - ▷ Any history of intracranial hemorrhage
    - ▷ Sustained blood pressure >185/110 mm Hg
    - ▷ Any current anticoagulation (warfarin or heparin)

4

▷ Platelet count <100,000/mm³
▷ NR >1.7
▷ Plasma glucose <50 mg/dL or >400 mg/dL

Site of Occlusive CVA and Expected Clinical Symptoms

Site of Occlusion	Clinical Findings
ACA	• Contralateral lower extremity weakness > upper extremity weakness • Contralateral lower extremity sensory denervation with or without incontinence and confusion
MCA	• Contralateral hemiparesis • Contralateral sensory denervation • Homonymous hemianopsia with deviation **toward** the lesion • If **dominant** hemisphere → **aphasia** • If **nondominant** hemisphere → confusion and **apraxia**
PCA	• Contralateral homonymous hemianopsia • Hallucination • Agnosia
Paramedian branches of basilar artery	• "Locked-in syndrome" • Only vertical eye movements remain intact
PICA	• Ipsilateral facial numbness • Contralateral body numbness • Horner syndrome • Vertigo • Ataxia and dysarthria
Ophthalmic artery	Complete blindness (amaurosis fugax); always due to **carotid embolization**

Abbreviations: anterior cerebral artery, ACA; cerebrovascular accident, CVA; middle cerebral artery, MCA; posterior cerebral artery, PCA; posterior inferior cerebellar artery, PICA

• Role of heparin drip in CVA—heparin drip is **not** a primary treatment for CVA; it has a role only in patients who are at high risk of a second CVA from thromboembolic phenomena; specifically, those with **A-fib or those with heart disease at risk of undiagnosed A-fib**

• Blood pressure control in CVA
  ▸ Drug of choice is IV labetalol

▶ In general, do not be aggressive with antihypertensives to keep systolic BP <140 mm Hg unless there is a clear indication to do so (e.g., acute heart failure, myocardial infarction), because it may cause cerebral hypoperfusion in the distribution of the stroke

Blood Pressure Control in CVA

Ischemic CVA	Hemorrhagic CVA
• Thrombolysis given—up to 185/110 mm Hg • Thrombolysis not given—up to 220/120 mm Hg	Up to 185/110 mm Hg

Further Management of TIA and Workup After Acute CVA

4

- Carotid duplex, Holter monitor, and 2-D echocardiogram should all be performed
- For test-taking—the choice of which test to do first must be based on presentation. Examples: in an 80-year-old woman with a history of CHF, do the Holter first (to rule out A-fib); but in a 50-year-old male smoker, check the carotids first (atherosclerotic disease is more likely)

Carotid Endarterectomy

- Indications for carotid endarterectomy
  - ▶ >70% occlusion **with** symptoms; **or**
  - ▶ >60% occlusion, age <60 years, and asymptomatic
- Contraindications for carotid endarterectomy
  - ▶ Prior CVA with irreversible focal deficits
  - ▶ 100% occlusion (risk outweighs benefits)

If A-fib Is Found on Holter

Warfarin, unless contraindicated; goal INR: 2–3

Stroke Prevention

- All patients with TIA or history of CVA should be on **aspirin** (start 24 hours after tPA)
  - ▸ If allergic to aspirin—use clopidogrel
  - ▸ If recurrent CVA on aspirin—**add** dipyridamole (Aggrenox® is the combination drug of acetylsalicylic acid [ASA]/dipyridamole) and instruct that it must be taken at the same time every day

Treatment of Post-CVA Spasticity

Dantrolene is the drug of choice; baclofen and benzodiazepines are second-line (increased risk of sedation).

TRIGEMINAL NEURALGIA

- Clinical—sudden onset of **severe paroxysmal lower jaw and facial pain** along the trigeminal nerve; worsened by any **touch, cold breeze, chewing, touching a cotton swab over lower jaw/cheek, or brushing teeth**
- Diagnosis—clinical
- Treatment—**carbamazepine** is the drug of choice; if it fails, then baclofen or gabapentin; alcohol injection of trigeminal nerve is last resort

MOVEMENT DISORDERS

Benign Essential Tremor

- Familial **hand** tremor that **worsens** with **action** (rarely seen in legs/feet); **less tremor at rest** (opposite of Parkinson disease); **head bobbing** and trembling voice also seen
- Autosomal dominant transmission with variable expression
- Characteristically **improves with alcohol** in two-thirds of patients
- Drug of choice is **propranolol**; if fails, try a benzodiazepine or primidone (preferred in the elderly)
  - ▸ Gabapentin and topiramate are second-line

Huntington Disease

- Autosomal dominant expansion of CGG trinucleotide repeats, progressively worsening with each generation
- Clinical—chorea and behavioral changes at age of **40** → progresses to ataxia → depression → severe dementia → death within 10–15 years of diagnosis
- Diagnosis—genetic testing is first-line; CT scan may show **atrophy of the caudate nucleus**
- Treatment—none; control behavioral changes/psychosis with antipsychotics (haloperidol also helps to control chorea)

Parkinson Disease

- Multiple insults deplete dopamine in basal ganglia; includes drugs, toxins, or tumor
- Clinical—**bradykinesia**, **lead-pipe rigidity**, instability, **resting tremor, which improves with action** (contrast to benign essential tremor), **masklike face**
  - ▸ Multiple system atrophy (formerly Shy-Drager syndrome) presents with a combination of Parkinsonism plus severe orthostatic hypotension (autonomic dysfunction) and ataxia
- Diagnosis—entirely clinical
- Treatment—carbidopa/levodopa is always reserved for severe functional impairment, secondary to tolerance of effects
  - ▸ If age <60 years
    - ▹ Drug of choice is anticholinergics—benztropine or trihexyphenidyl
  - ▸ If age >60 years
    - ▹ Drug of choice is amantadine
  - ▸ If severe impairment
    - ▹ Drug of choice is carbidopa/levodopa
      - – If significant fluctuations in response to therapy, add selegiline, a dopamine agonist (pramipexole, ropinirole), or a catechol-O-methyltransferase (COMT) inhibitor (tolcapone or entacapone)

4

- ► If medical treatment fails
    - ▷ Before changing medication, add a selective serotonin reuptake inhibitor (**SSRI**) (rate of depression high)
    - ▷ If all medical therapy is exhausted—pallidotomy or thalamotomy

Restless Legs Syndrome

- Clinical—**"creepy, crawly" feeling in legs at night** leads to insomnia and distress

- Diagnosis—clinical; often history of **bruising** secondary to movement during sleep

- Treatment
    - ► Must rule out **iron deficiency anemia or uremia**
    - ► Dopamine agonists are first-line—pramipexole or ropironole; second-line is benzodiazepines if no improvement; third-line is levodopa/carbidopa

SPINAL CORD DISEASE

Refresher on the spinal tracts:

- Dorsal column system—position and vibration sense, immediately contralateral

- Spinothalamic tracts—pain and temperature; ipsilateral at level of innervations and contralateral below

- Corticospinal tracts—muscular innervations; ipsilateral until level of pyramids (brain stem)

Spinal Cord Disease

Disease	Etiology	Symptoms	Treatment
Anterior spinal artery infarction	Embolism of artery supplying anterior two-thirds of spinal cord	Only **dorsal columns** remain intact → flaccid paresis progressing into spastic paresis below lesion	None
Brown-Sequard syndrome	Hemitransection of spinal cord—MCC trauma	Ipsilateral hemiparesis, loss of position and vibration sense, contralateral loss of pain and temperature sense	None
Syringomyelia	• Communicating: Arnold-Chiari MCC • Noncommunicating: tumors and trauma MCC	Only **dorsal columns** and **tactile touch** remain intact; usually at **cervical spinal cord**	Surgical
Subacute combined degeneration	Vitamin B-12 deficiency	Paresthesia, spastic paresis, and ataxia (complete loss of dorsal columns)	Vitamin B-12 replacement

Abbreviations: most common cause, MCC

DEMYELINATING DISEASE

Amyotrophic Lateral Sclerosis (ALS) (Lou Gehrig Disease)

- Pathology—degeneration of anterior horn cells and corticospinal tracts from demyelinating disease of both upper and lower motor neurons

- Clinical—combined upper and lower motor neuron disease with loss of cranial nerve function that usually starts in the **hands**; bowel/bladder and sexual function (autonomics) are **not affected**; ability to make decisions is also **not affected** (cognition remains intact); affects males > females

- Diagnosis—best initial tests are electromyogram (fibrillations; positive sharp waves; and large, long motor action potentials) and nerve conduction studies (decreased motor action potentials); CT/MRI and lumbar puncture (LP) are **normal**; creatinine phosphokinase (CPK) elevated

- Treatment—drug of choice is **riluzole**; treat spasticity with baclofen
  - ▸ Vitamin E helpful but has no effect on survival

Guillain-Barré Syndrome (GBS)

- Formation of antibodies to **myelin** 1–3 weeks after infection with *Campylobacter*, Epstein-Barr virus, HSV, Lyme disease, or cytomegalovirus (CMV), or polio vaccination

- **Ascending paralysis** (feet > arms) with **sensory loss** and total **loss of reflexes**; if severe → autonomic dysfunction
  - ▸ Miller Fisher variant—disease affects the brain stem first and presents with a **triad** of areflexia, ataxia, and ophthalmoplegia; look for a patient with diplopia and "wobbly" gait

- Diagnosis—first do LP → **increased protein and normal WBC count; confirm diagnosis with electromyography → demyelination pattern**
  - ▸ Positive for circulating **GQ1b antibodies** very useful

Management of Guillain-Barré Syndrome

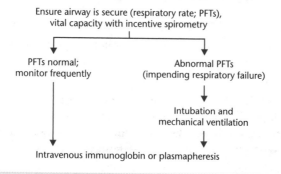

Ensure airway is secure (respiratory rate; PFTs), vital capacity with incentive spirometry

PFTs normal; monitor frequently

Abnormal PFTs (impending respiratory failure)

Intubation and mechanical ventilation

Intravenous immunoglobin or plasmapheresis

Abbreviations: pulmonary function tests, PFTs

Multiple Sclerosis (MS)

- Autoimmune destruction of myelin most common in **young females**; geographically **specific to the northern hemisphere**

- Clinical—multiple complaints; most often **ataxia and diplopia** which remitted prior to presentation; isolated weakness of one limb, etc.

  ▸ Four clinical subtypes (see Treatment of Multiple Sclerosis table)

  ▸ **Optic neuritis** seen in 25% of patients and is the initial presentation in 25% of patients

- Diagnosis—best initial test is **contrast-enhanced MRI**; shows characteristic increased T1 and T2 signal intensities in a **patchy distribution** (indicates active disease)

  ▸ If MRI negative and suspicion for disease is high → do **LP**, findings are:

    ▹ Increased protein and mildly increased WBCs with **oligoclonal IgG band pattern**

  ▸ Schumacher criteria for diagnosis of MS: 2 CNS lesions, 2 separate attacks or 6 months of progressive decline, symptoms must involve the white matter, objective deficits in the neurologic exam, and no other medical problem can explain the presentation

Treatment of Multiple Sclerosis

Type	Presentation	Acute Exacerbation	Disease Maintenance/ DOC	Second-Line
Relapsing remitting MS **(most common type)**	Exacerbations with complete or incomplete recovery of function; often worsens with each relapse	IV steroids followed by oral taper → plasma exchange therapy if unresponsive	IFN-beta-1a **or** IFN-beta-1b **or** Glatiramer acetate	Mitoxantrone*, IVIG, or other immunosuppressive agents

(continued)

Treatment of Multiple Sclerosis (continued)

Type	Presentation	Acute Exacerbation	Disease Maintenance/ DOC	Second-Line
Primary progressive MS	Steady decline in neurological function with no clear exacerbations; early complete disability	No approved treatment	No approved treatment	No approved treatment
Secondary progressive MS	Each exacerbation accompanied by progressively worsening function and incomplete recovery	IV steroids followed by oral taper → plasma exchange therapy if unresponsive	IFN-beta-1b	Mitoxantrone, IVIG, or other immunosuppressive agents
Progressive relapsing	Steady neurologic decline with episodic attacks	No approved treatment	No approved treatment	No approved treatment

Abbreviations: drug of choice, DOC; interferon, IFN; IV immunoglobulin, IVIG; multiple sclerosis, MS

*Must do 2-D echo to assess ejection fraction before treatment; very cardiotoxic

- Important points on MS in pregnancy:
  - ▸ All disease-modifying therapy must be stopped (IFN, glatiramer, and/or cytotoxic agents)
  - ▸ Rare exacerbation during pregnancy (usually **improves**) but common to have **exacerbations immediately after delivery**

NEUROMUSCULAR DISORDERS

Myasthenia Gravis

- Autoimmune formation of acetylcholine receptor antibodies destroys the neuromuscular junction

- Clinical—chief complaints are weakness, **fatigue, diplopia**, ptosis, weak voice, dysphagia; **normal reflexes**; if severe exacerbation → respiratory failure

- Incidence is bimodal—women in their 20s, men in their 40s; male-to-female ratio is 3:2

- Diagnosis
  - ▸ Best initial test is **acetylcholine receptor antibodies**, diagnostic if positive with typical symptoms → muscles fatigue with repetitive use, better with rest (ice packs also improve symptoms)
  - ▸ If doubtful, perform edrophonium challenge test → immediate improvement in muscular weakness (test will no longer be performed after current supplies run out on market)
  - ▸ Most sensitive and specific test—electromyography; shows **decrease** in muscle contractions with **repetitive** stimulation
  - ▸ Always **rule out thymoma** with **CT scan of chest** (may precipitate myasthenia)
    - ▹ Thymus hyperplasia with lymphocytic hyperplasia is seen in 65–75% of cases; thymoma seen in 15% of cases

Management of Myasthenia Gravis

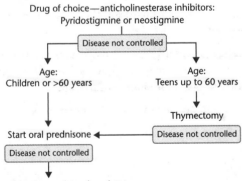

4

199

SEIZURE DISORDERS AND EPILEPSY

- New-onset seizures in patients under 10 years of age—most common cause idiopathic; second most common cause congenital

- New-onset seizures in a patient over 40 years of age—most common cause tumor; second most common cause ischemic or hemorrhagic stroke

  ► If you suspect tumor—get MRI of brain (chest x-ray indicated in **all** smokers)

  ► If you suspect stroke—get CT scan

- Always rule out organic causes first

- If seizure(s) unwitnessed—look for incontinence with or without tongue-biting (always **lateral**, never on the top); almost pathognomonic

- When to start anticonvulsant therapy—everyone is allowed to have one seizure in his or her lifetime; therapy is indicated after a single seizure only if tumor is present; other criteria include focal deficits, status epilepticus, abnormal EEG, and family history

- When can patient drive again? Must be seizure-free and/or on medication for at least **1 year** (but varies from state to state)

- When to stop anticonvulsant therapy—when seizure-free for 2–3 years

- Breakthrough seizures—even on maximal drug therapy, breakthrough seizures may occur every few months; this **does not indicate a need for change in therapy**

- Seizures in pregnancy—use carbamazepine

Management of Status Epilepticus

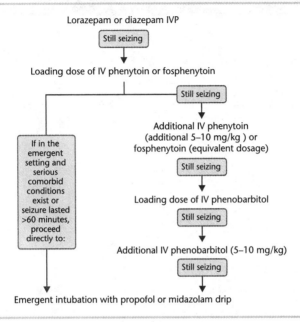

Lorazepam or diazepam IVP

Still seizing

Loading dose of IV phenytoin or fosphenytoin

Still seizing

If in the emergent setting and serious comorbid conditions exist or seizure lasted >60 minutes, proceed directly to:

Additional IV phenytoin (additional 5–10 mg/kg) or fosphenytoin (equivalent dosage)

Still seizing

Loading dose of IV phenobarbitol

Still seizing

Additional IV phenobarbitol (5–10 mg/kg)

Still seizing

Emergent intubation with propofol or midazolam drip

Abbreviations: IV push, IVP

Diagnosis and Long-Term Management of Seizure Disorders

Type	Features	Diagnosis	Treatment
Simple partial— no LOC	Unsynchronized tonic to clonic movements with or without aura; never postictal confusion	EEG: spike, sharp waves	DOC: carbamazepine or phenytoin
Complex partial— LOC but appear awake	Lip-smacking, GI upset, strange smells or increased salivation, plus altered consciousness	• EEG: temporal lobe spikes or sharp waves • MRI to rule out organic brain disease	DOC: carbamazepine or phenytoin

(continued)

Diagnosis and Long-Term Management of Seizure Disorders (continued)

Type	Features	Diagnosis	Treatment
Absence (petit mal), seen in pediatric patients	Classic "stare" with complete unresponsiveness; no aura and no postictal state	EEG: spike and wave 3-second activity	• DOC: ethosuximide • Alternative: valproic acid
Tonic-clonic (grand-mal)	Eyes roll back → unresponsive → rhythmic contractions → long postictal state (hours)	EEG: generalized seizure activity	• DOC: valproic acid • Second-line: lamotrigine, carbamazepine, or phenytoin
Tonic	Asymmetric increase in tone	EEG: generalized seizure activity	Multiple
Atonic	Sudden loss of tone in postural muscles leads to "drop attack"	EEG: low-voltage fast activity, poly-spike and wave pattern or electrodecrement	Multiple
Juvenile myoclonic epilepsy	Myoclonic jerks of head, trunk, and extremities → complete loss of tone → fall forward	EEG: varied	DOC: valproic acid

Abbreviations: drug of choice, DOC; loss of conciousness, LOC

VERTIGO AND "LIGHTHEADEDNESS"

- Most important in diagnosis is complete history—i.e., "What do you mean by 'dizzy'?"
  - ► Vertigo—sensation of spinning, or feeling as though person will fall backward; neurologic origin
    - ▷ Central vertigo—gradual onset with pure nystagmus; with symptoms of weakness and diplopia
    - ▷ Peripheral vertigo—sudden onset with mixed nystagmus and no other symptoms; symptoms tend to be worse than central vertigo
  - ► Presyncope—"lightheaded," or feeling as though person will "black out"; cardiac origin

▶ Loss of balance—cerebellar disease

▶ Unexplainable dizziness—check for anxiety and depression

Most Important Causes of Vertigo and Lightheadedness

Diagnosis	Symptoms	Treatment
Labyrinthitis	Sudden, severe vertigo with hearing loss and tinnitus lasting **days** following **URI**	Meclizine is first-line; diazepam if meclizine fails
Ménière disease	• Sudden severe vertigo, tinnitus, and hearing loss lasting **hours** at a time; seen in trauma and syphilis • **A diagnosis of exclusion**	Low-sodium diet and carbonic anhydrase inhibitors (acetazolamide) first-line; surgery if this fails
Benign paroxysmal vertigo	Sudden severe vertigo **exacerbated by any movement of the head;** lasts up to 1 minute and abates	Dix-Hallpike and Barany maneuver to dislodge otolith
Vasovagal (neurocardiogenic) syncope	Sudden "lightheadedness" and feeling of passing out, or history of syncope	Confirm diagnosis with tilt-table testing with and without pharmacologic stimulation (isoproterenol); no specific treatment

Abbreviations: upper respiratory infection, URI

NORMAL PRESSURE HYDROCEPHALUS

- Clinical—triad of urinary incontinence, dementia, and ataxia ("magnetic gait"); gait disturbance is usually the first finding on examination

- Diagnosis—CT scan shows dilated ventricles; confirm with high volume and increased opening pressure on LP (symptoms should improve after removing approximately 50 cc of CSF)

- Treatment—VP (ventriculoperitoneal) shunt if gait improves after removal of 20–50 mL of CSF during LP

HEADACHE

Primary Headaches

Diagnosis	Clues/ History	Pain	Keys to Diagnosis	Treatment
Tension-type	Most common HA, but often not severe enough to be the chief complaint	"Band-like" "Vise-like"	Does not usually interfere with the ability to work	NSAIDs
Migraine	Episodic, 1 to several per month	Progressively increasing in intensity	Not able to work (patient wants to stay still/go to bed) Photophobia Phonophobia	Triptans oral or SQ if vomiting
Migraine with aura	20% of migraine patients—focal neurologic event (visual, sensory, motor) preceding HA, less than 60 minutes duration. HA follows in 50% of cases. **Hemiplegic migraine**—gradual, **sequential progression** of a neurologic deficit (**e.g., left arm** weakness, **followed by left leg** weakness), whereas TIA is abrupt, spontaneous weakness of both limbs			
Cluster HA	Occur in clusters of daily headaches 2 to 3 months in duration, typically at the same times (**"alarm clock headache"**)	Unilateral, stabbing periorbital pain (10/10) with tearing or rhinorrhea **15 min to 3 hrs duration** So severe, some commit suicide	Restless, can't stay still (unlike migraine) **Alcohol** and **sleep** may precipitate	100% oxygen first step in management Chronically may try lithium, verapamil, triptans, or prednisone
Idiopathic intracranial hypertension (pseudotumor cerebri)	Increased intracranial pressure of unknown cause	Throbbing HA, **worse in mornings** Nausea, vomiting Tinnitus Diplopia (caused by abducens palsy)	All ages, but typically **young obese females** Lumbar puncture reveals **increased pressure Papilledema OCP use and** VitA toxicity linked to syndrome	First: **drain CSF** Second: **acetazolamide** (avoid in pregnancy) Optic nerve sheath fenestration Ventriculoperitoneal shunt if severe

(continued)

Secondary Headaches

Diagnosis	Clues/ History	Pain	Keys to Diagnosis	Treatment
Cold stimulus HA	"Brain freeze" Caused by consuming cold food or beverages More common in **migraineurs**	Short, severe, sharp, unilateral Lasts about **2 minutes**	Sudden cooling of the sympathetics around the carotid	Don't drink cold drinks or eat ice cream rapidly
Medication overuse HA	Caused by **withdrawal** from headache medication	Chronic headaches At least **15 days** per month	Frequent use of headache medications (e.g., triptans, narcotics, caffeine, NSAIDs)	Withdraw all pain medications
Chronic daily HA	At least **15** days/month for **3 months**	Daily or almost daily 4 hours or more	Depression, anxiety, or sleep disorder	Treat depression, anxiety, sleep disorder
Low CSF pressure or volume HA (CSF leak)	Typically after **lumbar puncture**, after **trauma**, or **spontaneously**	Severe, worse when **sitting up** Some spontaneous cases might describe a **"popping" sound** in the back	Pain worse with **postural changes** Chronic disease may lose the postural changes	Bed rest, **blood patch**, abdominal binder, **caffeine** Surgical repair if the leak is large
Temporal arteritis	>50 y/o, **average age = 75**	Unilateral (temporal area) Jaw claudication, visual defects, blindness	Elevated **ESR** Tender temporal artery Dx: **temporal artery biopsy**	Oral corticosteroids **Intravenous CS if visual symptoms** present ****Do not wait** for biopsy results to start treatment; can result in blindness
Trigeminal neuralgia	"Tic douloureux" when associated with facial spasm	**Brief paroxysms** of lancinating pain: maxilla or mandibular areas	Can be triggered by light touch	Carbamazepine

4

(continued)

Secondary Headaches (continued)

Diagnosis	Clues/ History	Pain	Keys to Diagnosis	Treatment
Subarachnoid hemorrhage	MCC: **berry aneurysm** Risk factors: HTN, smoking, alcohol abuse	**Thunderclap HA, maximum intensity within 1 minute HA absent (10%)**	HA, photo-phobia, miosis, nuchal rigidity, fever	**CT head** (nor-mal in 10%), if normal → **LP** to check for **xantochromia**
HA caused by metastasis	Cancer	Pressure-like, **constant HA**	Head CT or MRI	Dexametha-sone to decrease cere-bral edema

Abbreviations: cerebrospinal fluid, CSF; corticosteroids, CS; diagnosis, Dx; cerebrovascular accident, CVA; erythrocyte sedimentation rate, ESR; headache, HA; hypertension, HTN; lumbar puncture, LP; most common cause, MCC; non-steroidal anti-inflammatory drugs, NSAIDs; transient ischemic attack, TIA

4

Important Points about Headache

- Headache + fever—do LP first

- Headache + major trauma or focal findings—do CT scan first

- Headache + blindness + temporal point tenderness—immediate high-dose steroids

- Major contraindications to sumatriptan—ischemic heart disease (IHD), previous MI, angina, uncontrolled HTN, concurrent monoamine oxidase inhibitors (MAOIs), SSRIs, lithium therapy

IX. PULMONOLOGY

ROLE OF PULMONARY FUNCTION TESTING

Used to categorize lung disease into restrictive vs. obstructive, to determine the severity of lung disease, and to monitor response to treatment.

Common Pulmonary Function Tests

Measurement	Measuring	Normal Values
Total lung capacity (TLC)	Entire capacity of the lung, including dead space	80–120% of age and sex predicted value
Tidal volume (TV)	Volume of air expired during normal single breath	—
Vital capacity (VC)	Maximal volume expired after a maximal inspiration	—
Residual volume (RV)	Volume of air remaining in the lungs after a maximal expiration ("dead space")	—
Functional residual capacity (FRC)	Volume remaining in the lungs at the end of normal expiration	—
Forced expiratory volume (FEV1)	Volume of air in a forced expiration in the first second	—
Forced vital capacity (FVC)	Volume of air in a forced expiration for 6 seconds	—
FEV1/FVC ratio	Ratio between FEV1 and FVC	70–100% of predicted

In **obstructive** lung diseases the FEV1 is reduced more than the FVC. The FEV1/FVC ratio is less than 70% of that predicted for a normal patient with the same gender, height, and weight.

In **restrictive** lung diseases, the total lung volume is reduced, while both the FEV1 and FVC are reduced to approximately the same extent. The FEV1/FVC ratio is greater than 70% of that predicted.

Diffusing Capacity for Carbon Monoxide (DLCO)

DLCO measures the ability of the lung to **transfer of gas** across the **alveolar-capillary membrane**. DLCO is dependent on the **concentration and volume of hemoglobin**.

Decreased DLCO	Increased DLCO
Loss of effective capillary surface + interface	Excess hemoglobin
• Emphysema	• Polycythemia
• Pulmonary HTN	• Alveolar hemorrhage
Destruction and thickening of alveolar-capillary membrane	• Asthma
• Pulmonary fibrosis	
• ILD	

Causes of Hypoxemia*

	Examples	A-a gradient	Hypoxia corrected by 2L nasal cannula?
Low FI O_2	High altitude	Normal	Yes
Hypoventilation	Opiate overdose	Normal	Yes
Diffusion defect (with exertion)	Early interstitial lung diseases	Increased	Yes
V/Q mismatch	Pulmonary embolism, asthma, COPD, late ILD	Increased	Yes
Shunting	CHF, pneumonia, ARDS	Increased	No

Abbreviations: interstitial lung disease, ILD; fraction of inspired oxygen, FI O_2; chronic obstructive pulmonary disease, COPD; adult respiratory distress syndrome, ARDS; congestive heart failure, CHF; ventilation-perfusion, V/Q

*Note: Hypoxemia = PaO$_2$ <85 mm Hg on room air.

A-a Gradient

This measures **effectiveness of alveolar capillary unit** in oxygenation. Calculate as follows:

$A\text{-}a = (150 - [1.25 \times PaCO_2] - PaO_2)$

<20 = normal

>20 = possible disease

Ventilation-Perfusion Relationships

Ventilation (V) and perfusion (Q) of the lung both increase moving from the apex to the base of the lung, but perfusion increases more. The V/Q ratio is higher in the apices of the lungs, normally 3.0 in apices and 0.6 in the bases.

4

Ventilation-Perfusion Relationships

	Chronic Bronchitis	Emphysema	Pulmonary Fibrosis	Pulmonary Hypertension
FEV1/FVC	<0.70	<0.70	Increased	Normal
TLC	Normal	Increased	Decreased	Normal
DLCO	Normal or Decreased	Decreased	Decreased	Decreased

Flow Volume Loops

- Obstruction on expiration → intrathoracic (tracheal tumor, foreign body)

- Obstruction on inspiration → extrathoracic (vocal cord dysfunction, benign adenomas)

- Obstruction of both → fixed upper airway obstruction (tracheal stenosis)

PLEURAL EFFUSION

- Thoracocentesis indicated in all unilateral effusions; when bilateral, perform when new or not completely explained by degree of illness

  ▸ Choosing the correct method of thoracocentesis (see figure on page 210)

Management of Pleural Effusions

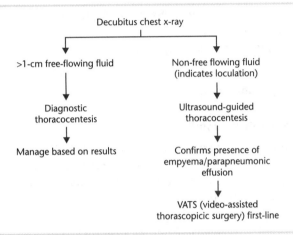

- Must measure serum and pleural fluid LDH and protein for Light criteria; if you suspect malignancy, also send for cytology

Origin of Pleural Effusions

Transudate—Bilateral and Symmetric on CXR	Exudate—Unilateral and Asymmetric on CXR
CHF	Pneumonia
Cirrhosis	Malignancy
Renal failure with fluid overload	Any infectious process
	Rheumatic disease

Abbreviations: congestive heart failure, CHF; chest x-ray, CXR
Note: Pulmonary embolism is the only effusion that may be either a transudate or an exudate.

Light Criteria

	Exudate	Transudate*
Pleural effusion LDH value	>200	<200
Pleural effusion LDH/serum ratio	>0.6	<0.6
Pleural effusion protein/serum ratio	>0.5	<0.5

Abbreviations: lactate dehydrogenase, LDH
Note: **All three values **must** be met to diagnose with transudate; otherwise, it is an exudate.*

Management of Acute Shortness of Breath

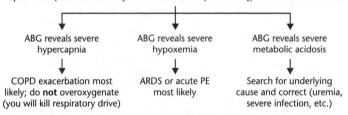

Rule out airway obstruction
↓

1. Check pulse oximetry
2. Get ABG
↓

Supplement oxygen in "step-up" fashion to keep pulse oximetry around 90–92%
if known, CO_2 retainer; if not known, keep O_2 sat 100%, if possible
Start with O_2 via nasal cannula (up to 4 L; maximum of ~30% FIO_2) → ventimask
up to 60% (max of 60% FIO_2 → non-rebreather (100% FIO_2) → intubate last resort

ABG reveals severe hypercapnia	ABG reveals severe hypoxemia	ABG reveals severe metabolic acidosis
↓	↓	↓
COPD exacerbation most likely; do **not** overoxygenate (you will kill respiratory drive)	ARDS or acute PE most likely	Search for underlying cause and correct (uremia, severe infection, etc.)

Abbreviations: arterial blood gas, ABG; acute respiratory distress syndrome, ARDS; chronic obstructive pulmonary disease, COPD; pulmonary embolism, PE; saturation, sat

RESTRICTIVE LUNG DISEASE

- Pulmonary function tests (PFTs) show forced expiratory volume in 1 second (FEV1) and FEV1/forced vital capacity (FVC) 80–120% of predicted; FEV1 is always reduced but the FEV1/FVC ratio could be normal to increased

- Decreased DLCO secondary to fibrosis and scarring of alveolar membranes

- Pulmonary HTN and cor pulmonale when severe

211

Restrictive Lung Diseases

Disease	Risk Factors	Presentation	Diagnosis	Treatment
Asbestosis	**Shipyard and construction workers, plumbers**	Dyspnea in an older patient with history of exposure	• CXR/CT shows fibrosis **plus evidence of pleural thickening, asbestos-related pleural plaques, and diaphragmatic calcifications*** • Definitive diagnosis: lung **biopsy** shows **barbell-shaped fibers**	• None; **smoking cessation** • High risk of adeno-carcinoma, squamous cell carci-noma, and mesothelioma
Coal-miners lung	**Coal miners**	Dyspnea in an older patient with history of exposure	• CXR/CT shows **circular densities in apical lung fields** • Labs: increased **IgA, IgG, ANA, and RF**	None
Idiopathic pulmonary fibrosis	None known	Dyspnea in a 40-year-old with coarse, dry crackles on exam	• CXR/CT shows **diffuse "ground-glass" opacities** • BAL shows increased macrophages	Oral prednisone with or without azathioprine
Pneumo-coniosis	**Metal mining or dust**	Dyspnea in an older male with history of exposure	CXR shows **irregu-lar opacities** and dense interstitial structures	None

(continued)

Restrictive Lung Diseases (continued)

Disease	Risk Factors	Presentation	Diagnosis	Treatment
Sarcoidosis	None known	Usually incidental; **African Americans age 20–45**; may have **Bell palsy**; acute polyarthritis, and erythema nodosum**	• CXR/CT scan shows **hilar adenopathy**; honeycombing in late disease • Labs: **hypercalcemia and hypercalciuria** • Gold standard: biopsy shows **noncaseating granulomas** (sites of choice are skin except EN, lacrimal gland, palpable lymph node or parotid gland; only biopsy lung if these are not possible)	• Oral prednisone only if **positive for uveitis, neurologic disease, hypercalcemia, or evidence of new infiltrates** • Monitor progression of disease with serum **ACE inhibitor** levels
Silicosis	**Jewel miners, glassworkers, sandblasters**	Dyspnea in patient with history of exposure; sometimes sudden onset with death in months	• CXR/CT shows 1 mm–1 cm **nodules in upper lobes with or without eggshell calcifications** • The only lung disease which may be restrictive or obstructive	• None • Increased risk of pulmonary tuberculosis; **yearly PPD and INH if positive**

Abbreviations: angiotensin-converting enzyme, ACE; antinuclear antibodies, ANA; bronchoalveolar lavage, BAL; chest x-ray, CXR; erythema nodosum, EN; isoniazid, INH; rheumatoid factor, RF

Notes:

* You may have lung findings indicative of asbestos **exposure** but no evidence of restrictive disease; this is called asbestos-related pleural plaques.

** The triad of hilar adenopathy, acute polyarthritis, and erythema nodosum is known as Löfgren syndrome; has overall good prognosis, and disease is self-limited.

4

OBSTRUCTIVE LUNG DISEASE

Reversible	Irreversible
Asthma	• COPD (emphysema, chronic bronchitis) • Bronchiectasis • Cystic fibrosis

Asthma

See Asthma, page 404.

Chronic Obstructive Pulmonary Disease (COPD)

- **Irreversible** airway obstruction
  - ▸ Emphysema = permanent dilation of alveoli with cartilage destruction
    - ▹ Alpha-1-antitrypsin deficiency—autosomal recessive trait causing **panacinar** emphysema and liver failure
  - ▸ Chronic bronchitis = hypertrophy of mucus cells causing productive cough × at least 3 consecutive months for at least 2 consecutive years
  - ▸ Most COPD patients have both emphysema and chronic bronchitis
  - ▸ 90% of COPD patients smoked; active smokers have 15% risk of developing COPD; most with >20-year history of 1 pack per day

- Clinical
  - ▸ Chronically decreased airway entry with or without wheezing and rhonchi; chest x-ray shows hyperinflation, diaphragmatic flattening, and rib flattening
  - ▸ **Tip: Most patients** with COPD have **both emphysema and chronic bronchitis.**

- Diagnosis—initial test of choice is PFTs
  - ▸ Bronchodilators cause **no change** in FEV1 or FEV1/FVC ratio
  - ▸ Increased residual volume (RV) and total lung capacity (TLC)

- DLCO
  - ▷ Chronic bronchitis—normal
  - ▷ Emphysema—decreased
- Pulse oximetry and arterial blood gas (ABG) shows hypoxemia

Stepwise Management of COPD

First-line—anticholingergic bronchodilators
Ipratropium is short-acting; use q 4–6 hours
Tiatropium is long-acting; use once daily

May add inhaled beta-adrenergic agonists (albuterol)
Avoid in CHF—or may try levalbuterol (more selective,
less tachycardia and induction of exacerbations)

Add theophylline (monitor serum levels)

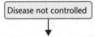

Check ABG and pulse ox:
If PO² <55 mm Hg or pulse ox <88%
Add **supplemental home oxygen (decreases mortality)**
And encourage to **quit smoking (decreases mortality)**

Abbreviations: arterial blood gas, ABG; congestive heart failure, CHF; pulse oximetry, pulse ox

- All should have the pneumococcal vaccine (every 5 years), influenza vaccine (yearly) and *Haemophilus influenzae* vaccine (once per lifetime)
- **FEV1** is the best long-term indicator of prognosis (the lower the FEV1, the higher the mortality)

Acute exacerbation of COPD (AECOPD)

AECOPD diagnosed when **one or more** of the following are present: increase in sputum volume, increase in sputum purulence, worsening of dyspnea, fever of no apparent cause, increase in wheezing and cough, increase in respiratory rate or heart rate by 20%. **Important points:**

- Peak flow has **no role** in the management of acute COPD; it is used only in acute asthma exacerbation

- Even if the chest x-ray is normal, you **still use IV antibiotics** (decreases mortality in the acute setting)

- **Do not sedate the patient** unless intubated (kills respiratory drive)

Management of Acute COPD Exacerbation

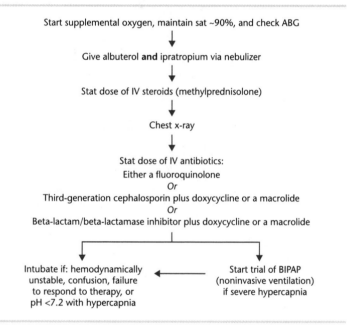

Start supplemental oxygen, maintain sat ~90%, and check ABG

↓

Give albuterol **and** ipratropium via nebulizer

↓

Stat dose of IV steroids (methylprednisolone)

↓

Chest x-ray

↓

Stat dose of IV antibiotics:
Either a fluoroquinolone
Or
Third-generation cephalosporin plus doxycycline or a macrolide
Or
Beta-lactam/beta-lactamase inhibitor plus doxycycline or a macrolide

Intubate if: hemodynamically unstable, confusion, failure to respond to therapy, or pH <7.2 with hypercapnia ← Start trial of BIPAP (noninvasive ventilation) if severe hypercapnia

Abbreviations: arterial blood gas, ABG; biphasic positive airway pressure, BIPAP; saturation, sat

ADULT RESPIRATORY DISTRESS SYNDROME (ARDS)

- Damage to the alveolar membrane → alveolar edema → impaired gas exchange → severe hypoxia

  ▸ Due to trauma, severe infection, prolonged use of high FIO_2 during mechanical ventilation, etc.

- Clinical—dyspnea, tachypnea, rales, and severe hypoxemia
  - ▸ Chest x-ray—**diffuse alveolar infiltrates** causing complete **"white-out"** of bilateral lung fields; **"ground-glass" pattern**
  - ▸ ABG—**severe hypoxemia with normal $PaCO_2$**
  - ▸ PaO_2-to-FIO_2 ratio >200 **required** for diagnosis
  - ▸ Swan-Ganz catheterization—**increased pulmonary artery pressure; all other values normal**
- Treatment—**mechanical ventilation with positive end-expiratory pressure (PEEP) of 6 cm** (higher PEEP associated with worse outcomes) **and permissive hypercapnia**; treat underlying causes

ATELECTASIS

- Collapse of small airways
- Most common cause is post-op pain → decreased inspiratory effort → post-op fever (**first 24 hours**) and focal or lower-lobe rales on physical exam
  - ▸ Others—foreign body, mucus plug (common in mechanical ventilation), or obstructing tumor
- May be incidental finding on chest x-ray
- Treatment—**incentive spirometry is first-line**; adequate pain control post-op; bronchoscopy if suction not effective for mucus plugs

BRONCHIECTASIS

- Permanent dilation of bronchi from either recurrent pneumonia/ infection or Kartagener syndrome (diffuse bronchiectasis + situs inversus + infertility + chronic sinusitis)
- Clinical—chronic productive cough with **foul-smelling** sputum, **recurrent pneumonia**
- Diagnosis—**high-resolution CT of the chest** is first-line; chest x-ray changes late in disease

4

- Treatment—**chest physiotherapy**; bronchodilators for dyspneic symptoms
  ► If any increase or change in quality of sputum production
    ▷ Outpatient—oral fluoroquinolone
    ▷ Inpatient—two IV antibiotics with antipseudomonal coverage
  ► If localized bronchiectasis and adequate PFTs—partial pneumonectomy

SOLITARY PULMONARY NODULE

- Usually an incidental finding on chest x-ray or CT scan done for some other clinical indication (see figure)

Management of Solitary Pulmonary Nodule

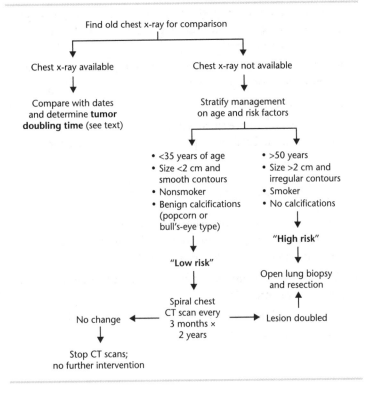

- Tumor doubling times—a doubling time of <1 month or >480 days usually means the lesion is benign (doubling measures volume and **not** diameter); any doubling time between 1 month and 480 days is suspicious for malignancy

LUNG CANCER

More than 90% of cases linked to smoking; risk increased with number of pack-years smoked

Lung Cancer Types and Characteristics

Tumor Class	Type	Location	Paraneoplastic Syndrome/ Characteristics
Non-small cell	Adenocarcinoma	Peripheral	• Most common tumor seen in **nonsmokers** and **with asbestos exposure** • If effusion: look for high **hyaluronidase levels** in analysis
	Large cell	Peripheral	**Cavitation**
	Mesothelioma	Peripheral	**Pleural plaques;** second most common tumor type in **asbestos** exposure
	Squamous cell	Central	• **Cavitary** • Secretes **PTH-like peptide → hypercalcemia**
Small-cell carcinoma	Small (oat) cell	Central	• **Eaton-Lambert** (myasthenic-like syndrome; look for muscle weakness in history) • **SIADH** • **Superior vena cava syndrome**

Abbreviations: parathyroid hormone, PTH; syndrome of inappropriate antidiuretic secretion, SIADH

4

Diagnosis and Management of Suspected Malignancy

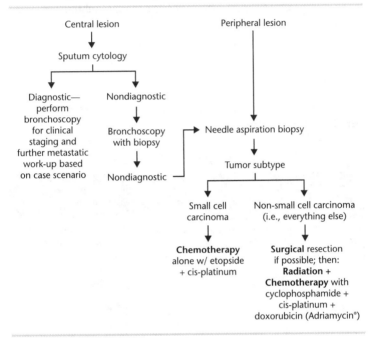

Criteria for Surgical Resection

- Must have tidal volume of >800 mL in the lung to be preserved on "split" lung testing (nuclear study)

- Not a surgical candidate if: local extension into surrounding tissue (includes anything from chest wall to evidence of superior vena cava syndrome), hoarseness, malignant effusion, or evidence of distant metastasis

Role of Video-Assisted Thoracoscopic Surgery (VATS) When Surgical Resection Is Indicated

- If the nodule is close enough to the periphery, VATS is the best choice for resection (less invasive than thoracotomy)

- Otherwise, open thoracotomy must be done

HEPATOPULMONARY SYNDROME

- Diagnosis—**desaturation** on pulse oximetry **with change in body position** along with **increased A-a gradient**
- Treatment—liver transplant most effective; supplemental oxygen if hypoxic

PULMONARY EMBOLISM (PE) AND DEEP VENOUS THROMBOSIS (DVT)

- DVTs **above the popliteal vein** are creators of PE (studies do **not** link DVT distal to the popliteal vein with PE, but most extend upward)
  - ▸ Sites of DVT in patient populations
    - ▹ Immobility—popliteal, femoral, and pelvic DVT
    - ▹ Pregnancy—pelvic DVT
    - ▹ Central and percutaneous inserted central catheter (PICC) lines—brachial and subclavian DVT

- Risk factors: immobility (recent surgery), malignancy, protein-losing nephropathy, pregnancy, hereditary hypercoagulable states
  - ▸ Look for hereditary causes in **young patients with family history or in young patients with rheumatologic disease**
  - ▸ Protein C, protein S, and factor V Leiden mutation or anticardiolipin antibodies

- Clinical—sudden onset of dyspnea, tachycardia, tachypnea, unilateral leg edema, pleuritic chest pain, and hemoptysis
  - ▸ Other findings
    - ▹ ABG—hypoxemia + **increased A-a gradient**
    - ▹ Chest x-ray—**normal** in majority; rare findings are Westermark sign (no vascular markings) and Hampton hump (wedge infiltrate above diaphragm)
    - ▹ ECG—**sinus tachycardia in majority**; rare S1, Q3, T3 sign (S wave in lead I and Q wave with T wave inversion in lead III)

4

- Diagnosis—determine **pretest probability**
  - ▶ Criteria: numerous scoring systems exist, and it is not necessary to know them all. Just know this: if more than two of the following are present, the pretest probably justifies doing the CT or V/Q scan first; if fewer than two are present, then d-dimer is the best initial test.
    - ▷ Clinical signs of likely DVT (leg swelling, etc.); heart rate >100/min; history of immobilization; history of DVT, PE, hypercoagulability, malignancy, or hemoptysis

4

Management of Pulmonary Embolism

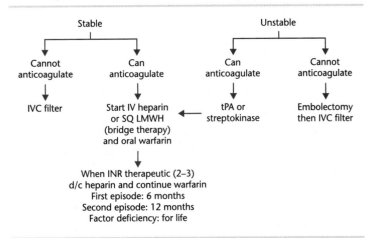

Abbreviations: international ratio, INR; inferior vena cava, IVC; low molecular-weight heparin, LMWH; tissue plasminogen activator, tPA

- IV heparin vs. low molecular-weight heparin (LMWH)
  - ▶ IV unfractionated heparin is associated with higher rates of bleeding and HIT syndrome and requires monitoring of the PTT every 6 hours until therapeutic; **must** reach therapeutic PTT within 24 hours or else physician is legally liable if adverse outcome occurs

> ► LMWH is injected SQ daily or twice/day, and is dose-adjusted according to the creatinine clearance; monitor with daily PT/PTT/INR
>> ▷ Most clinicians prefer using LMWH, but it is much more costly than IV heparin

- Management of DVT in the posterior tibial vein (below the knee)—anticoagulate for 3 months **or** serial duplex ultrasound exams

- Complications of DVT—post-thrombotic syndrome: pain, edema, and hyperpigmentation due to valvular obstruction; ulceration if severe; prevent with compression stockings

SLEEP APNEA

- Most common complaint is **daytime somnolence**; diagnose with **sleep study** (criteria: >15 episodes of >10 seconds of apnea with desaturation on pulse oximetry)

- Obstructive sleep apnea—**obesity** leads to difficult airflow during sleep; treatment of choice is **weight loss**; continuous positive airway pressure (CPAP) if ineffective

- Central sleep apnea—poor ventilatory drive; treatment with supplemental oxygen plus either acetazolamide, theophylline, or progesterone

X. RHEUMATOLOGY

APPROACH TO RHEUMATOLOGIC DISEASE

Key to diagnosing rheumatologic disease—number of joints, length of symptoms, presence or absence of systemic symptoms, and family history

Joint Fluid Aspirates

Diagnosis	WBC Count	Polarization	Crystals
Traumatic joint injury or degenerative joint disease	<2,000 cells/mm³	None	None
Inflammatory joint disease	5,000–50,000 cells/mm³	• Gout → negative birefringence • Pseudogout → positive birefringence	• Gout → needle-shaped • Pseudogout → rhomboid
Septic joint disease	>50,000 cells/mm³	None	None

Abbreviations: white blood cell, WBC

CRYSTAL ARTHROPATHIES

Gout

- Risk factors—alcohol abuse; steroid withdrawal; prescription drugs; foods that contain excess purine, including cheese; severe medical illness

- Clinical—sudden onset of severe pain (usually in the great toe) with erythema, edema, and extreme point tenderness; chronic gout leads to joint deformation, tophi, and renal stones

- Diagnosis—examination of joint fluid aspirates (serum uric acid has no role acutely)

- Treatment
  - ▶ Acute—depends on presence of comorbid conditions
    - ▷ If no comorbid conditions—NSAIDs (indomethacin) are the drugs of choice
    - ▷ Elderly (cannot tolerate NSAIDs)—colchicine every hour until diarrhea occurs
    - ▷ Renal failure—oral prednisone
  - ▶ Chronic—therapy indicated when other measures fail (good diet, avoidance of alcohol, etc.); serum uric acid can be used to monitor response to therapy
    - ▷ Probenecid used in "undersecretors"
    - ▷ "**All**opurinol is used in **all**": overproducers, undersecretors, renal failure, and renal stones; **do not** initiate during acute attack, but if the patient was already taking allopurinol, then continue it

4

Pseudogout (Calcium Pyrophosphate Deposition Disease; CPPD)

- Risk factors
  - ▶ If age >50, related to aging
  - ▶ If age <50, rule out hemochromatosis, hyperparathyroidism, hypomagnesemia, and/or hypophosphatemia
- Clinical/diagnosis—like gout, except usually involves the **knee**; joint aspirates are key to diagnosis (see Joint Fluid Aspirates on the preceding page); x-rays show linear radiodense deposits in cartilage (chondrocalcinosis)
- Treat the same as gout

DERMATOMYOSITIS AND MIXED CONNECTIVE TISSUE DISEASE

Dermatomyositis

- Pathophysiology—inflammatory myopathy causing progressive muscular weakness

- Clinical—affects **proximal muscle** groups, never affects facial muscles; **heliotrope rash** (purple-blue rash encircling the eyes); **Gottron sign** (scaly, erythematous lesions on the knuckles)
  - ▶ **Tip:** You **must** rule out malignancy in an elderly patient with new-onset dermatomyositis.

- Labs—elevated serum CPK and aldolase; positive **anti-Jo-1 antibodies**

- Diagnosis—EMG will show short-duration, low-amplitude movements; gold standard is **muscle biopsy**

- Treatment—oral steroids

Mixed Connective Tissue Disease

- Clinical—combination of multiple rheumatologic diseases without fitting one diagnosis; e.g., combination of SLE findings with muscle weakness (dermatomyositis)

- Labs—may have a combination of positive antibodies (ANA, rheumatoid factor [RF]); **anti-RNP (anti-ribonucleoprotein) is specific** for diagnosis

- Treatment—oral steroids

OSTEOARTHRITIS

- Pathophysiology—chronic wear and tear causes destruction of articular cartilage; most commonly involves the knee and **posterior interphalangeal (PIP) and distal interphalangeal (DIP) joints**

- Clinical—joint stiffness lasting **<20 minutes upon awakening**; joint crepitations, no signs of inflammation; pain **improves with rest**

- Labs—always normal

- Diagnosis—x-ray reveals osteophytes and irregular joint-space narrowing

- Treatment—drug of choice is **acetaminophen**; NSAIDs are second-line agents
  - ► If using an NSAID, COX-2 inhibitors (celecoxib) have fewer GI side effects and are safer in the elderly
  - ► Surgery is reserved for severe refractory disease (joint replacement)

POLYMYALGIA RHEUMATICA (PMR)

- Clinical—typically, patient age ≥50 years becomes acutely incapacitated with marked constitutional symptoms (fever, chills, night sweats, fatigue) and morning stiffness of the girdle (shoulders and hips)
  - ► **Tip:** 15% also have temporal arteritis, but 40% of temporal arteritis patients also have PMR.
- Labs—anemia of chronic disease, thrombocytosis
- Management—dramatic response to low-dose prednisone (15–20 mg)

RHEUMATOID ARTHRITIS (RA)

- Pathophysiology—inflammatory, symmetric synovitis with various degrees of systemic involvement causing eventual bony destruction of joints; mediated by T lymphocytes
- Risk factors—smoking, possible infectious trigger
- Diagnosis—requires four or more of the following: morning stiffness lasting >**1 hour**; swelling of symmetric joints for >**6 weeks**; swelling of more than three asymmetric joints for >6 weeks, or swelling of wrist, **posterior interphalangeal (PIP)**, and/or **metacarpophalangeal (MCP) joints** for >6 weeks; evidence of **joint erosions** on x-ray; **positive RF, rheumatoid nodules**
  - ► Hint—DIPs **never** affected in RA
  - ► Others—radial deviation, Boutonnière and swan-neck deformities, rheumatoid nodules
    - ▷ Felty syndrome = RA + splenomegaly + neutropenia

4

▷ Caplan syndrome = RA + pneumoconiosis

▷ Stills disease = RA + effervescent salmon-colored rash + high fever

► Diagnosis—no one single test

► Labs

▷ Almost all are **RF**-positive

– In **RF-negative RA**—get **anti-CCP** (citrulline-containing peptide) antibody

► Treatment—**NSAIDs** are the initial drug of choice

▷ Disease-modifying antirheumatic drugs (DMARDs) indicated: when NSAIDs fail, with steroid-dependent disease, or with radiographic evidence of joint disease

– DMARD of choice—**methotrexate**; second-line agents are hydroxychloroquine, gold, sulfasalazine, and tumor necrosis factor (TNF) inhibitors

▷ TNF inhibitors

– **PPD testing required before initiating therapy** (associated with reactivation of latent TB)

- Infliximab—requires adjunct methotrexate (prevents anti-infliximab antibody formation)

- Adalimumab

- Etanercept

– Monitor response to treatment with ESR, CRP, and degree of morning stiffness

▷ Complications—atlantoaxial instability of C1-C2: those requiring intubation must have lateral cervical spinal x-rays (otherwise → quadriplegia if not corrected); if present → neurosurgical evaluation is necessary

SCLERODERMA (SYSTEMIC SCLEROSIS)

• Pathophysiology—abnormal accumulation of connective tissue affecting all organ systems

• Clinical

► Skin—thickening with "shiny" appearance and small wrinkles; Raynaud phenomenon

- ▶ GI—esophageal dysmotility with chronic GERD; decreased motility → malabsorption and formation of diverticula
- ▶ Pulmonary—fibrosis → restrictive lung disease
- ▶ Renal—fibrosis → ESRD and malignant hypertension
  - ▷ Renal crisis—acute onset of malignant HTN progressing to acute renal failure; **drug of choice is ACE inhibitors**

- Two distinct syndromes exist
  - ▶ CREST syndrome ("limited scleroderma")
    - ▷ **C**hondrocalcinosis, **R**aynaud phenomenon, **e**sophageal dysmotility, **s**clerodactyly, and **t**elangiectasias
    - ▷ **ANA-positive** with **anticentromere** antibody pattern
    - ▷ Multiorgan involvement rare
  - ▶ Diffuse scleroderma
    - ▷ **ANA-positive** (nucleolar pattern) and **anti-Scl-70–positive**
    - ▷ **Multiorgan** involvement
      - – Must have monthly blood pressure checks

- Treatment
  - ▶ Skin abnormalities—D-penicillamine
  - ▶ Renal abnormalities and hypertension—ACE inhibitors (**not** used prophylactically for renal protection)
  - ▶ Raynaud phenomenon—CCBs

SPONDYLOARTHROPATHIES

Ankylosing Spondylitis

- Abnormal calcification of interspinal discs affecting **men** in their **20s** who are **HLA-B27–positive**

- Clinical—young male presents with **morning low-back stiffness for >1 hour, relieved with activity**
  - ▶ Beware of **anterior uveitis**, aortic valvular insufficiency, and heart block
  - ▶ Schober test—mark L5 disc upright and 10 cm superior → full flexion of spine → will be <15 cm distance on flexion (normal = >15 cm)

- Diagnosis—spinal and hip x-rays are first-line; **sacroiliitis and obliteration of intervertebral discs** ("bamboo spine")
- Treatment—**NSAIDs** and **encourage physical activity** (slows progression of disease)
  - ► Severe disease of spine—TNF inhibitors

Reactive Arthritis (Reiter Syndrome)

- Several causes
  - ► Infection with *Chlamydia*—**Reiter syndrome**
    - ▷ Arthritis, keratoderma blenorrhagica, balanitis, mucocutaneous ulcers, **uveitis**, and **conjunctivitis**
    - ▷ Treatment—**tetracycline plus NSAIDs**
  - ► After a bout of infectious diarrhea—most common cause is *Campylobacter*
    - ▷ Treatment—NSAIDs
  - ► Viral arthritis—most common cause is parvovirus B19
    - ▷ History of recent upper respiratory infection (URI), acute arthritis, and weakly positive RF
    - ▷ Treatment—NSAIDs

SJÖGREN SYNDROME

- Pathophysiology—lymphocytic infiltration of exocrine glands
- Clinical—everything dries up: dry eyes ("sandy feeling"), dry mouth (constant thirst, increased cavities), and esophageal dysmotility (dysphagia, oral thrush)
- Diagnosis
  - ► Clinical tests—Schemer test reveals decreased tear production, and Rose-Bengal stain reveals corneal ulcerations
  - ► Best initial test—**anti-Ro (SSA) and anti-La (SSB)** antibodies (anti-La is specific)
  - ► Confirmatory test—parotid gland biopsy (lymphocytic infiltration)
- Treatment—artificial tears, encourage frequent sips of water

SYSTEMIC LUPUS ERYTHEMATOSUS (SLE)

Pathophysiology—autoantibody destruction of multiple organ systems

Must-Know Antibodies in SLE

"Best Tests"	Serum Test	Role
Screening test	ANA (rim pattern)	Nonspecific; usually positive
Screening if ANA negative (3% of SLE)	Anti-Ro (SSA) antibody	Nonspecific
Confirmatory tests	Anti-ds-DNA and anti-Smith antibodies	Specific
Disease activity	Serum C3 levels	Decreased in lupus flare
	Anti-ds-DNA antibody	Increased in lupus flare and **lupus nephritis**

Abbreviations: antinuclear antibodies, ANA; double-stranded, ds; systemic lupus erythematosus, SLE

- Four of the following criteria are required for diagnosis: malar rash, discoid rash, photosensitivity, oral ulcers, arthritis, serositis, nephritis, neurologic symptoms, hematologic abnormalities, or positive antibody titers
  - ▸ Rash induced by **UV-B** light
  - ▸ Discoid lupus distinct from SLE—raised rim with central pallor; heals with scarring

- Fertility and pregnancy
  - ▸ Increased risk of recurrent spontaneous abortion from **antiphospholipid (anticardiolipin) antibodies** (also increased risk of DVT and PE)
    - ▹ Have increased PTT and false-positive rapid plasma reagin (RPR) and Venereal Disease Research Laboratory (VDRL)
    - ▹ Treatment of choice—aspirin plus LMWH
  - ▸ Increased risk of congenital heart block from transplacental passage of **anti-Ro (SSA) antibody**

- Treatment—no single drug of choice; symptomatic treatment
  - ▶ Arthritis and serositis—NSAIDs
  - ▶ Rash—topical corticosteroids
  - ▶ Any severe lupus or lupus flare—oral corticosteroids plus a cytotoxic agent (hydroxychloroquine, etc.)
  - ▶ Lupus nephritis—first step in management is renal biopsy to determine stage of involvement
    - ▷ Stage I or II proliferative glomerulonephritis (GN)—no treatment
    - ▷ Stage III or IV proliferative GN—IV methylprednisolone plus mycophenolate (cyclophosphamide is now second-line)
    - ▷ Sclerotic renal disease—no treatment
- Prognosis
  - ▶ Premature CAD is the most common cause of ACS in SLE
  - ▶ Lupus nephritis is most common cause of severe disability

DRUG-INDUCED SLE

- Most common causes—hydralazine, quinidine, procainamide, and isoniazid
- Diagnosis—positive ANA and **anti-histone antibodies**
- Treatment—stop the medication

VASCULITIDES

Diagnosis	Vessel Affected/ Symptoms	Diagnosis	Treatment
Churg-Strauss syndrome	Medium-vessel vasculitis affecting every organ, **including lungs (asthma, nasal polyps,** and **peripheral eosinophilia)**	• Best initial test: p-ANCA (myeloperoxidase antibody) • Most accurate test: lung biopsy shows eosinophils and noncaseating granulomas	Oral prednisone plus cyclophosphamide

(continued)

Vasculitides (continued)

Diagnosis	Vessel Affected/ Symptoms	Diagnosis	Treatment
Polyarteritis nodosa	• Medium-vessel vasculitis • Every organ system involved **except lungs** • **Abdominal pain** common, and mimics intestinal ischemia • Associated with **hepatitis B infection**	• Best initial test: **sural nerve biopsy** • When confirmed, perform **angiography** to rule out aneurysm formation (rupture common); **or** if symptoms of intestinal ischemia, do angiography first (will show aneurysm formation)	Oral prednisone plus cyclophosphamide
Temporal arteritis	• Large-vessel vasculitis affecting the **head** (headache, scalp tenderness, jaw claudication, blurry vision) • Associated with **polymyalgia rheumatica**	• Best initial test— ESR (>50 mm/hour >90% specific) • Confirm with temporal artery biopsy	Oral prednisone; **begin when ESR is high, do not wait** for biopsy to be done or for biopsy results to return; blindness if not treated promptly
Granulomatosis with polyangitis (formerly Wegener granulomatosis)	Small-vessel disease of **upper and lower respiratory tract** (rhinitis, sinusitis, dyspnea, and hemoptysis) **and kidneys** (hematuria)	• Best initial test: **c-ANCA** (anti-proteinase-3 antibody) • Then confirm with **biopsy of the nasal septum** (granulomas and vasculitis); renal biopsy is most specific but more invasive	Oral prednisone plus cyclophosphamide

Abbreviations: cytoplasmic antineutrophilic cytoplasmic antibody, c-ANCA; erythrocyte sedimentation rate, ESR; perinuclear antineutrophilic cytoplasmic antibody, p-ANCA

4

5

DERMATOLOGY

PEDIATRIC DERMATOLOGY

Atopic Dermatitis/Eczema

- Etiology
  - ▸ Inflammatory skin condition, often associated with asthma and allergic rhinitis. Many theories exist, but appears to be caused by a genetic defect in epidermal filaggrin resulting in dry and sensitive skin. The vast majority of cases are seen in children; 40% outgrow the disorder
  - ▸ *Staphylococcus aureus* colonization is common and plays a large role in superinfection and acute exacerbations
- Clinical
  - ▸ Infantile eczema (birth–2 years)—look for pruritic, red, scaly, and crusted lesions on the cheeks and/or scalp that **spare the diaper area** (in contrast to diaper dermatitis)
  - ▸ Childhood eczema (2–12 years)—look for lichenified plaques in the flexural surfaces of the antecubital and popliteal fossae, volar aspect of the wrists, ankles, and neck
  - ▸ Adult eczema (≥12 years)—look for lichenification of areas involved in typical infantile eczema and/or the hands, neck, flexural surfaces
- Management
  - ▸ Noninflammatory (skin is just dry and itchy)—therapy is primarily aimed at maintaining skin's moisture

- Suggest short, lukewarm showers and avoidance of hot or prolonged tub bathing, which depletes skin's moisture
- Follow with use of high-oil-content emollients (Vaseline®, Aquaphor®)
- Avoid stress and anxiety (known triggers for flare-ups)
- Use oral antihistamines for bothersome itching
- Intermittent use of topical steroids (e.g., twice per week) between flares can be used as a preventive strategy

- Inflammatory
  - When a flare-up occurs, change to *daily* application of a low-potency topical steroid (e.g., hydrocortisone) for mild cases and moderate- to high-potency for more severe cases
  - Once the flare-up has resolved, return to 2–3 times/week preventive applications
  - In those who are *intolerant* of steroid use or have atopy in areas at high *risk of skin atropy* (face, neck, skin folds), treat flares with topical calcineurin inhibitors (tacrolimus, pimecrolimus), but **use with extreme caution** and for the shortest time necessary (increased risk of skin cancer and lymphoma)
  - Difficult-to-manage or severe cases—refer to dermatology for potential oral immunosuppressive treatment such as oral cyclosporine or mycophenolate

Molluscum Contagiosum

- Etiology/clinical—infection with poxvirus results in **pearly-pink papules** with **central umbilication**; highly contagious; common in school-age children or immunosuppressed HIV-AIDS patients
- **Tip:** May mimic disseminated cryptococcosis in AIDS. Differentiate with serum cryptococcal antigen.
- Diagnosis—clinical; biopsy will show keratinocytes containing inclusion bodies
- Management—curettage (usually preferred), cryotherapy, or laser ablation

Lice or Pediculosis (Head and Pubic)

- Clinical—head louse is small, gray-white insect that attaches to hair, most common infection in elementary-school children; pubic louse is spread by sexual contact, is common in young adults, is 2–3 mm and translucent unless filled with blood

- Diagnosis—fine-toothed nit comb with visual inspection; most common symptom for both head and pubic lice is pruritus

- Treatment—topical permethrin, pyrethrin, or malathion are first-line therapies; repeat after 2 weeks if still infected

Warts

- Pathophysiology—there are >150 serotypes of the DNA virus that result in warts and cutaneous/squamous malignancies. Each serotype has a different tropism (i.e., the tissue it prefers to infect) for different body sites and varying degrees of predilection for malignancies. For example, high-risk HPV serotypes 16 and 18 are responsible for the majority of cervical cancer (see Cervical Neoplasia, page 300).

  ▸ Common warts—caused by HPV types 2 and 1; usually rough, irregular asymptomatic papules on the hands

  ▸ Plantar warts—caused by HPV types 1 and 2; spread easily in public swimming pools and shared shower spaces (like the gym); characteristically interrupt the skin's normal swirl/whirl pattern. At first asymptomatic, they grow *inward* and become painful under the pressure of walking

  ▸ Butcher's warts—caused by HPV types 2 and 7; seen in meat, poultry, and fish handlers

  ▸ Anogenital warts (condylomata)—caused by HPV types 6 and 11, spread by sexual contact; also asymptomatic unless large; may cause perianal/perivaginal itching and bleeding depending on site of inoculation

- Treatment—cryotherapy, salicylic acid, liquid nitrogen, or curettage. All methods are effective and are chosen based upon patient preference.

5

Scabies

- Etiology—infestation with *Sarcoptes scabiei,* which burrows into the skin to lay its eggs, resulting in an intense hypersensitivity reaction (type IV)

- Clinical—**intense pruritus**, primarily around the **fingers, toes, genital area**, and **breast creases** with superficial **burrows**

- Diagnosis—application of mineral oil to burrow with microscopic examination of skin scrapings, adhesive tape test (examination of tape under microscope), or dermoscopy

- Management—topical permethrin cream or oral ivermectin
  - ▸ Beware that symptoms may persist for weeks to months after successful eradication of the mite
  - ▸ **Tip:** Norwegian or crusted scabies is severe infection more often found in immunocompromised hosts. Preferred treatment is both topical permethrin and oral ivermectin.

Staphylococcal Scalded-Skin Syndrome (SSSS)

- Etiology/clinical presentation—newborn infants are susceptible to the exfoliative toxins in *Staphylococcus aureus.* Seen around 3–7 days of age starting as fever and blanching perioral erythema followed by flaccid blisters at areas of mechanical stress. Mucous membranes *are not* involved (unlike TEN)
  - ▸ **Tip:** Destruction is caused by toxin-mediated cleavage of the desmoglein-1 complex.
  - ▸ Diagnosis—usually clinical; skin biopsy in cases of clinical doubt will show characteristic cleavage plane in the lower stratum granulosum with minimal necrosis. Bullae are sterile.
  - ▸ Treatment—naficillin or oxacillin, but consider vancomycin as first-line treatment in areas with high prevalence of community-acquired MRSA

ADULT DERMATOLOGY

Acne Vulgaris

- Pathogenesis—four main factors are involved:
  - ▸ Follicular hyperkeratinization leads to increased desquamation in the hair follicle with increased sebum production and impaction
  - ▸ *Propionibacterium acnes* is a normal anaerobic skin flora. It thrives and multiples in the lipid-rich environment of impacted sebum, leading to cytokine release and inflammation of the surrounding skin
  - ▸ Increased androgens during puberty (DHEA) cause sebaceous gland growth and increased secretion; male adolescents are affected more than female
  - ▸ Diet's role remains controversial, but some studies have linked to increased acne to dairy-rich diets (due to increased IGF-1)
- Clinical lesions in order of increasing severity
  - ▸ Closed comedone—"whitehead"
  - ▸ Open comedone—"blackhead"
  - ▸ Inflammatory nodules—papules, pustules, and nodules (tender, >5 mm diameter)
  - ▸ Nodular or cystic acne—may form sinus tracts as lesions merge
- Management
  - ▸ Discourage picking/popping—causes secondary staphylococcal infections and repetitive microtrauma (related to worsened inflammatory acne)
  - ▸ **Tip:** All **female** patients taking **oral isotretinoin** must be on **oral contraceptive therapy**, and must be instructed to use **barrier contraception** and **spermicides** during intercourse (oral isotretinoin is highly teratogenic).
  - ▸ Drug therapies—see table, following page
    - ▹ Choose oral antibiotics (if applicable) based on side effects, cost, and patient profile (allergy history, etc.)
    - ▹ Limit oral antibiotic treatment to 12–18 weeks, to control acne; then change to topical maintenance treatment only

5

Everything You Need to Know about Acne

Classification*	Diagnosis	First-Line Treatment
Mild comedonal acne	<20 comedones *or* total lesion count lower <30	Topical **retinoid** (tretinoin, adaptalene, or tazarotene)
Mild papular/ pustular acne	<15 inflammatory lesions *or* total lesion count <30	Topical **retinoid** *plus* topical **benzoyl peroxide** and an **antimicrobial** (DOC : erythromycin and clindamycin; alternatives: topical sulfacetamide, topical dapsone)
Moderate acne	20–100 comedones *or* 15–50 inflammatory lesions *or* total lesion count 30–125	Topical **retinoid** with or without benzoyl peroxide *plus* **oral antibiotic** 12–18 weeks until remission (DOC: doxycycline; alternatives: minocycline, tetracycline, trimethoprim-sulfamethoxazole, erythromycin, azithromycin)
Severe acne	>5 cysts, >100 comedones, >50 inflammatory lesions, or >125 total lesions	Oral **isotretinoin**

Note: There are multiple different classification systems for acne.

ADVERSE DRUG ERUPTIONS

Erythema Multiforme

- Clinical
  - ► Characterized by erythematous targetoid lesions
  - ► Minor—start on hands or feet; **no mucosal involvement**
  - ► Major (a.k.a. Stevens-Johnson syndrome)—at least 2 mucosal surfaces must be involved; lesions become hemorrhagic, usually blistering around the mouth
- Etiology
  - ► Most common cause—infections (90%)
    - ▷ Most common viral cause: herpes simplex virus (HSV)
    - ▷ Most common bacterial cause: *Mycoplasma pneumoniae*

- ▶ Second most common cause—drugs (around 10%; sulfonamides, NSAIDs, antiepileptics)
- **Tip:** Pathogenesis is a cell-mediated immune response against antigens. Resolves spontaneously within 2 weeks. Recurrent erythema multiforme is rare; most often seen in HSV reactivation.

Erythema Nodosum

- Etiology—an immunologic response to a variety of different stimuli (most commonly tuberculosis, streptococcal infection, and sarcoidosis) resulting in inflammation of the fat cells under the skin → panniculitis
- Unknown etiology in 30–50% of cases
- Peak incidence—between 20 and 30 years of age, with women 3–6 times more affected than men
- Most common cause in young women—**oral contraceptive pills (OCPs)**
- May be seen in infections, inflammatory bowel disease (IBD), autoimmune disease, and pregnancy, and with some medications
- Clinical—**tender, red, raised nodules**, usually on both **shins**, with a **smooth and shiny** appearance; frequently associated with fever, malaise, and pain and inflammation of joints
  - ▶ Usually resolves within 3–6 weeks after the inciting event without scarring
  - ▶ May occur anywhere there is fat under the skin, including thighs, arms, trunk, face, and neck
  - ▶ 1–10 cm in diameter and may coalesce
  - ▶ As the nodules age, they become bluish-purple, brownish, yellowish, and finally green (similar to a resolving bruise)
- Diagnosis—clinical; biopsy when the diagnosis is unclear
  - ▶ Determine the underlying cause (may use CBC, erythrocyte sedimentation rate [ESR], anti-streptolysin O [ASO] titers, urinalysis, cultures, and chest x-ray)

5

- Management—treat underlying cause; symptoms can be treated with bed rest, leg elevation, compressive bandages, wet dressings, and **nonsteroidal anti-inflammatory drugs** (NSAIDs; usually more effective acutely than with chronic disease)
  - ▸ Corticosteroids in severe cases

Fixed Drug Eruption

- Common; **recurs at the same site with each exposure** to a particular medication
- Medications inducing fixed drug eruptions are usually taken intermittently; typical causes are tetracyclines and sulfonamides

Urticaria

- Etiology—release of inflammatory mediators including histamine → local fluid leakage, superficial edema, and a skin rash known for dark-red, raised, itchy bumps
- Hives are frequently caused by allergic reactions; however, there are many nonallergic causes
- Acute urticaria—**lasts less than 6 weeks** and is usually the result of an allergic trigger
  - ▸ Acute viral infection or viral exanthems; others include friction, pressure, temperature extremes, exercise, and sunlight
  - ▸ Wheals may be pinpoint-size, or several inches in diameter
  - ▸ Drug-induced urticaria
- Chronic urticaria—hives **lasting longer than 6 weeks**, with majority of cases being idiopathic or autoimmune
  - ▸ Dermatographism—benign appearance of linear hives when the skin is stroked
  - ▸ Physical urticarias are categorized as follows:
    - ▹ Adrenergic—reaction to adrenaline/noradrenaline
    - ▹ Aquagenic—rare reaction to water
    - ▹ Cholinergic—reaction to exercising or hot showers
    - ▹ Cold-induced—worsens with sudden change in temperature

▷ Delayed pressure—reaction to standing for long periods, bra straps, elastic bands on undergarments, or belts

▷ Heat—rare reaction to hot food or objects

▷ Solar—more common in fair-skinned persons

▷ Vibration—rare

- Management

  ▸ Chronic urticaria is difficult to treat; avoid known triggers; some forms have several known triggers

  ▸ First-line therapy—histamine H_1 antagonists, including diphenhydramine and hydroxyzine acutely; newer H_1 antagonists such as loratadine, cetirizine, or fexofenadine chronically (less sedating)

  ▸ Second-line therapy—histamine H_2 antagonists (cimetidine and ranitidine); they also have been shown to have a synergistic effect when taken with an H_1 antagonist

  ▸ Oral corticosteroids or cyclosporine for very severe outbreaks

- Angioedema is similar to urticaria, but swelling occurs in the lower layers of the dermis and subcutaneous tissue

  ▸ May be hereditary from C1 esterase deficiency or acquired (angiotensin-converting enzyme-I [ACE-I])

  ▸ Usually affects the mouth, throat, abdomen, but may occasionally occur in other locations

  ▸ Urticaria and angioedema may occur simultaneously

  ▸ Angioedema of the throat may be fatal

  ▸ Management—C1 esterase inhibitor replacement protein is first-line; if not available, use fresh frozen plasma (FFP)

Morbilliform Rash

- Etiology—most common cutaneous drug eruption; characterized by a **measles-like viral exanthem** starting in dependent areas → becomes generalized

- Clinical—begins 2–10 days after initiation of the drug and up to 14 days after the drug is stopped

- ▸ Frequently related to antimicrobial therapy with high frequency in **Epstein-Barr virus** or **cytomegalovirus** treated with **ampicillin**, and in **HIV** infection when using **sulfa drugs**
- ▸ Fever, leukemoid reaction, interstitial nephritis, or, rarely, elevated serum transaminases
- Management—discontinue the offending drug, use topical or systemic antihistamines, and, if severe, administer 2 weeks of systemic corticosteroids
- Most morbilliform rashes resolve with some degree of superficial skin desquamation

Stevens-Johnson Syndrome (SJS)

- Etiology—life-threatening hypersensitivity reaction resulting in cell death and complete separation of the epidermis from the dermis involving the **skin and mucous membranes**
  - ▸ Most cases due to medications, followed by infections and cancers
- Clinical—milder than toxic epidermal necrolysis with **<10% of total body surface** area involved
- Management—ICU/burn unit care; intubation if respiratory tract involvement

Toxic Epidermal Necrolysis (TEN)

- Etiology—same mechanism as SJS, mortality rate 25–35%
  - ▸ Most common cause—phenytoin, sulfonamides, allopurinol, and NSAIDs
- Clinical—**more than 30% of body surface area (BSA) is involved**
  - ▸ Erosions with positive Nikolsky sign (rubbing the skin results in blisters) → skin peels off
- Diagnosis—clinical; skin biopsy is the gold standard → complete necrosis
- Management—must be admitted to a **burn unit** with supportive care, treat secondary infection; high mortality

► IV immunoglobulin (IVIG) for just 4 days is thought to halt progression of disease; high-dose short-term steroids in **adults only**

► Baseline and routine ophthalmologic exam; lubricating eye drops

► **Tip:** Up to 40% of TEN survivors will develop sicca syndrome.

ALOPECIA AREATA

• Etiology—immune-mediated hair loss from some or all areas of the body, usually from the scalp; affects females > males; more commonly occurs during childhood or young adulthood

• Clinical—smooth, shiny, noninflammatory patchy hair loss can spread to the entire scalp (alopecia totalis) or to the entire epidermis (alopecia universalis); does **not** cause scarring in contrast to lupus

• Management—intralesional corticosteroid injections for isolated disease; topical immunotherapy for extensive disease

PEMPHIGUS

A rare group of autoimmune blistering diseases that affect the skin and mucous membranes.

Pemphigous and Bullous Pemphigoid

Disease and Presentation	Associations	Diagnosis	Treatment
Pemphigus vulgaris • Painful, flaccid bullae with positive Nikolsky sign • Oral ulcers	• Most common in the US • Ashkenazi Jews (esp. HLA-DR4 haplotype)	• Punch biopsy shows intraepithelial acantholysis **without** disruption of the basement membrane and IgG deposits • ELISA shows antibodies against desmoglein-3 +/– desmoglein-1	• First-line: oral corticosteroids • Can add cyclophosphamide, azathioprine, or mycophenolate (steroid-sparing agents)

(continued)

Pemphigous and Bullous Pemphigoid (continued)

Disease and Presentation	Associations	Diagnosis	Treatment
Pemphigus foliaceus • Less severe: **erosions** instead of blisters, **no** oral ulcers • Erythema, scaling (dermatitis-like), and crusting on **face and scalp** progresses to chest and back	• More common in Africa • Can be drug induced (penicillamine, ACE-I, antibiotics)	• Punch biopsy similar to vulgaris but more superficial involvement • ELISA shows antibodies against desmoglein-1 only	• Same as above • Withdraw offending drug if applicable
Paraneoplastic pemphigus • **Severe, painful** sores in the **mouth**, lips, and esophagus • Polymorphous skin lesions +/– bronchiolitis obliterans	• Non-Hodgkin lymphoma • Castleman disease • CLL	• Variable histopathology • ELISA shows anti-envoplakin and anti-periplakin antibodies	• Surgical removal of tumor, if possible (in Castleman or thymoma), is curative • If not resectable, steroids are first-line • Consider rituximab and steroid-sparing agents as above
Bullous pemphigoid Localized or generalized blistering of the skin that are **tense and pruritic**	Age 70s–80s	• Perilesional punch biopsy shows linear IgG and/or C3 along the basement membrane • Autoantibodies to BP180 and BP230	• First-line: high-potency topical steroids • If disease is extensive or refractory: oral steroids and (if needed) steroid-sparing agents

Abbreviations: angiotensin-converting enzyme inhibitor, ACE-I; chronic leukocytic leukemia, CLL; enzyme-linked immunosorbent assay, ELISA; immunoglobulin G antibodies, IgG

BACTERIAL SKIN INFECTIONS

Impetigo

- Etiology—superficial skin infection with *Staphylococcus aureus* (most commonly) or *Streptococcus pyogenes,* affecting children age 2–6 years; spread by direct contact with skin lesions or nasal carriers

  ▸ **Tip:** *S. aureus* exfoliative toxin is responsible for targeting desmoglein-1 protein → bullous impetigo.

- Clinical

  ▸ Nonbullous impetigo—**honey-colored scabs and crusts** found on the arms, legs, or face

  ▸ Bullous impetigo affects infants and children <2 years and causes painless, pruritic, fluid-filled **blisters** with **surrounding erythema** that appear on the trunk, arms, and legs and **scab over with a honey-colored crust**

  ▸ Ecthyma is a more extensive form of impetigo that extends into the dermis. **Painful fluid- or pus-filled sores** → deep **ulcers** on the legs and feet → covered with **hard, thick, gray-yellow crust** → regional **lymphadenopathy**.

- Diagnosis—clinical
- Management

  ▸ Get cultures for sensitivities if empiric therapy fails

  ▸ Localized disease without bullae—topical mupirocin is first-line therapy

  ▸ Extensive disease or bullae formation—oral dicloxacillin, cephalexin, or clindamycin; all are acceptable

  ▸ Risk factors for MRSA—clindamycin, doxycycline, minocycline, [226] trimethoprim-sulfamethoxazole

Folliculitis

- Etiology—inflammation from damage of one or more hair follicles (insect bite, shaving, or clothing) causing a rash and pustule formation most commonly on the neck, axilla, or groin

- Most cases due to *Staph. aureus* infection
- Iron deficiency anemia is associated with chronic cases
- Hot-tub folliculitis is due to *Pseudomonas aeruginosa* infection of exposed body parts; usually the legs, hips, and buttocks, especially the areas where the bathing suit was worn
- Management
  - Topical warm compresses are first-line and inflammation almost always resolves spontaneously
  - If infection persists, use topical mupirocin for suspected *Staph. aureus*

Furuncles

- Small skin abscesses caused by staphylococcal infection of a hair follicle and surrounding tissue, most often in sites of friction: neck, face, axillae, buttocks
- Management
  - Warm compresses, and incision and drainage (I&D), with cultures for larger lesions
  - Given higher incidence of MRSA, coverage should probably account for this organism in high-prevalence regions: clindamycin, doxycycline or minocycline, trimethoprim-sulfamethoxazole, linezolid

Carbuncles

- **Clusters** of furuncles connected **subcutaneously**, causing deeper suppuration and scarring
- Management
  - I&D is first-line therapy (send cultures), plus any of the oral antibiotics noted above for furuncles
  - Consider hospitalization and IV antibiotics (vancomycin) if systemic symptoms/findings (high WBC, positive left shift, fever)

> **Important:** Sensitivities vary widely in all staphylococcal skin infections, so obtaining culture and sensitivities is a **must**.

Cellulitis and Erysipelas

- Cellulitis
  - ▸ Etiology—diffuse infection of connective tissue with severe inflammation of the dermis and subcutaneous fat; caused most commonly by Group A *Streptococcus* and *Staph. aureus*
  - ▸ Occurs where the skin has previously been broken: cracks, cuts, blisters, burns, insect bites, wounds, especially the face (known as erysipelas), or lower legs

- Erysipelas
  - ▸ Etiology—infection of the upper dermis and superficial lymphatics with very clear lines of demarcation and superficial edema; usually due to Group A **beta-hemolytic *Streptococcus***
  - ▸ Affects the very young and the very old

- Diagnosis—clinical, cultures often not helpful

- Management
  - ▸ Erysipelas—IV ceftriaxone or cefazolin
  - ▸ Nontoxic cellulitis (no systemic signs)—oral dicloxacillin, cephalexin, or clindamycin are all acceptable for outpatient therapy
  - ▸ Toxic-appearing cellulitis—IV nafcillin or cefazolin is first-line; IV vancomycin if from area of high prevalence of CA-MRSA (prisoners, nursing home, etc.) or purulent cellulitis
    - ▹ If toxicity is severe and pain is out of proportion to the clinical findings, you *must consider* necrotizing fasciitis—emergency debridement is required if confirmed. Get a surgical consult with or without CT scan immediately.

5

DECUBITUS ULCERS

Caused by unrelieved pressure in bedbound patients, particularly at the bony prominences (e.g., sacrum, heel), which damages the underlying tissue. Prevent by frequently turning bedbound patients and by offloading mattresses.

Stages of Decubitus Ulcers

Stage 1	Skin is reddened	Apply a local transparent dressing *and* intensify measures to prevent further development
Stage 2	Partial-thickness injury with dermal loss—results in a shallow red ulcer or blistering	Apply an occlusive, semipermeable dressing to maintain a moist environment
Stage 3	Full-thickness injury through the dermis into the subcutaneous tissue—results in an ulcer with exposed **subcutaneous tissue**	• Assess for signs of infection including redness, calor around the site, pus, foul smelling exudates, significant change in pain • Dressing depends on type of wound—it is not necessary to know all of them • Remember that dressing should keep wound moist to promote epithelization and healing while preventing complete maceration
Stage 4	Full-thickness injury with exposed **bone, tendon, or muscle**	As above; assess for underlying osteomyelitis
Unstageable	Full-thickness tissue loss in which the base of the ulcer is covered by slough (yellow, tan, gray, green, or brown) and/or eschar (tan, brown, or black) making staging impossible to determine	• Most need some type of debridement • Consultation with wound care experts is recommended

- Key concepts
  - ▶ Pressure ulcers can be excruciating, particularly in more advanced wounds. Ensure adequate pain relief in all patients, and be alert for pain in those unable to communicate (grimacing, moaning, tachycardia)
  - ▶ Nutrition
    - ▷ Assess caloric intake (30 kcal/kg/day) and protein intake (1.5 g/kg/day)

▷ Ensure both goals are met since **this is vital for healing**

► Despite common practice, there is *no* convincing data that vitamin C or zinc supplementation is efficacious

► Support surfaces/powered beds are most effective in decreasing length of stay in those who would otherwise be discharged. They are *significantly* more expensive than standard hospital mattresses.

DERMATOPHYTOSES

• Tinea = superficial dermatophyte infection

• Fungal infections of the skin—three types: *Trichophytin, Microsporum, Epidermophyton*

• Tinea capitis—located on the head

• Tinea cruris—located on the groin

• Tinea pedis—located on the feet

• Tinea versicolor—**hypo- or hyperpigmented patches** with **scaling** due to lipophilic yeast, *Pityrosporum orbiculare* (*Malassezia furfur* is the filamentous form), present in the hair follicle

► KOH prep—yields classic "**spaghetti-and-meatballs**" appearance

• Onychomycosis—infection of the toenails causing **brittleness and yellow discoloration**; predisposes to secondary cellulitis (always rule out and treat **onychomycosis and tinea pedis** in a patient with cellulitis of the lower extremities)

• Management

► Localized skin disease—**topical** "-azoles" (ketoconazole, clotrimazole, etc.)

► Extensive skin disease, onychomycosis, or tinea capitis must be treated with **systemic** therapy

▷ Tinea capitis—griseofulvin is the drug of choice (DOC)

▷ Onychomycosis or widespread skin disease—terbinafine or itraconazole are the DOCs

HERPES SIMPLEX

- Etiology—herpes simplex virus-1 (HSV-1) and HSV-2 infection
- Categorized by the site of infection
  - ▸ Oral herpes (cold sores)—infects the face and mouth and is the most common form of infection; due to HSV-1 in the majority of cases
  - ▸ Genital herpes—second most common form of herpes; due to HSV-2 in the majority of cases; often asymptomatic with active viral shedding
  - ▸ Herpetic whitlow—sometimes seen in dentists and transmitted during active oral herpes outbreaks; due to HSV-1
  - ▸ Herpes keratitis—infects the ocular nerve and may result in blindness; due to HSV-1
  - ▸ Herpes encephalitis presents with characteristic mood disturbances (primarily affects the temporal lobes) and features of encephalitis, largely due to HSV-1. HSV-2 can cause aseptic meningitis, but encephalitis is unusual.
  - ▸ Severe, widespread herpes infection in immature or suppressed immune system
- Herpes viruses cycle between periods of active disease—present as blisters containing infectious virus particles → last for 2–21 days → remission → virus moves to sensory nerves → resides as lifelong latent virus in the ganglion
  - ▸ Diagnose prior exposure and latent infection with HSV-1 and HSV-2 serology
  - ▸ Tzanck prep of active lesions shows multinucleated keratinocytes. Nowadays, direct immunofluorescence of scraping can give results in hours if the diagnosis is in question. Otherwise reactivation is generally a clinical diagnosis.
  - ▸ Episodes of active disease reduce in frequency with time
- Transmission
  - ▸ Easily transmitted by direct contact with a lesion or bodily fluids, but most transmission occurs during asymptomatic shedding

> ▸ Skin-to-skin contact during periods of asymptomatic shedding
>> ▷ **Tip:** In genital herpes, antiviral therapy decreases viral shedding by up to **95%,** reducing transmission to sexual partners.
>
> ▸ Barrier protection methods (gloves and condoms) help but transmission may still occur

- Management—no cure and no vaccine currently available
  - ▸ Oral acyclovir, famciclovir, or valacyclovir can decrease viral shedding and speed healing time during active outbreaks
  - ▸ Suppressive therapy recommended in the immunosuppressed and in those with severe, frequent outbreaks
  - ▸ Must add steroids if evidence of herpes ocularis
  - ▸ Acyclovir-resistant herpes is treated with foscarnet

5

HERPES ZOSTER

- Etiology—due to prior varicella virus infection (chickenpox)
- Clinical—**painful groups of vesicles** on an erythematous base along a **dermatomal distribution**
  - ▸ Approximately 20% of cases result in painful postherpetic neuralgia, especially in the elderly and the immunosuppressed
  - ▸ If zoster occurs on the **nose**, refer to ophthalmologist because of high incidence of **herpes zoster ophthalmicus**; look for **dendritic lesions** → may result in blindness
  - ▸ Watch for Ramsay Hunt syndrome → triad of ipsilateral facial paralysis, ear pain, and vesicles in the auricle and auditory canal. Reactivation of varicella zoster virus in geniculate ganglion frequently involves cranial nerves V, IX, and X.
- Diagnosis—clinical, but can confirm with direct immuno-fluorescence testing of skin scrapings (preferred acutely), viral culture, or PCR
- Management
  - ▸ Acyclovir, famciclovir, or valacyclovir most effective within the **first 72 hours of symptoms** if patient >**50 years of age or**

immunocompromised. All patients with eye involvement or Ramsay Hunt should be treated.

- ▸ Oral amitriptyline or nortriptyline for treatment of post-herpetic neuralgia as first-line therapy; if ineffective, may try gabapentin or opioids

PARONYCHIA

- Clinical—tender and painful local infection where the nail meets the skin. Seen in nail-biters, thumb-suckers, dishwashers, those with excessive manicures.
  - ▸ Acute paronychia is usually caused by bacteria; treat with antistaphylococcal antibiotics, cream or oral, and/or I&D if local abscess formation
  - ▸ Chronic paronychia starts gradually, most often caused by *Candida* infection
- Management—oral dicloxacillin or erythromycin (if penicillin-allergic) covers methicillin-sensitive *Staph. aureus* (MSSA); or TMP-SMX if high incidence of CM-MRSA
  - ▸ Hot-water soak 2–3 times daily
  - ▸ In chronic cases, can use topical antifungal or topical steroid to relieve the pain and inflammation; always rule out diabetes, and advise to avoid excessive exposure to water or moisture

PITYRIASIS ROSEA

- Clinical—acute, self-limiting skin eruption; starts as a **"herald" patch** (may be preceded by a sore throat), followed after 1–2 weeks by a generalized secondary rash with a typical **"Christmas-tree" distribution**
  - ▸ Numerous oval patches start on the chest, following the rib line → small, circular patches appear on the back and neck several days later, lasting up to 6 weeks
  - ▸ It is unusual for lesions to form on the face, but they may appear on the cheeks or at the hairline and last for about 6 weeks

- About 25% of patients have mild to severe symptomatic **itching**
- Rash may be accompanied by low-grade headache, fever, nausea, and fatigue
- Management—none; disease is self-limited and resolves in 1–3 months; natural sunlight helps to speed up the disappearance of lesions

PREMALIGNANT AND MALIGNANT LESIONS

- Actinic keratosis
  - ▶ Clinical—**nontender** erythematous macules with **brown to gray scales** in **sun-exposed areas**; may also present with classic **cutaneous horn** most often seen on the **ear**
  - ▶ Diagnosis
    - ▷ Most often clinical—appearance and feel of lesion (rough, scaly)
    - ▷ Biopsy recommended to rule out squamous cell carcinoma if diagnosis in question or if lesion is painful, indurated, or diameter ≥1 cm
  - ▶ Management—cryotherapy, electrodesiccation, curettage, or topical 5-fluorouracil (5-FU) are all acceptable (no best therapy)

- Seborrheic keratosis
  - ▶ Clinical—**greasy, brown, crusty lesions** with classic **"stuck-on"** appearance affecting face and scalp
  - ▶ Common in the **elderly**
  - ▶ Diagnosis—based on clinical appearance in most cases. Shave biopsy is recommended for questionable lesions.
  - ▶ Management—electrodesiccation, cryotherapy, or excision is acceptable but indicated only if lesions are bothersome (they are **benign**)

- Basal cell carcinoma
  - ▶ Most common skin cancer in Caucasians

5

- Clinical—**pearly papule** with surrounding **telangiectasia** and may extend through skin into the bone
- Management—most clinicians prefer surgical excision by means of Mohs micrographic surgery; electrodesiccation or cryotherapy are also acceptable

- Kaposi sarcoma
  - Clinical—**purple plaques and nodules** occurring anywhere on the skin due to **human herpesvirus (HHV 8)** infection; seen in the elderly and the immunosuppressed (especially **AIDS patients or transplant recipients**)
  - Management—control underlying HIV infection and decrease immunosuppression if applicable (transplant patients) first; if cosmetically bothersome or involving underlying organs, may use chemotherapy and/or radiation

- Squamous cell carcinoma
  - Most common skin cancer in African Americans
  - Clinical—**ulcerated, nodular mass** that **bleeds easily**; chronic **burns, scars,** draining sinuses, areas of chronic infection and trauma are at especially high risk (the carcinoma often develops on top of them)
  - Management—excision is curative in most

- Malignant melanoma
  - Etiology—malignancy of melanocytes, with Caucasians at highest risk
  - Clinical—most common on sun-exposed areas, and occurs within **nevi** (especially dysplastic nevi)
  - ABCDE (determining suspicion of underlying melanoma in a nevus)
    - **A**symmetry
    - **B**order is irregular
    - **C**olor is varied; red-tan or black or changed
    - **D**iameter >6 mm
    - **E**nlarging or elevating lesion

- ▸ Superficial spreading form is the most common type
- ▸ Diagnosis—depth of invasion is the most important prognostic factor (depth used to divide melanoma into stage I–IV); serum S-100 is an antibody used to differentiate the melanocyte form
- ▸ Management—excision is first-line and curative in most cases without invasion of the basement membrane. In metastasis, combine metastasectomy (if possible) with immunotherapy (IL-2, ipilimumab) with or without radiation therapy.

PSORIASIS

- Etiology—autoimmune disease causing increased proliferation in the epidermis
- Clinical—**shiny**, **silvery** scales, especially on the **cheeks in children** and on the **extensor surfaces, elbows, and knees in adults**
  - ▸ May have nail changes, including **pitting**, onycholysis, yellowing, and subungual debris
  - ▸ Geographic tongue—"maplike" appearance of the tongue
  - ▸ Köbner phenomenon—occurrence of lesions at sites of trauma
  - ▸ Auspitz sign—punctuate bleeding when a little bit of scale is pulled off
- Guttate psoriasis—**droplike** scaly plaques on the trunk and extremities most commonly seen in children and young adults; very responsive to UV-B phototherapy
- Pustular psoriasis—localized to **hands and feet**; pustules are **sterile**
- Psoriatic arthritis can affect distal interphalangeals causing severe erosion of joints; may have classic **sausage-shaped digits** in males; spondylitis is also commonly seen
- Management
  - ▸ Skin psoriasis
    - ▹ Mild–moderate disease—topical emollients, corticosteroids, and calcipotriene used in combination is preferred

5

> ▷ Moderate–severe disease—try phototherapy first; if this fails or response is incomplete, add systemic therapy with methotrexate, cyclosporine, anti-TNF agents (etanercept, infliximab, adalimumab)

- ▸ Psoriatic arthritis—NSAIDs are first-line; if this fails, then systemic disease-modifying antirheumatic drugs (DMARDs; cyclosporin, methotrexate, hydroxyurea, etc.)
  - ▷ Systemic tumor necrosis factor (TNF) inhibitors are also very effective

SEBORRHEIC DERMATITIS

- Etiology—due to superficial lipophilic yeast infection with *Malassezia* sp. (formerly *Pityrosporum ovale*)

- Clinical—**erythematous patch** with **greasy, yellow scales** usually in **glabella, eyebrows, nasolabial fold, mustache, beard, or scalp**

- **Tip:** If seborrheic dermatitis starts suddenly with extensive lesions, you should rule out **AIDS**.

- Management—ketoconazole cream or shampoo is the treatment of choice. May also use a low-potency steroid for facial involvement until remission of lesions.

STASIS DERMATITIS

- Clinical—associated with abnormal venous flow causing varicose veins → develops erythema with reddish-brown hue, edema, vesiculation, scaling occurring on the medial leg → progresses to involve the feet and shins (so called **"brawny discoloration"**)

- Management of uncomplicated cases—topical steroids
  - ▸ Antibiotics only if secondary infection present
  - ▸ Elevation of the legs and use of compression stockings are also important (increases venous return)

GENERAL SURGERY

SKIN AND SOFT TISSUE

Necrotizing infections of the skin and fascia include necrotizing forms of cellulitis and fasciitis.

Gas Gangrene/Clostridial Myositis

- Etiology—rapidly developing, life-threatening muscular infection caused by *Clostridium perfringens* (most common bacterial cause) and group A *Streptococcus* (GAS; *Strep. pyogenes*) due to alpha toxin–mediated destruction
  - ► Most common portal of entry is traumatic; look for necrosis 24–36 hours after injury

- Clinical—severe pain followed by skin changes, including shiny pallor → rubor → purple with or without bullae
  - ► Systemic toxicity and rhabdomyolysis develop quickly, leading to multiorgan failure; kidneys are affected first

- Diagnosis—gas in the soft tissue can be felt as crepitus on physical exam; confirm with x-ray first (gas in the soft tissues), then CT or MRI to identify extent of injury

- Management—immediate surgical debridement plus IV penicillin and clindamycin
  - ► Surgical exploration shows very edematous muscle that does not bleed or contract on stimulation
  - ► Extensive surgical debridement improves survival

- ► Penicillin is the drug of choice; combination therapy with penicillin and clindamycin is now being recommended as first-line therapy
- ► If you are asked to choose between the two (antibiotics vs. surgical debridement), pick surgical debridement first; in clinical practice, both are done simultaneously
- ► Use of hyperbaric oxygen is controversial

Necrotizing Fasciitis

- Etiology—deep-seated infection of the subcutaneous tissue, resulting in destruction of fascia and fat, but usually spares skin; most common organisms are GAS, methicillin-resistant *Staphylococcus aureus* (MRSA)
  - ► Have a high level of suspicion in diabetic patients; it can be fatal

- **Fournier gangrene**—rapid and aggressive, affecting the perineal and genital areas
- Occurs through a break in the GI or GU tract (urethral mucosa, most commonly) by enteric organisms
- Clinical—gas in the soft tissue can be identified by physical exam as crepitus, but is rarely seen
  - ► Systemic toxicity is usually rapidly progressive and a bad prognostic indicator

- Diagnosis—x-ray, CT, or MRI
- Management—early aggressive surgical debridement and IV antibiotics
  - ► Ampicillin/ampicillin-sulbactam combined with metronidazole or clindamycin, or monotherapy with piperacillin-tazobactam or ticarcillin-clavulanate; all are acceptable

- IV antibiotics are important but surgical debridement is the best initial step
- Even with optimal therapy, necrotizing fasciitis has a high mortality

TOXIC INGESTIONS

- Most occur in children and in psychotic, suicidal, and alcoholic patients

- The severity and extent of esophageal and gastric damage resulting from a caustic ingestion depend on the corrosive properties of the ingested substance (alkali/acid); the amount, concentration, and physical form (solid or liquid) of the agent; and the duration of contact with the mucosa

- Alkali—worse injuries than acids; cause deep liquefaction necrosis and are more likely to cause cancer

  ▸ Button batteries (used in hearing aids, calculators, and watches) contain highly concentrated alkaline solutions. Damage can occur from release of the alkali, and direct pressure necrosis from the foreign body

  ▸ When alkali is lodged in the esophagus, burns can occur within 4 hours and perforation within 6 hours; urgent endoscopy is indicated in this setting

- Acid—causes coagulation necrosis

- Clinical manifestations—**oropharyngeal** and/or **retrosternal pain**, dysphagia, **hypersalivation**

- Diagnosis—chest x-ray (rule out pneumomediastinum) and abdominal x-ray (rule out free air under diaphragm)

- Management—strict NPO (nil per os, or nothing by mouth), do not induce vomiting, and **no nasogastric tube** (may cause perforation)

  ▸ Endoscopy within the first 24–48 hours to assess the lesion and guide therapy—do not go past site of injury, due to risk of perforation

  ▸ Endoscopy is absolutely contraindicated if you suspect perforation or if the patient is hemodynamically unstable, in severe respiratory distress, or exhibiting signs of severe oropharyngeal or glottic edema

6

- Assessing the degree of injury
  - ▶ Primary burns → hyperemia, edema, and hemorrhage; treat with observation and conservative management (NPO, IV fluids, spitting, antibiotics); patient may usually restart diet in 4–5 days
  - ▶ Secondary burns → exudates, ulceration, and sloughing of the mucosa; high probability of stricture due to scarring (granulation and fibroblastic reaction); treat with prolonged observation and conservative management → surgery only if signs of peritonitis, sepsis, mediastinitis, or perforation (free air)
  - ▶ Tertiary burns → deep ulcers, narrowing of the esophageal lumen, and perforation; treat as above, but surgery is usually necessary (esophagectomy with gastric pull-up or colonic interposition)

GI TRACT

Esophageal Perforation

- Most common cause—esophagogastroduodenoscopy
- Most common site—near the cricopharyngeal muscle (cervical esophagus)
- Clinical—dysphagia, pain, respiratory distress, fever, and tachycardia
- Diagnosis—best initial test is diatrizoic acid (Gastrografin®) CT scan of chest and abdomen or swallow study followed by thin barium swallow, if no evidence of perforation
- Management
  - ▶ If perforation is contained and self-draining, and patient is without systemic effects → nonsurgical treatment
    - ▷ No nasogastric tube; treat with NPO, spit, IV fluids, and antibiotics
    - ▷ Repeat diatrizoic acid study in 7–10 days
  - ▶ Free perforations (i.e., noncontained)
    - ▷ If <24 hrs with minimal contamination → attempt primary surgical repair (intercostal muscle flap), drain with chest tubes

▷ If >24 hrs with systemic effects → cervical esophagostomy with wash out and placement of chest tube and jejunostomy tube

- Keep patient NPO for 7–10 days, then repeat barium swallow to rule out stricture formation (uncommon)
- Distal feeding tube or TPN may be indicated for nutritional support
- Leave drains in place until patient is on a regular diet without increased drain output

Management of Suspected Esophageal Perforation

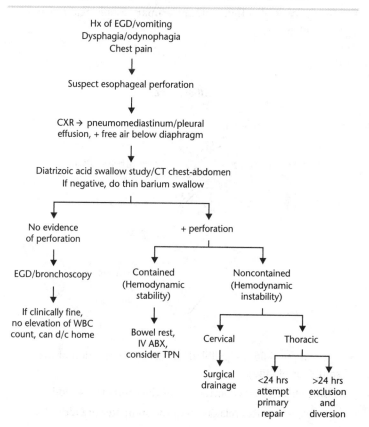

Abbreviations: antibiotics, ABX; chest x-ray, CXR; discharge, d/c; esophagogastro-duodenoscopy, EGD; history, Hx

Boerhaave Syndrome

- Risk factors—look for a history of **alcoholism**, gastric or duodenal ulcer

- Etiology—severe **retching and/or forceful vomiting** results in **tearing of the esophageal mucosa** → perforation most commonly occurs on the lateral left wall of the esophagogastric (EG) junction

- Clinical—hematemesis with retrosternal and upper abdominal pain (epigastric); shock can develop soon thereafter

- Diagnosis—diatrizoic acid swallow study

- Management—left thoracotomy, primary esophageal repair, and chest tubes

Gallbladder

Biliary Tree

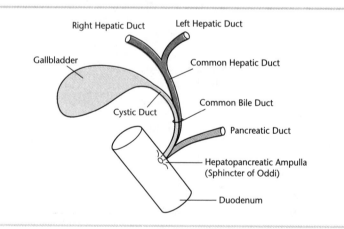

- Normal physiology—gallbladder fills by contraction of the sphincter of Oddi

  ► Morphine causes contraction of the sphincter of Oddi

  ► Glucagon causes relaxation of the sphincter of Oddi

- Most common cause of pathology is gallstones
  - ▶ Nonpigmented stones—most common type in the United States (75%); exclusive to the gallbladder and due to cholesterol insolubilization → yellow
  - ▶ Pigmented stones—most common worldwide → calcium bilirubinate
    - ▷ Black—total parenteral nutrition (TPN), ileal resection, hemolytic disorders
    - ▷ Brown—primary common bile duct (CBD) stones and infections (*Escherichia coli*)
- Cholesterol stones found in the CBD are secondary CBD stones

Biliary colic

Right-upper quadrant (RUQ) and epigastric **discomfort** that is often **not accompanied by any clinical signs** → due to transient obstruction of the cystic duct during passage of a gallstone → usually resolves in 4–6 hours

Cholecystitis

- Pathophysiology—inflammation of the gallbladder most commonly due to obstruction of the cystic duct by gallstones (cholelithiasis) **resulting in gallbladder wall distention and inflammation**
- 90% of cases are due to stones in the cystic duct (i.e., calculous cholecystitis)
- The other 10% of cases are due to bile stasis → acalculous cholecystitis (think of trauma, sepsis, diabetes mellitus [DM], sickle cell disease, TPN)
- Symptoms—**colicky RUQ pain**, pain referred to the **right shoulder or scapula**, with nausea and vomiting and **leukocytosis**
- Risk factors—age >40, female, obesity, pregnancy, ileal resection(s), rapid weight loss
- Mnemonic for calculous cholecystitis—the "4 F's": fat, female, forty, and fertile

6

- Most common organisms are *E. coli*, *Klebsiella,* and *Enterococcus*

- Diagnosis—**RUQ ultrasonography**; provides >95% sensitivity and specificity for the diagnosis of gallstones
  - ▸ **Tip:** This is the **best initial evaluation for any patient with RUQ pain and jaundice.**
  - ▸ Findings—hyperechoic focus, **pericholecystic fluid, gallbladder wall thickening >4 mm,** and sonographic **Murphy sign** (inspiratory arrest with RUQ pressure)

- If RUQ ultrasound is **nondiagnostic**, get a HIDA scan (technetium taken up by the liver and excreted into the biliary tract)
  - ▸ HIDA scan is positive if the gallbladder is not visualized → obstruction of the cystic duct from edema or stones (can be positive in calculous or acalculous cholecystitis (edema/sludge)

- Management
  - ▸ 72 hours or less since pain began → emergent cholecystectomy is the treatment of choice
  - ▸ >72 hours after the pain began → allow a **cool-off period** with NPO → IV fluids, IV antibiotics; then do cholecystectomy in 4–6 weeks
    - ▹ If patient does not improve with conservative management, or if there is persistence of RUQ pain, fever, and/or high white blood cell (WBC) count → take patient to the operating room (OR) for laparoscopic cholecystectomy
    - ▹ Cholecystostomy tube placement in severely ill patients
    - ▹ Indications: pre-op endoscopic retrograde cholangiopancreatography (ERCP)—jaundice, gallstone pancreatitis, elevated liver function tests (LFTs), elevated bilirubin, cholangitis, or stones in CBD

Cholangitis

- Pathophysiology—an infection of the biliary tract with significant morbidity and mortality

- Choledocholithiasis (biliary tract obstruction) is the most common cause

- In the past 10 years, biliary tract manipulations/interventions and stents are becoming more common causes of cholangitis

- Hepatobiliary malignancies are a less common cause of biliary tract obstruction and subsequent bile contamination

- Clinical
  - ▸ Charcot triad—**RUQ pain, fever, and jaundice**
  - ▸ Raynaud pentad—Charcot triad **plus mental status changes** (predictor of poor outcome) **and shock**

- Diagnosis—best initial step is ultrasound to look for CBD dilation and stones
  - ▸ Also obtain CBC, LFTs, and blood cultures → common laboratory findings include leukocytosis, hyperbilirubinemia, and elevated alkaline phosphatase levels with or without elevated transaminases

- Management—the mainstay of therapy is antibiotics (ampicillin-sulbactam or piperacillin-tazobactam plus metronidazole) with fluid resuscitation and establishing biliary drainage
  - ▸ The following procedures may be used for diagnostic and therapeutic purposes—start with ERCP; if this fails, get percutaneous transhepatic cholangiography (PTC)

6

Obstructive jaundice

- Evaluation always begins with a RUQ ultrasound

- ERCP—presence of stones, without evidence of a mass

- ERCP is also useful in the presence of a mass (especially cholangiocarcinoma)

- CT/MRI—presence of a mass, without evidence of stones

- Endoscopic ultrasound—becoming more popular, but results are operator-dependent

Diagnosis and Management of Gallbladder and Pancreatic Disorders

Diagnosis	Choledocholithiasis	Cholangiocarcinoma (Klatskin Tumor)	Pancreatic Cancer
Symptoms	RUQ **pain** and jaundice	**Painless** jaundice and weight loss	**Painless** jaundice and weight loss
Risk factors	Gallstones, primary CBD stones (in the Asian population, think of *Ascaris lumbricoides*)	*Clonorchis sinensis*, choledochal cysts, PSC, ulcerative colitis	Tobacco, obesity, genetic predominance
Location	Anywhere along the biliary tree	Upper third of the biliary tree, **confluence of right and left hepatic ducts**	70% in the **head of the pancreas**
Labs	Conjugated hyperbilirubinemia, high alkaline phosphatase, GGT	Conjugated hyperbilirubinemia, high alkaline phosphatase, GGT	Conjugated hyperbilirubinemia, high alkaline phosphatase
Tumor markers	None	Elevated CEA, CA 19-9 (not specific)	Elevated CA 19-9
Nonsurgical management	ERCP with Dormia basket/Fogarty catheter stone extraction	ERCP with stent placement; if this fails, then PTC	ERCP with stent placement; if this fails, then PTC
Surgical management	Cholecystectomy after successful ERCP **or** Cholecystectomy with CBD exploration (choledochotomy) if ERCP fails	Resection, diverting hepaticojejunostomy for early disease	Resection (Whipple procedure)

Abbreviations: common bile duct, CBD; carcinoembryonic antigen, CEA; endoscopic retrograde cholangiopancreatography, ERCP; gamma-glutamyltransferase, GGT; primary sclerosing cholangitis, PSC; percutaneous transhepatic cholangiogram, PTC; right-upper quadrant, RUQ

Appendicitis

- The most common cause of abdominal pain requiring surgical intervention

- Etiology—obstruction of the appendicial lumen due to fecalith, lymphoid hyperplasia (most common cause in children), tumors, or foreign bodies

- Most common organisms associated with appendicitis—*Bacteroides fragilis, E. coli, Pseudomonas*

- Clinical—**constant, sharp periumbilical pain** lasting 6–8 hours then localizing to the right lower quadrant (RLQ; somatic pain) with symptoms of anorexia, nausea/vomiting, and fever

- Diagnosis—80% of cases can be diagnosed clinically
  - ▶ Exam
    - ▷ Local tenderness at McBurney point
    - ▷ Rovsing sign is pathognomonic when present → referred tenderness to the RLQ when left-lower quadrant (LLQ) is palpated
    - ▷ Psoas sign—RLQ pain with hyperextension of the right hip joint
  - ▶ Labs—leukocytosis (11,000–16,000/mm^3) with a left shift (WBCs can be normal even with perforated appendicitis, so it is better to remove a normal appendix if the clinical suspicion is high)
  - ▶ Imaging studies
    - ▷ Ultrasound—useful in children and pregnancy; noncompressible, distended appendix >7 mm
    - ▷ CT—96% sensitive; get this for inconclusive or atypical presentations only; will show appendix that is >6 mm in diameter, has thickened walls, and does not fill with oral contrast (due to obstruction)

- Management—surgical removal is first-line, plus NPO, IV fluids, IV antibiotics, while preparing open or laparoscopic appendectomy
  - ▶ Laparoscopy preferred if no evidence of perforation—lower rates of wound infection and abscess formation
  - ▶ Open approach mandatory if perforation—peritoneal washout required

6

Mesenteric Ischemia

- Pathophysiology—due to reduced intestinal blood flow from occlusion, vasospasm, and/or hypoperfusion of the mesenteric vasculature

Management of Suspected Mesenteric Ischemia

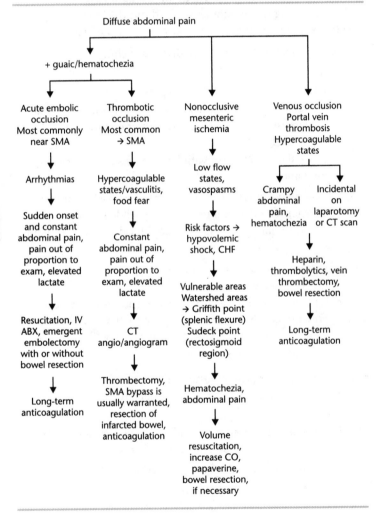

Abbreviations: antibiotics, ABX; cardiac output, CO; congestive heart failure, CHF; superior mesenteric artery, SMA

- Most common causes—acute embolic occlusion, thrombotic occlusion (acute), low flow states (can be acute due to hypoperfusion such as in trauma or chronic due to atherosclerosis), and venous thrombosis (acute)

- Acute mesenteric ischemia
  - ▸ Symptoms—**sudden onset** of **diffuse, severe abdominal pain**, hematochezia (bloody diarrhea) with **normal physical examination**
  - ▸ **Tip:** Look for this in an elderly patient with a history of atrial fibrillation.

- Chronic mesenteric ischemia
  - ▸ Symptoms—**postprandial** epigastric and periumbilical **abdominal pain** with bloating **30–60 minutes after meals** (intestinal angina)
  - ▸ **Tip:** Look for an elderly patient with history that includes weight loss from **fear of eating**.
  - ▸ 95% due to atherosclerosis—usually have history of other cardiovascular disease

6

Small-Bowel Obstruction (SBO)

- Etiology—the most frequent causes of SBO are **postoperative adhesions and hernias**, which cause extrinsic compression of the intestines; next most common cause is tumor or strictures of the small bowel, but these are much less common

- Pathophysiology—obstruction leads to dilation of the stomach and small intestine proximal to the blockage with decompression of the distal small bowel and colon

- Clinical—**abdominal distension**, **nausea**, **vomiting**, and **crampy** abdominal pain; obstipation (inability to pass flatus) may or may not be present
  - ▸ **Proximal** obstruction—**frequent nonbilious** vomiting → obstruction is proximal to the ampulla of Vater; will have colicky pain at frequent intervals with minimal to absent abdominal distension

▷ Obstipation occurs late in the course

▶ **Distal** obstruction—vomiting is **bilious** and **less frequent** (can be feculent if obstruction is longstanding) → colicky pain is less intense and less frequent but there is often a "constant ache" with gradual abdominal distension

▶ As the small bowel dilates, its blood flow becomes compromised → ischemia and necrosis, strangulation, and/or sepsis

- Diagnosis
  ▶ Best initial test is abdominal x-ray—two views: flat and upright → air–fluid levels, multiple distended loops of bowel, absence of air in the rectum (or distal to the obstruction)

  ▶ Most sensitive test is CT scan—90% specific for detecting SBO; useful in making an early diagnosis of strangulated obstruction and in delineating the myriad other causes of acute abdominal pain, especially when clinical and radiographic findings are inconclusive
    ▷ **Tip:** CT scanning is the study of choice if the patient has fever, tachycardia, localized abdominal pain, and/or leukocytosis.
    ▷ CT will show the transition point (site of obstruction)—dilated proximal small bowel → transition point → collapsed distal bowel

  ▶ Upper GI series with small-bowel followthrough—barium is the contrast of choice, but should be avoided if perforation is suspected; upper GI series is falling out of favor due to higher accuracy and ease of CT scans

- Management—NPO (bowel rest), nasogastric tube to suction, IV fluids with aggressive hydration, and IV antibiotics
  ▶ Surgery to release the obstruction if no clinical improvement or signs of ischemia (metabolic acidosis, lactic acidosis)

  ▶ Unfortunately, there is no reliable sign or symptom differentiating patients with strangulation or impending strangulation. This makes the diagnosis quite challenging unless the above are present, and by then, the prognosis is usually poor.

Management of Small-Bowel Obstruction

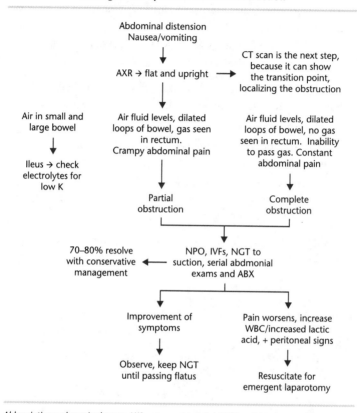

Abbreviations: abnominal x-ray, AXR; nasogastric tube, NGT; nothing by mouth, NPO

Large-Bowel Obstruction

- Etiology—Most common cause is **tumors**, volvulus, diverticulitis, and pseudoobstruction (Ogilvie)
  - ▸ Ogilvie syndrome—think of this in an elderly male patient with no abdominal scars, hernias, or palpable masses and with sudden, massive abdominal distention
    - ▹ **Tip: Always rule out hypokalemia** (most common electrolyte abnormality associated with ileus).

273

- Clinical—abdominal pain, inability to pass flatus, constipation, nausea, vomiting, and gradual abdominal distension (tympany to percussion)
  - ► If peritoneal signs are present (abdominal rigidity and rebound tenderness), emergent laparotomy is warranted

- Diagnosis—flat and upright abdominal x-ray → dilated small bowel, air–fluid levels, no air in the distal colon/rectum
  - ► CT with rectal contrast—study of choice
  - ► Rigid sigmoidoscopy—helps rule out mass lesions in rectum and sigmoid
  - ► Gastrografin enema—best choice if perforation is suspected; will show cut-off point and is also a good way to rule out partial vs. complete obstruction

- Management—NPO, nasogastric tube to suction, IV fluids for aggressive hydration, broad-spectrum IV antibiotics → surgery for decompressive colostomy

TRAUMA

- The initial evaluation of a patient who is critically injured from multiple traumas is a challenging task, and every minute can make the difference between life and death

- Early trauma deaths result from failed oxygenation of the vital organs, massive injury to the central nervous system (CNS), or both

- The ABCDEs identify life-threatening conditions, and are part of the primary survey

A = Airway Maintenance with Cervical Spine Control

- Always assess this first

- Ascertain patency of the airway (ability to respond verbally) and rule out obstruction (inspect for fractures and foreign bodies)

- Establish a patent airway with the chin lift/jaw thrust technique. All of this must be done while protecting the cervical spine (C-spine). **Always assume a C-spine injury is present in any patient with trauma and in those with altered mental status**.

- Patients with Glasgow coma scale (**GCS**) <8 **usually require a definitive airway** (intubation/surgical airway); these must be recognized promptly

- Constant reevaluation of the airway is important to identify those patients who cannot or will not maintain their airway

B = Breathing and Ventilation

- Adequate ventilation is necessary for proper gas exchange

- Good lung function and a normal chest wall are necessary for ventilation, and should be rapidly assessed

- Certain injuries can acutely compromise ventilation—flail chest (apply sandbags), tension pneumothorax (needle decompression), massive hemothorax (chest tube), and pulmonary contusion (supportive care)

C = Circulation and Hemorrhage Control

- Rapid assessment of the hemodynamic status is essential

- Hypovolemic hypotension (shock) should always be considered first until proven otherwise

- Evaluate pulse (weak and rapid), skin color (ashen/gray), and level of consciousness (decreased cerebral perfusion causing altered mental status)

- External hemorrhage should be quickly identified with application of manual compression to the wound

- Avoid tourniquets; they cause distal ischemia

- Patients can bleed profusely into the chest, abdomen, pelvis, and thighs; intracranial bleeds **cannot** cause hypovolemic hypotension

6

D = Disability

- Rapid neurologic evaluation with GCS to establish the level of consciousness

- Rule out hypoxia and hypovolemia as causes of altered mental status first, then consider CNS injury as the origin

- Keep in mind that alcohol and other drugs can also cause an altered mental status

E = Exposure/Environment

- Patient's body should be completely exposed to allow adequate inspection for other injuries

- Beware of hypothermia, especially in hypovolemic patients

> It is generally good practice to reassess the ABCs every 15 minutes until patient is completely stable.
>
> If any hemodynamic changes occur (decreased blood pressure, altered mental status, tachycardia), always go back and reassess the ABCs.

CHEST TRAUMA

Pneumothorax

- Pathophysiology—results in a collection of air in the space between the visceral and parietal pleura, collapsing the lung parenchyma. This causes a V/Q (ventilation-perfusion) shunt/mismatch.

- May be caused by blunt or penetrating trauma

- Tension pneumothorax—one-way valve that allows air to move into the pleural space without being able to exit, subsequently collapsing the lung

- Etiology—most common cause is lung laceration with an air leak, usually from blunt trauma

- Clinical—decreased or absent breath sounds and hyperresonance to percussion on the affected side
  - ► Other features include: respiratory distress, tachypnea, hyperexpansion of the chest wall, jugular venous distension, and hypotension secondary to decreased venous return (affects preload)
- Diagnosis—clinical; do not waste time with a chest x-ray; diagnosis is critical and must be made quickly
  - ► If taken, chest x-ray may show a collapsed lung with tracheal deviation to the opposite side
- Management—immediate decompression with a 14-gauge needle into the second intercostal space at the midclavicular line
  - ► After initial decompression, definitive treatment is with a chest tube in the fourth or fifth intercostal space anterior to the midaxillary line

Hemothorax

- Etiology—most common cause is lung laceration or laceration of an intercostal vessel
- Clinical—decreased breath sounds with dullness to percussion
- Management—placement of a large-caliber chest tube (32 French or greater)
- Indications for performing a thoracotomy:
  - ► >1,500 cc of drainage after initial insertion
  - ► >250 cc/hour for 3 hours
  - ► >2,500 cc in 24 hours
- If blood is not evacuated, fibrothorax or infected hemothorax may occur

Traumatic Aortic Injury

- Aortic rupture (transection) is the most common cause of sudden death after a fall from a height >20 feet or from a motor vehicle collision at speeds >45 mph

6

- Site of tear—ligamentum arteriosum, distal to the subclavian takeoff

- Clinical—usually asymptomatic, although patients may complain of chest pain/interscapular pain → look for upper-extremity hypertension
  - ▸ A high index of suspicion is required, and the mechanism of injury (deceleration) is what should alert the clinician to the diagnosis

- Radiographic signs—**widening of the mediastinum**, loss of aortic contour, left hemothorax, first-rib fractures, depression of the left main stem bronchus

- Diagnosis—best initial test is **CT angiogram of the chest**, transesophageal echocardiogram (can be done but is operator-dependent); aortogram is the gold standard

- Management—must control blood pressure with IV labetalol, esmolol, or nitroprusside
  - ▸ Always address life-threatening injuries first, then aortic rupture can be treated
  - ▸ Surgial repair through a left thoracotomy is the management of choice

ABDOMINAL TRAUMA

- Penetrating trauma—stab wounds or gunshot wounds (GSWs)
  - ▸ Stab wounds—40% involve the liver, 30% involve the small bowel, and 20% perforate the diaphragm
    - ▹ 30–40% of stab wounds do not penetrate the peritoneum; if there is suspicion of a tangential wound or a wound superficial to the aponeurotic layer, **local wound exploration** can be done by extending the wound with your finger and tracking it down through all the layers
  - ▸ GSWs—50% involve the small bowel, 40% involve the colon, and 30% involve the liver
    - ▹ **Remember: All GSWs to the abdomen go to the OR**; do not waste time exploring the wound

- Blunt trauma—causes crushing injury to the abdomen → hollow viscus and solid organs can deform and rupture → most common organs affected are the spleen (40–55%) and liver (35–45%); formation of retroperitoneal hematomas is also common
- Evaluation of abdominal trauma
  - Diagnostic peritoneal lavage (DPL) is indicated in hemodynamically unstable patients
    - Limitation—cannot identify retroperitoneal bleeds and hematomas
    - Criteria for positive DPL: >10 cc of gross blood, 100,000 red blood cells (RBCs)/cc, >500 WBCs or food particles or bacteria → exploratory laparotomy is the best next step
  - Focused abdominal sonography for trauma (FAST) is noninvasive and has the same sensitivity and specificity as DPL
    - Pitfalls—obesity obstructs view, and FAST is operator-dependent; small amounts of fluid can be missed (<80 mL)
    - Blood collects in four areas—perisplenic and perihepatic fossa, pericardium, and pelvis
    - Can be repeated to detect interval changes in hemoperitoneum
    - Can miss retroperitoneal bleeds or hollow viscus injury
  - CT scan is a time-consuming study that is indicated only in hemodynamically stable patients
    - Pitfalls—can miss diaphragmatic, bowel, and pancreatic injuries
    - Rules out retroperitoneal bleeds/hematomas
- Indications for exploratory laparotomy in trauma patients:
  - Transient response to fluid resuscitation in blunt trauma
  - Blunt trauma with positive DPL/FAST
  - Evidence of free air (indicates bowel rupture)
  - Signs of peritonitis
  - All abdominal GSWs

6

UROLOGY

Testicular Torsion

- Most commonly seen in neonates and postpubertal boys (peaks at 15 years of age)

- Clinical—sudden onset of pain (e.g., awakening with scrotal pain), and may occur several hours after vigorous physical activity or minor testicular trauma

- Diagnosis—classic physical finding is an **asymmetrically high-riding testis on the affected side** with the long axis of the testis oriented **transversely** (normally is longitudinal)

- Color Doppler ultrasonography is the diagnostic and confirmatory test of choice

- Management
  - ▸ If testicle is viable—bilateral orchiopexy
  - ▸ If testicle is not viable—resection with orchiopexy of the contralateral testis

6

Urethral Trauma

- Etiology—most commonly associated with pelvic fractures; the membranous urethra is at highest risk of transection

- Clinical—look for new, bright-red hematuria or **blood at the meatus**; floating prostate; **perineal ecchymosis**

- Diagnosis—**retrograde urethrogram** is the best initial test

- Management—**do not** place Foley catheter if injury is suspected → call urology stat
  - ▸ Safest and best method of treatment—place a suprapubic catheter for bladder drainage, with delayed repair in 8–12 weeks

Ureteral Trauma

- Background—the ureters are protected by the retroperitoneum, and injuries are usually due to iatrogenic injury (gynecologic and colorectal surgery), external trauma (GSWs, stab wounds) and blunt trauma (deceleration injuries)

- Clinical—**flank pain**, fever, and signs of sepsis; physical exam may reveal **costovertebral angle (CVA) tenderness**, evidence of a mass and/or peritoneal signs
  - Hematuria is not a reliable finding
- Diagnosis—in the acute setting, contrast-enhanced CT scan is the best initial test
  - IV pyelograms and retrograde urethrograms are also useful
- Management
  - Small ureteral segment injury is <2 cm → attempt primary repair and place stent
  - Injuries >2 cm
    - Injuries in the lower third → bladder reimplantation should be attempted
    - Injuries in the upper two-thirds → temporizing nephrostomy is best (tie off ureteral ends) with ureteroureterostomy at a later date

NEUROSURGERY

Subdural Hematoma (SDH)

- Pathophysiology—forms between the dura and the arachnoid membrane and caused by **torn bridging veins**; has a **crescent shape** on noncontrast head CT
- Higher rate of mortality than epidural hematomas; may be acute (after blunt trauma) or chronic (look for the alcoholic person with altered mental status a week after falling)

Epidural Hematoma (EDH)

- Pathophysiology—forms between the dura and the skull and is caused by a tear of the **middle meningeal artery → lens or "lentiform" shape** on noncontrast head CT, usually with midline deviation (always acute)
- Classic presentation—initial loss of consciousness → lucid interval → recurrent loss of consciousness

- Acutely symptomatic SDHs/EDHs are neurologic emergencies that require surgical decompression. Otherwise, rapid hematoma expansion causes increased intracranial pressure, brain herniation, and death.
- Chronic subdural hematomas may be intervally followed and do not require surgical intervention

Spinal Cord Compression Syndrome

- 31 segments in the spinal cord, with anterior (motor) and posterior (sensory) nerve roots
  - ▸ Ventral nerve roots—efferent, motor fibers
  - ▸ Dorsal nerve roots—afferent, sensory fibers
  - ▸ Spinothalamic tract—pain and sensory neurons
  - ▸ Corticospinal tract—motor neurons

- Injury can cause devastating and sometimes permanent neurologic disabilities
  - ▸ Most spinal cord injuries are associated with injuries to the vertebral column
  - ▸ The injury reflects the force and direction of the traumatic event, which produces pathologic flexion, rotation, extension, and/or compression of the spine. Most vertebral injuries in adults involve both fracture and dislocation.

- Etiology
  - ▸ Most common cause—bony fragments penetrating the spinal cord from fracture or penetrating injury
  - ▸ Trauma causing transection or mechanical disruption; usually due to fracture or dislocation of vertebral bodies, but can also occur from penetrating injuries (GSWs/stab wounds)
  - ▸ EDH from blunt or penetrating trauma
  - ▸ Epidural abscess formation from IV drug abuse, hematogenous infection, vertebral osteomyelitis → *Staphylococcus aureus* is the leading pathogen
  - ▸ Primary neoplastic disease—neuroblastoma, multiple myeloma, renal cell carcinoma

- ► Metastatic disease to the vertebral bodies—prostate, breast, or lung are most common; remember that metastatic disease is far more common than primary neoplastic disease

- Clinical—pain, motor, and sensory deficits with bladder and bowel dysfunction

- Diagnosis—standard films have been replaced by CT scan and MRI
  - ► CT—delineates bony structures → coronal and sagittal reconstructions are very sensitive in identifying fractures
  - ► CT myelogram is not used since the introduction of the MRI
  - ► MRI—the best initial test for spinal cord injuries, ligamentous, and soft-tissue injuries

- Management—remember the ABCs
  - ► The goal is to make a quick diagnosis and initiate treatment to avoid further injury
  - ► Use of steroids is still controversial but most physicians still favor their use
  - ► Current recommendations—IV steroids (methylprednisolone) should be instituted within 8 hours of injury; initial bolus followed by continuous infusion

6

Spinal Shock

- Occurs immediately after cord injury
- Clinical—triad of **hypotension, bradycardia, and warm extremities** (due to vasodilatation from loss of sympathetic tone)
  - ► Flaccid paralysis, areflexia, and autonomic paralysis below the level of the lesion; priapism may occur in males
- Management—initially treat with IV fluid resuscitation; may need vasopressors to maintain blood pressure
- Prognosis—physiologic effects revert in a matter of weeks; patients may fully recover

Spinal Cord Injuries

Disease	Etiology	Symptoms	Treatment
Complete cord transection	Blunt trauma— causing traction and compression forces	• High lesion: respiratory insufficiency, quadriplegia, areflexia, anesthesia - Loss of bladder and rectal tone - Horner syndrome may be present • Lower lesions: hemiplegia, spares respiratory muscles	High-dose corticosteroids
Anterior spinal artery infarction	• MCC is acutely ruptured disc (disc retropulsion/ bone fragments) • Embolism of artery supplying anterior two-thirds of spinal cord	• Only dorsal columns remain intact → flaccid paralysis progressing into spastic paralysis • Bilateral loss of pain, motor, and temperature sensation	• If evidence of ruptured disc: surgical repair • Otherwise, no good treatment options
Brown-Sequard syndrome	Hemitranssection of spinal cord; MCC is penetrating trauma	Loss of contralateral pain and temperature, with loss of ipsilateral motor function	• **High-dose corticosteroids** only if evidence of **neurologic deficit** • New treatments have improved recovery rates, good prognosis with high rates of ambulation
Syringomyelia	• Communicating: MCC is Arnold-Chiari • Noncommunicating: MCC is tumors and trauma	Only dorsal columns and tactile touch remain intact; usually at cervical spinal cord	Surgical

Abbreviations: most common cause, MCC

Remember: In traumatic cord injury with deficits, initial intervention includes high-dose steroids to decrease inflammation.

ORTHOPEDICS

Compartment Syndrome

- Limb-threatening—tissue pressure exceeds perfusion pressure in a closed anatomic space

- Etiology—most common cause is fractures; other causes include GSWs, snake bites, crush injuries, wearing a cast, and burns; reperfusion injury after vascular surgery/insult often overlooked

- Clinical—look for the "5 P's" → **pain, paresthesia, pallor, paralysis,** and **pulselessness** with or without poikilothermia (cold extremity)

  ▸ Pulses may be present and are usually the last to disappear

  ▸ **Limb that is tender to passive motion** is one of the most important findings

  ▸ Limb is tense, edematous with shiny skin

- Diagnosis—based on clinical suspicion; then confirm with measuring compartment pressure; >20–30 mm Hg is abnormal

- Management—fasciotomy remains the treatment of choice

  ▸ Compartment pressures >30 mm Hg are diagnostic and need rapid intervention

  ▸ The use and timing of fasciotomy have been debated: Fasciotomy extends hospital stay and converts a closed injury to an open injury → increases the risk of infection

  ▸ Fasciotomy must be done within 6 hours to avoid necrosis and irreversible tissue damage

Pelvic Fractures

- Etiology

  ▸ Most common cause in the elderly is falling from a standing position

  ▸ Most common causes in younger patients—motor vehicle collisions, falls from great height, crush injuries

- Pelvic fractures can be a major source of blood loss, and are associated with high morbidity and mortality

6

- Clinical—if there is history of blunt trauma, keep a high index of suspicion
  - ► Instability, laxity, and tenderness upon palpation of the pelvis
  - ► Beware of hypotension; patients can lose >2 L of blood
  - ► Avoid extensive manipulation → increases pain and bleeding
  - ► Instability on hip adduction suggests acetabular fracture with or without pelvic fracture
  - ► Evidence of vaginal bleeding or blood in the meatus with or without a high-riding, boggy prostate is suggestive of pelvic instability

- Diagnosis—anteroposterior plain radiograph is the initial test of choice; reveals 90–95% of fractures
  - ► CT scan is the test of choice in trauma patients; it is the best study to delineate pelvic anatomy and the presence of intra-peritoneal and retroperitoneal bleeding
  - ► FAST can identify blood in the pelvis, suggesting pelvic fracture
  - ► Other tests—arteriography and cystourethrography

- Management—start the evaluation with the ABCs to assess for life-threatening conditions
  - ► Application of external compression devices
  - ► If blood pressure is low and there is a negative DPL and chest x-ray and no other sources of blood loss → get angiography
  - ► Bleeding is mostly venous (from anterior pelvic fractures) and difficult to control with laparotomy
  - ► If pelvic hematoma is encountered, leave it alone unless it is expanding or the patient is hemodynamically unstable; if in the OR, most surgeons will pack the pelvis and then go to angiography for embolization

Hip Dislocation

- Etiology—falls and motor vehicle collisions
- Anterior dislocation—there is external rotation and abduction of the lower extremity

- ▸ Risk of injury to the femoral artery and avascular necrosis of the femoral head
- Posterior dislocation—evidence of internal rotation and adduction of the lower extremity
  - ▸ Risk of sciatic nerve injury
  - ▸ **Tip:** Look for a history of a patient in a motor vehicle collision whose legs hit the dashboard in the front passenger seat (most common mechanism of dislocation).
- Management—closed reduction

Ligamentous Injuries

- Anterior cruciate ligament (ACL)—most common ligament injury, due to high physical activity
  - ▸ Swelling, pain that is more severe with pivoting action, knee effusion
  - ▸ Positive anterior drawer test—anterior dislocation of the tibia when it is gripped with both hands
  - ▸ Best test is MRI
  - ▸ High-level athletes—primary early repair is recommended; otherwise, leg-strengthening exercises and physical therapy
- Posterior cruciate ligament (PCL)—less common
  - ▸ Swelling, knee pain, and effusion
  - ▸ Posterior drawer test—posterior dislocation of the tibia when it is gripped with both hands
  - ▸ MRI is best test
  - ▸ Conservative therapy initially, leg-strengthening exercises, surgery if medical management fails
- Lateral knee trauma—lesion of the ACL, midclavicular ligament (MCL), and medial meniscus

BURNS

- More than 50,000 patients are hospitalized for burn injuries each year, causing approximately 5,000 burn-related deaths

- Etiology
  - ▶ Scald burns (most common)—if seen in children, suspect abuse or neglect
  - ▶ Flame/explosion burns are most likely to cause hospital admission—suspect coexisting inhalation injuries (burned nasal hairs, soot in the mouth)
  - ▶ Chemical burns—alkalis produce deeper burns than acids
  - ▶ Electric burns—always fourth-degree burns → cardiac monitoring and serum creatinine phosphokinase (CPK) to rule out rhabdomyolysis and compartmental syndromes

Diagnosis of Burn Severity

Severity	Layers Involved	Description
First-degree	Epidermis	Erythema, pain
Second-degree superficial	Epidermis to the papillary dermis	Painful, blisters and blebs, pink and moist, **blanches** on palpation
Second-degree deep	Epidermis to the reticular dermis	Decreased sensation, loss of hair follicles, mottled appearance
Third-degree	Down to subcutaneous fat	Leathery-grey, **painless** due to destruction of nerves, surrounding tissues are very sensitive
Fourth-degree	Down to muscle and bone	Exposure of tissue, **painless**

> First-degree burns are not treated with the Parkland formula; there is no need for aggressive resuscitation.

- Management—initial evaluation is with ABCs
  - ▶ Smoke inhalation causes more than 60% of fire-related deaths; these patients require aggressive airway intervention
  - ▶ Direct thermal injuries to the upper airway may be due to toxic smoke or super-heated air

- If the patient is breathing spontaneously → place on 100% nonrebreather; must have a low threshold to secure airway with intubation
- Patients with facial burns, singeing of the eyebrows/nasal hairs, voice changes, stridor/wheezing, carbonaceous sputum, and/or altered mental status—suspect upper airway lesions; best next step is to visualize directly with laryngoscopy → intubation → inspect tracheobronchial tree with bronchoscopy
- "Rule of nines"—used to estimate the total body surface area (TBSA) burned; each of the 11 following areas is considered 9% of TBSA: head, chest, abdomen, upper back, lower back, each arm, each leg (below the knee), each thigh (leg above the knee) = 99%. The genitals make up the remaining 1%.

Rule of Nines

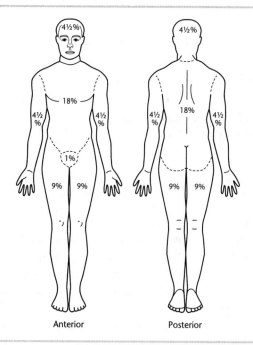

Anterior   Posterior

6

- Parkland formula—apply if greater than 20% of TBSA has been burned
  - ► Use lactated Ringer solution only in the first 24 hours; colloids (albumin) can be given after 24 hours
  - ► First, calculate total fluid needed—4 cc × patient's body weight in kg × % TBSA burned = total fluid volume needed
  - ► Administer half of the total fluid volume in the first 8 hours since the burn occurred and the other half in the following 16 hours
    - ▷ Example: A 110-lb (50-kg) woman has burns over 50% TBSA. Calculate: 4 cc × 50 kg × 50 TBSA = 10,000 cc fluid needed. Give the first 5,000 cc in 8 hours, and the other 5,000 cc over the next 16 hours.

- Maintain urine output >0.5–1 cc/kg/hour in adults and >2–4 cc/kg/hour in children; this is the best way to measure resuscitation

- Escharotomy—in the presence of circumferential burns, patients may need fasciotomy if compartment syndrome develops

- Criteria for admission to hospital
  - ► **All** inhalation injuries
  - ► Second- and third-degree burns in patients <10 or >50 years of age with >10% TBSA
  - ► Second- and third-degree burns with >20% TBSA in all ages
  - ► Third-degree burns with >5% TBSA in all ages
  - ► Electrical burns

- Complications
  - ► Infections—*Pseudomonas aeruginosa* is most common organism; use topical silver sulfadiazine creams on healing burns to prevent secondary bacterial infection, and wrap with sterile dressings
  - ► Pneumonia—most common infection and also the most common cause of death
  - ► Electrical burns—transverse myelitis, pancreatitis, liver necrosis, polyneuritis

7

GYNECOLOGY AND OBSTETRICS

I. GYNECOLOGY

VAGINAL DISCHARGE

Diagnosis and Management of Vaginal Discharge

Disorder	Symptoms/ Speculum Exam	Diagnosis	Treatment	Pregnancy
Bacterial vaginosis	Thin, **grayish-white** discharge with **"fishy"** odor; no inflammatory symptoms	Wet prep reveals **clue cells** (epithelial cells coated with bacteria yielding blurring of cell membrane); positive **"whiff test"** (fishy odor with application of KOH); vaginal pH >4.5	Metronida-zole intravagi-nally or orally	Oral metro-nidazole (safe during all trimesters)
Vaginal candidiasis	Thick white clumpy discharge, itching	Pseudohyphae and budding yeast on light microscopy (*Candida albicans*)	Topical nystatin, topical ketoconazole, or oral fluconazole	Topical nystatin or ketoconazole

(continued)

291

Diagnosis and Management of Vaginal Discharge (continued)

Disorder	Symptoms/ Speculum Exam	Diagnosis	Treatment	Pregnancy
Physiologic discharge	Thin, watery, cervical mucus discharge due to **estrogen effect**; seen especially during **ovulation**, increased during **pregnancy**; no inflammatory symptoms	Thin, watery discharge on speculum exam; no odor; normal exam and normal vaginal pH (<4.5); wet mount normal	Treatment of underlying cause, if applicable (e.g., PCOS) with oral contraceptives containing **cyclic progestins**	Normal during pregnancy
Trichomonas vaginitis	Profuse, watery, **frothy, greenish discharge** with inflammatory changes; strawberry cervix (cervical petechiae)	Wet prep reveals **motile, flagellated trichomonads (poor sensitivity); gold standard is PCR or NAAT**	DOC is **oral** metronidazole for patient and partner (intravaginal route associated with high failure rate)	Oral metronidazole
Neisseria gonorrhea	Purulent vaginal discharge with cervical motion tenderness	May see Gram-negative diplococci on microscopic examination of discharge; run **PCR-DNA**	Ceftriaxone IM once, or oral cefexime once	IM or IV ceftriaxone or other oral cephalosporin (desensitize if allergic)
Chlamydia	Clinically indistinguishable from gonorrhea in females	**PCR-DNA** as for gonorrhea	Oral doxycycline BID for 7 days, or a single large dose of azithromycin	PO azithromycin or amoxicillin; IV if required

Abbreviations: drug of choice, DOC; polycystic ovarian syndrome, PCOS; polymerase chain reaction, PCR

- **Tip:** Gonorrhea may cause pharyngitis or proctitis after unprotected oral or anal intercourse.

Additional Comments on Vaginal Discharge

Bacterial vaginosis risk factors—smoking, decreased estrogen production; **not a sexually transmitted disease (STD)** but associated with frequent intercourse.

PELVIC INFLAMMATORY DISEASE (PID)

- Pathophysiology: broad spectrum of infectious processes involving the female reproductive system (see Pathophysiology of PID below)

- Risk factors: promiscuity, adolescent females, and intrauterine devices (IUDs)

- Pathogens: gonorrhea and *Chlamydia*, anaerobes, and gram-negative enteric organisms

Pathophysiology of PID

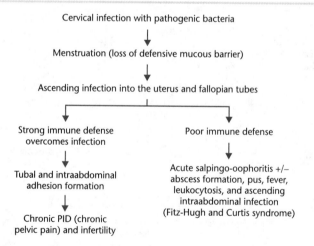

Cervical infection with pathogenic bacteria
↓
Menstruation (loss of defensive mucous barrier)
↓
Ascending infection into the uterus and fallopian tubes

Strong immune defense overcomes infection
↓
Tubal and intraabdominal adhesion formation
↓
Chronic PID (chronic pelvic pain) and infertility

Poor immune defense
↓
Acute salpingo-oophoritis +/− abscess formation, pus, fever, leukocytosis, and ascending intraabdominal infection (Fitz-Hugh and Curtis syndrome)

7

DIAGNOSIS AND MANAGEMENT OF ACUTE PELVIC INFECTION

Disease	Clinical Presentation	Diagnosis	Management
Simple cervicitis	Mucopurulent vaginal discharge; normal labs and afebrile	See Vaginal Discharge, page 291	Based upon etiology; empiric coverage if unknown: ceftriaxone *or* cefixime **plus** doxycycline
Acute salpingo-oophoritis*	Mucopurulent cervical discharge, bilateral **pelvic pain, cervical motion tenderness,** and guarding	• First-line: clinical with cervical examination • Cultures and sensitivity of discharge indicated • Gold standard is laparoscopy revealing pus within oviducts/cul-de-sac	• Outpatient: IM ceftriaxone **or** cefoxitin + oral probenecid **plus** oral doxycycline **with or without** oral metronidazole • Inpatient: IV cefotetan or cefoxitin **plus** doxycycline **or** IV clindamycin **plus** gentamicin
Tubal or ovarian abscess	**Severe** lower abdominal pain with **toxic** appearance; nausea/vomiting, high **fever**; rebound tenderness with guarding and **palpable adnexal mass**	• First-line: pelvic **ultrasound** (or CT scan) will show **complex, loculated pelvic masses** • Other findings: leukocytosis, fever, positive cervical cultures	• First-line: empiric IV antibiotics: clindamycin **plus** gentamicin • Second-line: if **no response** after 24–48 hours, **exploratory laparotomy** with excision of abscess with or without tubal excision
Chronic PID	Chronic lower abdominal/pelvic pain; **absence** of mucopurulent discharge, motion tenderness, fever, or systemic findings	• First-line: pelvic sonogram reveals complex cystic pelvic mass(es) • Gold standard: laparoscopy reveals **pelvic adhesions**	• First-line: analgesics (ibuprofen or aetaminophen) • Second-line (pain unremitting): laparoscopy with lysis of adhesions

Abbreviations: pelvic inflammatory disease, PID

* See Management of Acute Salpingo-oophoritis section on the following page regarding inpatient versus outpatient management.

Management of Acute Salpingo-oophoritis

- Outpatient: appropriate in the nontoxic appearing patient who will reliably follow up
- Inpatient: criteria include fever >102.2°F (>39°C), adolescent (reliability for follow-up is poor), unclear diagnosis, toxic-appearing or failure of previous outpatient management

UTERINE AND BOWEL PROLAPSE

- Pathophysiology—laxity of pelvic ligaments in multiparous women leads to varying degrees of organ prolapse; may involve the vagina, uterus, bladder, and/or bowel

- Clinical—**older, multiparous** woman presents with sensation of **pelvic pressure** and back pain

- Diagnosis—physical examination reveals prolapsed pelvic organs when patient is asked to "bear down"
  - ▸ Uterine prolapse—cervix descends into the vaginal canal (five grades of severity)
  - ▸ Cystocele—bladder is seen bulging into the anterior wall of the vagina
  - ▸ Enterocele—complete herniation of the pouch of Douglas into the vagina
  - ▸ Rectocele—bowel bulges into the posterior wall of the vagina

- Management
  - ▸ First-line (less severe prolapse)—Kegel exercises, physical therapy with biofeedback
  - ▸ Second-line—vaginal pessary (object inserted into the vaginal to support pelvic viscera)
  - ▸ Third-line (or first-line if severe prolapse; e.g., procidentia)—surgical repair

7

DIAGNOSIS AND MANAGEMENT OF URINARY INCONTINENCE

Diagnosis	Clinical Presentation	Diagnosis	Management
Stress incontinence	Loss of small amounts of urine with **coughing, sneezing**; secondary to pelvic ligament laxity	History plus **Q-tip test** (insert Q-tip into urethra → rotation of >30 degrees of tip is diagnostic	• First-line: Kegel exercises plus estrogen replacement • Second-line: vaginal tape repair or urethropexy
Urge incontinence	Increased bladder pressure → sudden urgency with loss of urine; occurs day and night	Cystometry → **normal residual volume** and involuntary detrusor contractions	• First-line: anticholinergics (oxybutynin, tolterodine) • Second-line or with history of glaucoma: TCAs (imipramine, dicyclomine, hyoscyamine)
Overflow incontinence	• Patients complain of **pelvic fullness** with loss of small amounts of urine **day and night** • Loss of neurologic function leads to bladder distention with overflow **when bladder pressure equals urethral pressure** (common in diabetes and patients with neurologic disease)	Cystometry → **increased residual volume** (>200 cc)	Start intermittent self-catheterization plus cholinergic agonist (bethanechol or neostigmine) → recheck post-void residual after ~1 week; if acceptable, may discontinue intermittent catheterization and continue pharmacologic therapy

Abbreviations: tricyclic antidepressants, TCAs

VULVAR DISEASE

- Any postmenopausal female with complaints of **vulvar itching** or a **new lesion** must have a Keyes **punch biopsy** to rule out malignant disease

- Squamous cell carcinoma of the vulva is caused by infection with **human papillomavirus (HPV) (types 16 and 18)**

- Diagnosis of vulvar dystrophy

  - ► Squamous hyperplasia—white focal to diffuse; **firm** and **cartilaginous** areas appreciated on palpation and histologically characterized by keratin and squamous epithelial proliferation

    - ▷ Treatment with topical fluorinated corticosteroid cream

  - ► Lichen sclerosis—blue-white papules coalescing into white plaques appreciated as **thin** and **parchment-like** on palpation, and histologically characterized by thinning of the epithelium

    - ▷ Treatment with topical clobetasol cream → increases epithelium → decreases symptoms

- Premalignant vulvar disease

  - ► Squamous dysplasia—multiple white, red, or pigmented lesions with cellular atypia of the epithelium **without invasion of the basement membrane**

    - ▷ Treatment with local surgical excision

  - ► Carcinoma in situ—clinically identical to dysplasia and distinguished only **histologically** with full-thickness epithelial atypia **without invasion of the basement membrane**

    - ▷ Treatment with laser vaporization

- Malignant vulvar disease

  - ► Squamous cell carcinoma—**most common cause of malignant vulvar disease**

    - ▷ Treatment options

      - Radical vulvectomy—not preferred because of **significant morbidity, mortality, and loss of sexual function**

7

- Modified radical vulvectomy—preferred over radical vulvectomy in select patients
- Lymphadenectomy—indicated in all patients with invasion >1 mm in depth; unilateral or bilateral, depending on location of lesion
- Radical local excision—preferred if lesion is <2 cm in diameter with <1 mm invasion

▶ Melanoma—**second most common** type of vulvar cancer; most important factor is **depth of invasion**; suspect in those with family history and changing mole, or dark, black lesions with irregular borders and/or ulceration

▷ Treatment—**excisional biopsy is indicated** in any suspected melanoma, *not* **shave biopsy** (does not allow accurate assessment of depth of invasion and creates scar tissue, obscuring subsequent histologic exam)

▶ Paget disease of the vulva—**red lesion** in **postmenopausal** women; may or may not invade basement membrane; associated with **other organ malignancies**

Diagnosis and Management of Vulvar Lesions

Disease	Cause	Symptoms	Diagnosis	Treatment
Molluscum contagiosum	Poxvirus infection	Wartlike, **pearly papule with central umbilication**	Clinical; waxy material may be expressed from center of lesions	Multiple options: observation, curettage, cryotherapy, laser ablation
Condylomata acuminata	HPV types 6 and 11	**Cauliflower-like lesions** may itch or bleed when large	Clinical	As above

(continued)

Diagnosis and Management of Vulvar Lesions (continued)

Disease	Cause	Symptoms	Diagnosis	Treatment
Bartholin gland cyst or abscess	Obstruction of Bartholin gland	• Cyst: large, palpable, **painless** mass lateral to introitus • Abscess: super-infection with large, palpable, **painful** mass; erythema and edema lateral to introitus	Clinical	• Cyst: treated if pressure symptoms develop; clear fluid on aspiration (versus abscess, which is infected) • Abscess: **acute** treatment with I&D followed by insertion of a **Word catheter** until resolution • Marsupialization • Excision of gland if >40 years, bloody discharge, or recurrence
New-onset itchy lesion in post-menopausal woman	Benign, premalig-nant, or malignant	Itching with or without identifiable lesion	Histological through **punch biopsy**	Based upon patho-logical report

Abbreviations: human papillomavirus, HPV; incision and drainage, I&D

7

Cervical Disease

Disease	Symptoms	Diagnosis	Treatment
Cervicitis	Mucopurulent vaginal discharge is most common; may also be due to infection with HPV (noted on colposcopy with normal histology or only signs of inflammation)	Directed toward suspected cause; PCR-DNA for STDs and/or HPV typing	Based upon cause

(continued)

Cervical Disease (continued)

Disease	Symptoms	Diagnosis	Treatment
Cervical polyp	Postcoital bleeding, and bleeding between menstrual cycles	Speculum exam reveals red-to-purple, **finger-like** growths protruding through the cervix	Removal with laser ablation, polyp forceps in the office, or electrocautery; send tissue for pathology
Nabothian cyst(s)	No clinical symptoms; noted on speculum exam in reproductive-age females	Smooth, round cervical bumps filled with mucoid material, also referred to as **"pimple-like"** lesions	None usually necessary; if indicated (multiple lesions with bleeding or cervical enlargement), outpatient electrocautery or laser ablation

Abbreviations: human papillomavirus, HPV; polymerase chain reaction, PCR; sexually transmitted disease, STD

CERVICAL NEOPLASIA

Gardasil® Vaccination

- Recommended in **all females age 9–26 years**, with most vaccinations occurring at age 11–12 years

- **Protects against HPV types 6, 11, 16, and 18** derived from purified capsular proteins

  ‣ HPV types 6 and 11 are responsible for 90% of genital warts

  ‣ HPV types 16 and 18 are responsible for **70% of cervical cancers**; types 31, 33, and 35 account for another 20%

    ▷ Therefore, **regular Pap-smear screening is still recommended regardless of vaccination status**

- Vaccine is most effective before exposure to HPV occurs; however, screening for infection prior to vaccination is not recommended or routinely available

- Vaccination may still be given to those with confirmed HPV infection (for example, a sexually active female with an atypical squamous cells of undetermined significance [ASCUS] Pap smear and confirmed high-risk HPV), although efficacy may be reduced

- Vaccination is **not recommended** in the following patients: pregnant, lactating, or immunosuppressed females
- Vaccination is administered in three doses: 0, 2, and 6 months
- It is safe to administer Gardasil® concomitantly with the hepatitis B vaccine; however, safety with other vaccines has not been studied
- Use of oral contraceptive pills (OCPs) does not alter efficacy
- Gardasil® does not contain preservatives or antibiotic derivatives

PAP SMEAR

- Recommended in all females at age 21 regardless of sexual activity
  - ▸ Screen every 3 years up to age 30 using conventional method (spatula), or every 2 years if using liquid-based methods (ThinPrep®)
  - ▸ When patient is >30 years of age, add HPV cotesting and extend interval to every 5 years
  - ▸ When to discontinue screening:
    - ▹ Age >65 years with an adequate screening history
    - ▹ After a total hysterectomy for any reason (cervix and uterus have been completely removed)
- Screening recommendations **are the same** for both heterosexual and homosexual females, although homosexual females are **less likely** to acquire the HPV virus
- Any visible lesion on the cervix that appears abnormal (friable, cauliflowerlike, or otherwise) should be biopsied **regardless of Pap-smear histology**
- A "satisfactory" Pap smear samples **both** endocervical and ectocervical cells
- Pap-smear and colposcopy findings (from best to worst)— normal → ASCUS → low-grade dysplasia → high-grade dysplasia or carcinoma in situ → cervical cancer
- **Tip:** Under these guidelines many women will test positive for high-risk HPV **but** have normal cytology. You should simply repeat the Pap and HPV cotest in 12 months.

7

Interpretation and Management of Pap-Smear Pathology Report

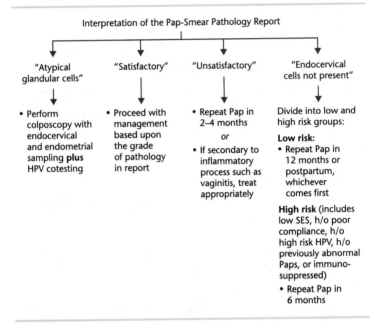

Interpretation of the Pap-Smear Pathology Report

"Atypical glandular cells"

- Perform colposcopy with endocervical and endometrial sampling **plus** HPV cotesting

"Satisfactory"

- Proceed with management based upon the grade of pathology in report

"Unsatisfactory"

- Repeat Pap in 2–4 months

  or

- If secondary to inflammatory process such as vaginitis, treat appropriately

"Endocervical cells not present"

Divide into low and high risk groups:

Low risk:
- Repeat Pap in 12 months or postpartum, whichever comes first

High risk (includes low SES, h/o poor compliance, h/o high risk HPV, h/o previously abnormal Paps, or immunosuppressed)
- Repeat Pap in 6 months

Abbreviations: history of, h/o; socioeconomic status, SES

Note: Omit endometrial and endocervical sampling in any pregnant woman.

Interpretation and Management of ASCUS Pap-Smear Results

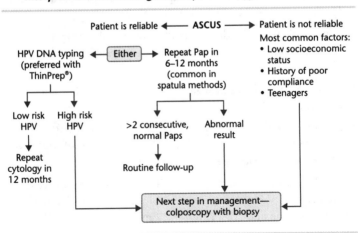

Patient is reliable ⟵ **ASCUS** ⟶ Patient is not reliable

Most common factors:
- Low socioeconomic status
- History of poor compliance
- Teenagers

HPV DNA typing (preferred with ThinPrep®) ⟵ **Either** ⟶ Repeat Pap in 6–12 months (common in spatula methods)

Low risk HPV

High risk HPV

>2 consecutive, normal Paps

Abnormal result

Low risk HPV → Repeat cytology in 12 months

>2 consecutive, normal Paps → Routine follow-up

Next step in management— colposcopy with biopsy

Management of Dysplastic Pap-Smear Result

Lesions may be low-grade squamous intraepithelial lesions (LSIL) or high-grade squamous intraepithelial lesions (HSIL); any degree of dysplasia from the Pap smear warrants proceeding to **colposcopy with biopsy** to determine depth of invasion, identify possible extension into the endocervical canal, and confirm the grade of dysplasia

Management of the Colposcopy Pathology Report

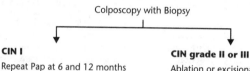

Colposcopy with Biopsy

CIN I
Repeat Pap at 6 and 12 months
OR
Repeat Pap with colposcopy in 12 months
OR
HPV-DNA typing in 12 months
OR
Ablation or excision

*All methods are acceptable, and method is chosen based on patient circumstances (reliability, etc.)

CIN grade II or III
Ablation or excisional therapy with any of the following:

• Laser conization
• LEEP (loop electrosurgical excision procedure)
• Cold knife cone biopsy

• All methods are acceptable; you will not be required to choose between them
• LEEP is preferred by most clinicians because of low rates of bleeding and infection

7

MANAGEMENT OF INVASIVE CERVICAL CANCER

• After confirming diagnosis through colposcopy with biopsy, start metastatic workup (chest x-ray, cystoscopy, sigmoidoscopy)

• Staging is **clinical**

• Preferred treatment is a radical hysterectomy. Radiation therapy with chemotherapy is an alternative.

• Follow-up after definitive treatment:

  ‣ Careful physical exam every 3 months for 2 years, then every 6 months for 3 years

  ‣ Annual Pap smear

Management of Cervical Carcinoma

Stage	Description	Management
IA1	≤3 mm invasion past the cervical basement membrane	Simple hysterectomy or cold knife cone
IA2	3–5 mm invasion past the cervical basement membrane	Modified radical hysterectomy
IB or IIA	>5 mm cervical invasion; spread into upper two-thirds of vagina	Radical hysterectomy plus: • Premenopausal: pelvic and paraaortic lymphadenectomy • Postmenopausal: peritoneal washing and/or pelvic radiation therapy
IIB or greater	Extends into the parametria, or distant metastasis	Radiation and chemotherapy (cisplatin is the most effective agent)

MANAGEMENT OF CERVICAL DYSPLASIA DURING PREGNANCY

- Pregnancy is **not** a contraindication to colposcopy; any pregnant patient with an abnormal Pap smear should undergo the same normal care as for a nonpregnant patient **except**:
  - ► Due to increased risk of bleeding and perforation of membranes, endocervical curettage **is contraindicated**; however, ectocervical biopsy is still performed
- Confirmed cervical intraepithelial neoplasia (CIN) during pregnancy—follow with Pap and colposcopy every 3 months until delivery, then 2 months postpartum
- Microinvasive cervical carcinoma—perform cone biopsy
  - ► If no frank invasion, follow as above for CIN
- Invasive cervical cancer—treatment based upon gestational age
  - ► Less than 24 weeks' gestation—recommend termination with hysterectomy or radiation
  - ► Greater than 24 weeks' gestation—follow until 32–33 weeks, then deliver by cesarean and perform hysterectomy

OVARIAN TUMORS

- For simplicity: divide into prepubertal, reproductive, and post-menopausal categories

- Prepubertal masses
  - Are **always** considered **abnormal**
  - Clinical—nonspecific abdominal pain or palpable pelvic mass; **germ cell tumors** are the most common cause
  - Diagnosis—first step should be basic laboratory tests and tumor markers, followed by pelvic ultrasound

Diagnosis of Prepubertal Ovarian Malignancy

Laboratory Finding	Diagnosis
High LDH	Dysgerminoma
High beta-hCG	Choriocarcinoma
High AFP	Endodermal sinus tumor

Abbreviations: alpha-fetoprotein, AFP; human chorionic gonadotropin, hCG; lactate dehydrogenase, LDH

  - Management
    - All should undergo laparoscopic surgery (or laparotomy if indicated)
    - Further management based on histology
    - Benign—cystectomy and annual follow-up
    - Malignant—salpingo-oophorectomy and staging; treat germ cell tumors with postoperative chemotherapy

- Reproductive masses
  - First step in management of **any** reproductive-age female with a pelvic mass is serum beta-human chorionic gonadotropin (beta-hCG) → rule out pregnancy (most common cause)

Diagnosis and Management of Ovarian Masses in Reproductive-Aged Females

Diagnosis	Risk Factors	Clinical Findings	Ultrasound Findings	Laboratory Data	Management
Functional ovarian cyst	Normal menses	Painless, mobile pelvic mass on routine examination	**Simple, fluid-filled cyst**	Beta-hCG negative	• <7 cm: routine follow-up • >7 cm: surgical removal with or without oral contraceptives (suppresses ovulation)
Ovarian torsion	Large, functional cyst or pelvic mass	**Sudden onset of severe** lower abdominal pain	Ovarian mass twists around normal axis, resulting in **decreased to absent vascular flow on color Doppler**	Beta-hCG usually negative	Immediate **surgical exploration**: • If adequate perfusion after untwisting: cystectomy • If evidence of necrosis: oophorectomy
PCOS	Increased androgens, insulin resistance	Obese, anovulatory female with evidence of hirsutism and acanthosis nigrans	**"String of pearls"** pattern on ovaries (multiple small, fluid-filled peripheral ovarian cysts)	LH:FSH ratio of **3:1** (normal is 1.5:1)	• Oligomenorrhea: OCPs • Hirsutism: spironolactone (inhibits 5-alpha reductase) • Infertility: clomiphene citrate with or without metformin • Insulin resistance: metformin
Teratoma	N/A	**Vague lower-abdominal pain** with palpable, **mobile pelvic mass**	**Irregular, complex** mass with evidence of **calcification**	Beta-hCG negative	Surgical removal and histology (10% may be malignant and 10% are bilateral)
Tubo-ovarian abscess	Unsafe sex, multiple sexual partners, young females	Fever with or without signs of sepsis, lower abdominal pain, **palpable and painful pelvic mass with guarding**	Complex, **septated mass** with **fluid** (pus) in the **cul-de-sac**	Leukocytosis; with or without positive gonorrhea or chlamydia titers	Broad-spectrum IV antibiotics are first-line; if no response, then surgical removal is indicated

Abbreviations: follicle-stimulating hormone, FSH; human chorionic gonadotropin, hCG; luteinizing hormone, LH; oral contraceptive pill, OCP; polycystic ovarian syndrome, PCOS

- Postmenopausal masses
  - ▸ Most common cause is **ovarian epithelial carcinoma**; usually presents late in course with widespread peritoneal metastasis and ascites
  - ▸ Risk factors—unopposed estrogen, nulliparity, obesity, smoking, talcum powder use
  - ▸ Risk-factor reduction—OCP use, multiparity, progesterone supplementation, tubal ligation, and breast-feeding
  - ▸ Clinical—most common complaint is **increased abdominal girth**, distention, and pain; an adnexal mass is usually palpable and fixed on physical exam
  - ▸ Diagnosis—first step in evaluation is a **pelvic ultrasound** and **serum CA-125**; CA-125 is elevated in 80% of cases and useful in monitoring response to therapy
  - ▸ Treatment—**debulking surgery** is the treatment of choice

GESTATIONAL TROPHOBLASTIC NEOPLASIA

- Pathophysiology—due to benign or malignant proliferation of the trophoblast and syncytiotrophoblast
- Risk factors—**Taiwanese or Philippine descent**, folate deficiency, and very young or older reproductive-age women
- Clinical presentation—first-trimester bleeding with passage of **vesicles**; pelvic exam reveals **uterus larger than dates**, and ultrasound examination reveals **"snowstorm"** pattern and **absent fetal heart tones**
- Diagnosis and management

7

> Whether benign or malignant trophoblastic disease is diagnosed, women **must be advised to avoid pregnancy and take OCPs** until the beta-hCG titers are **negative** for the recommended time lines.

Management of Trophoblastic Neoplasia

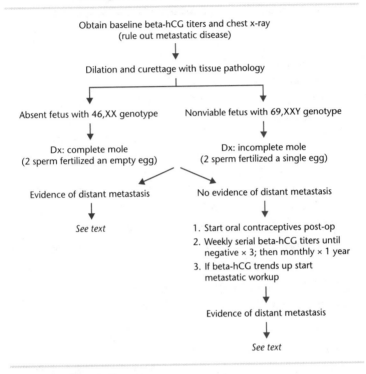

Obtain baseline beta-hCG titers and chest x-ray
(rule out metastatic disease)

↓

Dilation and curettage with tissue pathology

Absent fetus with 46,XX genotype   Nonviable fetus with 69,XXY genotype

↓   ↓

Dx: complete mole   Dx: incomplete mole
(2 sperm fertilized an empty egg)   (2 sperm fertilized a single egg)

Evidence of distant metastasis   No evidence of distant metastasis

↓   ↓

See text

1. Start oral contraceptives post-op
2. Weekly serial beta-hCG titers until
   negative × 3; then monthly × 1 year
3. If beta-hCG trends up start
   metastatic workup

↓

Evidence of distant metastasis

↓

See text

Abbreviations: diagnosis, Dx

Malignant Trophoblastic Disease

- Prognosis
  - ► Confined to uterus → 100% cure rate
  - ► Pelvic extension or lung metastasis → 95% cure rate
  - ► Brain or liver metastasis → 65% cure rate

- Treatment
  - ► No metastasis **or** local extension **or** lung metastasis → methotrexate **or** actinomycin D until beta-hCG is zero → start OCPs → beta-hCG titers every month for 1 year

► Evidence of brain or liver metastasis → methotrexate **plus** actinomycin D **plus** cyclophosphamide until beta-hCG is zero → start OCPs → beta-hCG titers every month for 2 years, then every 3 months for 3 years

CONTRACEPTION

- Multiple extremely effective options available; best choice will depend on patient's history, desired length of contraception, and future desire for pregnancy
- Condoms—extremely effective if used correctly; high failure rate due to improper usage (especially in teenagers/young adults); protects against STDs
- Vaginal diaphragm—inserted 30 minutes before intercourse; must be fitted by a physician; does not protect against STDs
- Spermicides—foam, lubricant, or jelly located on condoms or inserted into the vagina before intercourse; CDC warning: does not protect against STDs
- Estrogen and progestin contraceptives
  - ► Multiple types available (see Sex Steroid Contraception table on p. 310)
  - ► Contraindications to sex steroid contraceptives
    - ▷ Absolute—pregnancy; severe or acute liver disease; history of deep venous thrombosis (DVT), pulmonary embolism (PE), or cardiovascular accident (CVA); smokers >35 years; uncontrolled hypertension (HTN); migraines; thrombophilia or known hypercoagulable state (advanced cancer or hormonally mediated tumors)
    - ▷ Relative—migraines, depression, diabetes mellitus (DM), HTN, hyperlipidemia
  - ► Proven benefits of oral contraceptives
    - ▷ Decreases risk of ovarian cancer, endometrial cancer, dysfunctional uterine bleeding, PID, and ectopic pregnancy

7

Sex Steroid Contraception

Type of Contraception	Best Suited For	Disadvantages
Estrogen-progestin OCPs	One who desires regular and predictable menses	Requires taking pills every day at the same time
Transdermal estrogen-progestin patch	Low-maintenance contraception; applied weekly	Higher incidence of thromboembolic events (60% higher concentration of steroids)
Vaginal estrogen-progestin ring	Low-maintenance contraception; inserted every 4 weeks	Some may find it uncomfortable
Progestin-only OCPs ("minipills")	Breast-feeding mothers (does not affect lactation)	Breakthrough bleeding
Progestin-only injection (Depo-Provera®)	Low maintenance; injected every 3 months	Breakthrough bleeding
Progestin-only implants (Implanon®)	Long-term pregnancy prevention (effective for 3 years)	Breakthrough bleeding

Abbreviations: oral contraceptive pills, OCPs

- Intrauterine devices (IUDs)
  - ▸ Very effective long-term contraception for women in **monogamous relationships** (increased incidence of pelvic infections)
  - ▸ Contraindications—pregnancy, pelvic malignancy or mass, salpingitis or active pelvic infection, history of PID
  - ▸ Relative contraindications—history of ectopic pregnancy or abnormal Pap smears
  - ▸ **Note:** Nulligravidity is no longer a contraindication to use, but rate of spontaneous expulsion is higher than in multiparous women
  - ▸ Two types available
    - ▹ Copper IUD—effective for 10 years
    - ▹ Progestin IUD—effective for 5 years

- Natural family planning
  - ▶ Avoid intercourse around the time of ovulation, requires high degree of compliance on behalf of both partners (monitoring temperature, cervical mucus consistency, and menstrual timing)
  - ▶ Failure rate is highest with this method; usually preferred for religious reasons

- Permanent sterilization
  - ▶ In women: ligation, cutting, or clipping of the fallopian tubes (tubal ligation); in men: ligation and removal of the vas deferens (vasectomy); both are methods for permanent contraception
  - ▶ Best suited for those who have completed childbearing
  - ▶ Low failure rate (if failure occurs, think of recanalization)

MANAGEMENT OF MENORRHAGIA

- Acute menorrhagia
  - ▶ Hemodynamically unstable—place Foley catheter (to tamponade bleeding) and start high-dose IV estrogen first, then dilation and curettage when stabilized; hysterectomy as a last resort
  - ▶ Hemodynamically stable—outpatient high-dose oral estrogens are first-line; dilation and curettage if this fails

- Chronic menorrhagia
  - ▶ Desire to preserve childbearing—either oral contraceptives or levonorgestrel IUD
    - ▷ If hormonal therapy contraindicated (history of DVT, PE)—nonsteroidal anti-inflammatory drugs (NSAIDs) are first-line
  - ▶ No desire for childbearing—endometrial ablation usually first-line; hysterectomy is definitive

7

ENDOMETRIOSIS

- Pathophysiology—presence of endometrial glands and stroma **outside** the endometrial cavity; idiopathic, although many theories exist

- Clinical—classic history of **dyspareunia, painful** bowel movements, **cyclic** pelvic pain, dysmenorrhea, and **infertility**

- Diagnosis
  - ▶ Physical exam—**nodularity** of **uterosacral ligaments**, painful and tender nodularities in the cul-de-sac and pain with motion of uterus
  - ▶ Definitive/gold standard—laparoscopic visualization of ectopic implants ("gunshot" or "bluish" lesions within the pelvic cavity) or hemorrhagic cysts

- Treatment—based upon severity of symptoms and desire for fertility
  - ▶ Mild symptoms—NSAIDs with or without OCPs
  - ▶ Moderate symptoms or failure of above—gonadotropin-releasing hormone (GnRH) agonists (leuprolide) are first-line
  - ▶ Chief complaint of infertility, pelvic mass, or failure of above—laparoscopy with ablation/excisional therapy

VAGINAL BLEEDING IN CHILDREN

- Most common cause—**foreign body**
  - ▶ Best initial step—full pelvic examination (with sedation if necessary) with removal of object

- Other causes should be suspected based upon case scenario
  - ▶ Sexual abuse—child will be either **withdrawn and scared** or **overly sexual** for age (frequent touching, groping of other children or adults); pelvic examination shows breakage of the hymen with or without **scarring** of introitus and/or anus
  - ▶ Sarcoma botryoides—**"bag of grapes"** neoplasm protruding from the cervix or vaginal wall

► Precocious puberty—**breasts** usually developed; if pelvic examination is normal, get CT or MRI of the head to rule out pituitary adenoma

AMENORRHEA

Primary Amenorrhea

The absence of menses *and* secondary sexual development (breasts, pubic hair) by the age of 14 **or** the absence of menses by the age of 16 years *with* evidence of secondary sexual development.

Anatomic Causes of Primary Amenorrhea

Diagnosis	Physical Findings	Cause	Treatment
Imperforate hymen	Cyclic pelvic pain: exam shows **bulging, discolored, purple membrane** (hematocolpos) at the **introitus**	Thick, imperforate hymen	Surgical opening and resection
Transverse vaginal septum	Cyclic pelvic pain: exam reveals **vagina ending in blind pouch** at any level of the vagina with or without bulging membranes (hematocolpos)	Failure of the urogenital sinus to fuse or canalize during fetal development	Surgical repair
MRKH syndrome or vaginal agenesis	Primary amenorrhea with or without cyclic pelvic pain: exam shows **vaginal dimple**, and ultrasound confirms normal ovaries and variable uterine anomalies	Hypoplasia or complete agenesis of the müllerian duct	• First-line: self-dilation to create a functional vagina • Second-line: surgical repair if first-line fails

Abbreviations: Mayer-Rokitansky-Küster-Hauser, MRKH
Note: All of the above presentations have **normal** secondary sexual development.

Complete androgen insensitivity syndrome

- X-linked defect in 46,XY genotype—androgen receptor is **completely insensitive** to **normal** levels of **testosterone** → genotypic males fail to develop male secondary sexual characteristics with **estrogen domination**

- Physical examination—breasts with **pale areola** and **sparse** axillary and pubic hair, female-appearing genitalia and blind or short vagina; no uterus, fallopian tubes (Müllerian inhibitory factor is not affected, so these structures regress during fetal development)

- Treatment—removal of testes (high risk of malignancy, never fully descended); serial vaginal dilations for sexual preservation and estrogen supplementation to further secondary sexual characteristics

Kallmann syndrome

- Failure of GnRH production in the hypothalamus **plus** complete **anosmia**

- Failure of secondary sexual characteristics to develop—ultrasound examination will reveal anatomically normal uterus, fallopian tubes, and ovaries

- Treatment—supplemental estrogen and progesterone

Secondary Amenorrhea

The absence of menses for **at least 6 months** in a woman with previously normal menstruation

Treatment of secondary amenorrhea

- Hyperprolactinemia due to pituitary adenoma—oral bromocriptine if <1 cm; surgical resection if >1 cm in diameter

- Anovulation—oral contraceptives to regulate the menstrual cycle; oral clomiphene citrate if pregnancy is desired

- Ovarian failure—oral contraceptives to regulate menses and prevent early osteoporosis (if premature); in vitro fertilization or surrogacy if children are desired

Approach to the Diagnosis of Secondary Amenorrhea

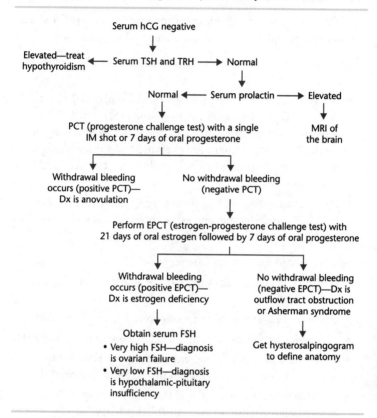

Abbreviations: diagnosis, Dx; estrogen-progesterone challenge test, EPCT; follicle-stimulating hormone, FSH; human chorionic gonadotropin, hCG; progesterone challenge test, PCT; thyroid-releasing hormone, TRH; thyroid-stimulating hormone, TSH

- Hypothalamic-pituitary failure—obtain brain MRI to rule out tumor; if negative, oral contraceptives

- Outflow tract obstruction—surgical repair

- Asherman syndrome—no treatment available

INFERTILITY

- Definition—inability to achieve pregnancy after **1 year** of frequent and unprotected intercourse in a woman <35 years of age

- First step in management—adequate history and physical examination
  - ▶ 30–40% due to male factors—get semen analysis; if normal → serum thyroid-stimulating hormone (TSH), FSH, LH, prolactin → if normal, get midcycle spinnbarkeit testing of cervical mucus (normal >10 cm elasticity) → if normal, get hysterosalpingogram to anatomically evaluate uterus and fallopian tubes
  - ▶ If oligomenorrhea or anovulatory—get serum TSH, prolactin, FSH, LH, progesterone, and estradiol levels; depending on the case, may need to order only one of these levels

- Best next steps for popular case scenarios:
  - ▶ If history of cold intolerance, hair loss, fatigue, and dry skin— serum TSH
  - ▶ If history of galactorrhea—serum prolactin
  - ▶ If an older reproductive-age female (40–50 years)—serum FSH
  - ▶ If there is a history of recurrent spontaneous abortions— hysterosalpingogram to rule out intrauterine abnormalities
  - ▶ If all lab values are normal and there is history of PID— hysterosalpingogram to evaluate tubal patency
  - ▶ History of pelvic pain, dyspareunia, and/or painful bowel movements—laparoscopy with lysis of endometrial implants, if present (may restore fertility)

OSTEOPOROSIS PREVENTION AND MANAGEMENT

- Risk factors for osteoporosis—Caucasian or Asian ethnicity, smoking, alcohol consumption, previous fragility fracture, chronic corticosteroids, low body weight, excess caffeine consumption, inactivity, anorexia, and advanced age

- Screening—**DEXA** (bone densitometry) scans recommended by the U.S. Preventative Services Task Force (USPSTF) starting at **age 65** in **postmenopausal** women; in postmenopausal women age **60–64 with significant risk factors**; and in men >80 years of age with no prior history of fractures or >65 years with risk factors
  - ▸ Interval screening—no consensus exists for the optimal interval between normal screens
    - ▹ If **drug therapy** is started, DEXA scan should be **repeated** in **1–2 years**
    - ▹ If on **chronic oral corticosteroids**, should screen **every 6 months** and start treatment if evidence of osteoporosis is found
- Diagnosis
  - ▸ The T-score is the standard deviation from the mean matched to **young, healthy adults** of the same ethnicity
    - ▹ T-score of –1 or greater—normal
    - ▹ T-score of –1 to –2.5—osteopenia
    - ▹ T-score of ≤2.5—osteoporosis
    - ▹ T-score of ≤2.5 plus evidence of one or more fragility fractures—severe or established osteoporosis
  - ▸ The Z-score is the standard deviation from the mean matched to adults of the **same age and race**
    - ▹ Z-score <1.5—the diagnosis is primary osteoporosis and is considered age-related and expected
    - ▹ Z-score >1.5—the diagnosis is secondary osteoporosis and is due to some underlying cause (smoking, endocrine abnormalities, chronic steroids, etc.)
- Prevention
  - ▸ Oral calcium and vitamin D supplementation are indicated in **all postmenopausal women** as **primary prevention**
  - ▸ Weight-bearing exercise is associated with improved bone density scores and should be encouraged in all who can tolerate exercise

7

▸ Encourage patients to quit smoking and reduce/eliminate excessive alcohol consumption

- Treatment
  ▸ Any evidence of osteoporosis is an indication for **bisphosphonates** (alendronate, risedronate, or ibandronate) as first-line therapy
    ▹ Caution regarding **erosive esophagitis**—advise to drink copious amounts of water and remain upright for at least 30 minutes after oral administration
    ▹ If patient cannot tolerate oral bisphosphonates secondary to reflux—IV zoledronic acid is first-line (the only IV bisphosphonate)
      – **Tip**: IV zoledronic acid is associated with **osteonecrosis of the jaw**; must get a routine dental examination before treatment.
  ▸ Raloxifene is an alternative in women unable to tolerate any bisphosphonate therapy—decreases risk of **vertebral fractures only**
  ▸ If recurrent fragility fracture despite bisphosphonates, human recombinant parathyroid hormone (PTH) may be used

7

II. OBSTETRICS

SPONTANEOUS ABORTION

- Multiple risk factors: maternal anatomic anomalies, fetal chromosomal anomalies, drugs, smoking, excessive caffeine consumption, and others

- 20% of pregnancies are lost to spontaneous abortions; risk increases with advanced maternal age

- Types of spontaneous abortion
  - ▸ Threatened abortion—positive fetal heart tones and closed cervical os; management is expectant
  - ▸ Inevitable abortion—fetal heart tones may or may not be present, intact fetus and dilated cervical os; management is supportive
  - ▸ Incomplete abortion—absent fetal heart tones, some retained products of conception on ultrasound; management is dilation and curettage
  - ▸ Complete abortion—absent fetal heart tones, no intrauterine products of conception, and dilated cervical os; management is supportive
  - ▸ Missed abortion—absent fetal heart tones with intact fetus and closed cervical os; management is dilation and curettage or dilation and evacuation

ECTOPIC PREGNANCY

- Clinical—classic **triad** of **amenorrhea** followed by **lower abdominal pain** (may radiate to the shoulder) and vaginal **spotting/bleeding**

- Next steps in management (diagnosis)
  - ▸ Transvaginal ultrasound—**no** evidence of intrauterine pregnancy and complex tubal mass that may or may not have fetal heart tones

7

▶ Serum hCG concentration (see the Clinical Management of Ectopic Pregnancy algorithm below)—management determined according to titer levels

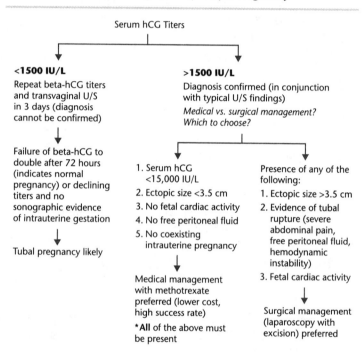

Clinical Management of Ectopic Pregnancy

Serum hCG Titers

<1500 IU/L
Repeat beta-hCG titers and transvaginal U/S in 3 days (diagnosis cannot be confirmed)

↓

Failure of beta-hCG to double after 72 hours (indicates normal pregnancy) or declining titers and no sonographic evidence of intrauterine gestation

↓

Tubal pregnancy likely

>1500 IU/L
Diagnosis confirmed (in conjunction with typical U/S findings)
Medical vs. surgical management? Which to choose?

1. Serum hCG <15,000 IU/L
2. Ectopic size <3.5 cm
3. No fetal cardiac activity
4. No free peritoneal fluid
5. No coexisting intrauterine pregnancy

↓

Medical management with methotrexate preferred (lower cost, high success rate)

*All of the above must be present

Presence of any of the following:
1. Ectopic size >3.5 cm
2. Evidence of tubal rupture (severe abdominal pain, free peritoneal fluid, hemodynamic instability)
3. Fetal cardiac activity

↓

Surgical management (laparoscopy with excision) preferred

Abbreviations: human chorionic gonadotropin, hCG; ultrasound, U/S

Post-Treatment Follow-up after Methotrexate

• Mild abdominal pain and cramping for 1 week after treatment is common, drug of choice (DOC) is oral acetaminophen (avoid NSAIDs secondary to drug–drug interactions); if pain is severe, get transvaginal ultrasound and admit for closer hemodynamic monitoring

- Preferred regimen is single-dose therapy, but multiple doses may be required (based on rate of beta-hCG decline); it is not necessary to know this for the exam

CERVICAL INCOMPETENCE

- Pathophysiology—**painless cervical dilation** during the **second trimester** with complete fetal loss; due to previous cervical trauma (repeated dilation and curettage [D&C], cervical laceration, or overly aggressive conization) or anatomic anomalies (diethylstilbestrol [DES] exposure in-utero)
- Management
  - ▶ Offer **elective cervical cerclage** placement at **13–16 weeks'** gestation
  - ▶ Emergent cerclage placement if early diagnosis and viable pregnancy
  - ▶ Complications—most common complication is infection
    - ▷ Remove at 36–37 weeks' gestation, after fetal lung maturity is confirmed

INDUCED ABORTION

May be performed for personal reasons, socioeconomic factors, or confirmed chromosomal anomalies (through chorionic villus sampling or amniocentesis)

- Mifepristone and misoprostol—indicated for gestational age <49 days; both agents are used together for 92% efficacy; incomplete abortions will require D&C
- Less than 20 weeks' gestation—D&C
- Greater than 20 weeks' gestation—dilation and evacuation (D&E)

7

PRENATAL MANAGEMENT

Prenatal Screening

The first prenatal visit

- Type, Rh status, and antibody screen—identify those at risk of isoimmunization

  ▸ RhD-negative mothers with positive antibody screen (indirect Coombs test positive)—methods to diagnose fetal anemia or potential hydrops fetalis should be offered

  ▸ RhD-negative mothers with **absence** of antibodies—provide **vaccination** with rho(d) immune globulin (RhoGAM®) at **28 weeks** and **immediately following delivery**; also vaccinate **at any point** you suspect maternal-fetal blood mixing (intrapartum vaginal bleeding, elective or spontaneous abortion, placental abruption, etc.)

- CBC—normal Hg 10–12 mg/dL (dilutional effect of increased plasma volume), normal white blood cell (WBC) count up to 16,000/mm³ (some margination occurs) with increased polymorphonuclear cells (PMNs)

- Rubella antibody titers—if negative, advise mothers to avoid exposure to persons with new rash or known cases, and offer the measles, mumps, rubella (MMR) vaccine **after delivery** (live attenuated vaccines are contraindicated in pregnancy)

- Rapid plasma reagin (RPR) or Venereal Disease Research Laboratory (VDRL)—confirm with fluorescent treponemal antibody absorption test (FTA-ABS) and treat if positive; all penicillin-allergic patients will require inpatient **desensitization, regardless of gestational age**

- Hepatitis screening—if positive for hepatitis B surface antigen **(HBsAg)** or hepatitis C virus **(HCV)**, risk of vertical transmission is high → must **encourage cesarean delivery** at term and **advise against breast-feeding**

- HIV screening—initiate highly active antiretroviral therapy (HAART) as soon as possible, recommend cesarean delivery (reduces vertical transmission), advise against breast-feeding (HIV-RNA secreted in breast milk), and obtain HIV viral load and CD4 count every trimester

- ▸ HIV treatment in pregnancy—previously recommended monotherapy with zidovudine (ZDV) in pregnancy is now considered suboptimal; all pregnant women with HIV infection should receive **three-drug antiretroviral therapy**
- ▸ The following antiretrovirals **should not** be used in pregnancy:
  - ▹ Efavirenz—documented neural tube defects when used in the first trimester
  - ▹ Didanosine and stavudine—higher risk of fetal lactic acidosis
  - ▹ Nevirapine—fetal hepatotoxicity
- Routine Pap smear and STD screening (see page 301)
- PPD (tuberculosis skin test)—recommendations are the same as for the nonpregnant patient

Gestation: 11–13 weeks

- First part of sequential screening
- Nuchal translucency screen and two serum markers

Gestation: 16 weeks

Second part of sequential screening.

Gestation: 16–20 weeks

- Quad screen is indicated if no sequential screening
- Includes maternal serum AFP, serum estriol, and serum beta-hCG, inhibin-A
  - ▸ Maternal serum AFP—accuracy of pregnancy dating is imperative to accurate interpretation; gestational age dating error is the most common cause of an abnormal AFP; also ensure a live, singleton fetus
    - ▹ High AFP → defined as >2.5 MoM (multiples of the median)
      - If 2.5–7.0 MoM—repeat the AFP → normal values are reassuring for a normal pregnancy

7

- If >7.0 or previous history of neural tube defects—
  perform obstetric ultrasound (rule out dating error or
  visible defects); if normal, recommend amniocentesis
  - Send amniotic fluid for **acetylcholinesterase levels**—
    if high, neural tube defect likely (most sensitive test)
▷ Low AFP is defined as <0.85 MoM
- Next step in management is obstetrical ultrasound
  - If ultrasound rules out dating error, repeat the AFP;
    normal levels = false alarm
  - If ultrasound confirms correct gestational age, next step
    in management is amniocentesis for fetal karyotyping
    (Down syndrome likely)

Interpretation of the Quad Screen

Diagnosis	Maternal Serum AFP	Maternal Serum Estriol	Maternal Serum hCG	Inhibin-A
Neural tube defect, omphalocele, or gastroschisis	High	Normal	Normal	Normal
Down syndrome (Trisomy 21)	Low	Low	High	High
Edwards syndrome (Trisomy 18)	Low	Low	Low	Normal

Abbreviations: alpha-fetoprotein, AFP; human chorionic gonadotropin, hCG

Gestation: 18–20 weeks

Fetal anatomy ultrasound to screen for anatomic defects.

Gestation: 24–28 weeks

- Screening for gestational diabetes with the 1-hour oral glucose
  tolerance test
- Administration of Tdap vaccine

Pathophysiology and management of gestational diabetes

- Pathophysiology—largely due to increased levels of **human
  placental lactogen (HPL)** and other pregnancy hormones

- Initial management consists of strict dietary therapy and, if the patient is capable of tolerating it, moderate exercise

Interpretation and Management of the Oral Glucose Tolerance Test

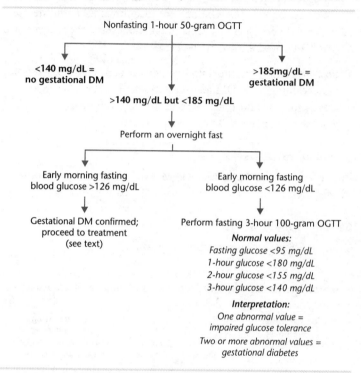

Abbreviations: diabetes mellitus, DM; oral glucose tolerance test, OGTT

- Insulin therapy is recommended if the following are observed on two separate occasions after 2 weeks of dietary therapy
  - ► Fasting blood glucose ≥90 mg/dL or 1-hour postprandial blood glucose ≥120 mg/dL
  - ► NPH insulin is recommended as a nighttime dose to control basal blood glucose levels; and rapid-acting insulin lispro, or aspart for elevated postprandial levels
    - ▷ **Avoid using ultralong-acting insulin glargine or detemir in pregnancy** (safety guidelines have not been established)

- Use of oral hypoglycemics in pregnancy
  - ▶ Although some studies have not shown a significant increase in morbidity with the use of glyburide, metformin, or acarbose in pregnancy, the American College of Obstetricians and Gynecologists (ACOG) **does not** recommend the routine use of oral hypoglycemic agents in pregnancy and these agents are not approved for use by the FDA

- Post-pregnancy monitoring—women are at **30% increased risk** of developing overt DM after gestational diabetes, should be closely followed postpartum, and should receive a 2-hour oral glucose tolerance test 3–4 weeks postpartum

Gestation: 28–30 weeks

Rho(d) immune globulin (RhoGAM®) vaccination, if the mother is Rh-negative.

Gestation: 36–37 weeks

Group B *Streptococcus* screening (if possible).

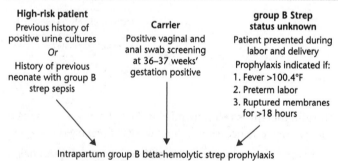

Indications for Intrapartum Prophylaxis of group B Streptococcus

High-risk patient	Carrier	group B Strep status unknown
Previous history of positive urine cultures *Or* History of previous neonate with group B strep sepsis	Positive vaginal and anal swab screening at 36–37 weeks' gestation positive	Patient presented during labor and delivery Prophylaxis indicated if: 1. Fever >100.4°F 2. Preterm labor 3. Ruptured membranes for >18 hours

Intrapartum group B beta-hemolytic strep prophylaxis
Drug of choice is **IV penicillin G**
If pen-allergic: IV cefazolin (if low-risk for cross-reactivity)
If pen-allergic and high risk for cross-reactivity: sensitivity of isolates required—use clindamycin if susceptible; otherwise, IV vancomycin is recommended

Abbreviations: penicillin-allergic, pen-allergic

BLEEDING DURING PREGNANCY

Most Common Causes of Bleeding During Pregnancy

Diagnosis	Pathophysiology	Clinical Presentation	Management
Placenta previa	Dislodgement of a low-lying placenta (near the cervical os)	• **Painless** late-term vaginal bleeding (**maternal** source); physical exam is unremarkable • Confirm with obstetrical ultrasound	• Hemodynamically unstable: emergent cesarean section • Hemodynamically stable: bed rest until fetal lung maturity
Placenta accreta, percreta, increta	• Accreta: placental villi invade through the decidua basalis • Increta: villi invade through the myometrium • Percreta: villi invade though the serosa or surrounding pelvic organs	• Painless, **massive hemorrhage** at time of delivery when **manual placental dislodgement** is attempted (**maternal** source) • Some cases may be diagnosed via obstetrical ultrasound	• Scheduled cesarean hysterectomy at 35–37 weeks (if diagnosed via obstetrical ultrasound) • Otherwise, blood transfusions and emergent hysterectomy are indicated

Placental abruption	**Trauma, severe hypertension,** or those with history of previous abruption or drug abuse (especially **cocaine**): dislodgement of a normally lying placenta from the uterine wall	**Painful** vaginal bleeding (**maternal** source); ultrasound confirms a normally implanted placenta with or without signs of retroplacental hematoma formation	• Hemodynamically unstable: emergency cesarean section
			• Hemodynamically stable:
			  – Preterm: inpatient observation and bed rest
			  – Term: vaginal or cesarean delivery, depending on clinical circumstance

Vasa previa	Fetal vessels within the placental membrane overlie the **cervical os**	**Painless** vaginal bleeding from **fetal blood loss** with **fetal bradycardia**; typical case is hemorrhage noted immediately **after amniotomy**	Blood transfusion and emergent cesarean section; otherwise, rapid fetal exsanguination and death

7

MANAGEMENT OF OBSTETRICAL COMPLICATIONS AND HIGH-RISK PREGNANCY

Preterm Labor

- Risk factors—multiple gestations, previous preterm pregnancy, premature rupture of membranes, maternal infection, excessive physical activity, smoking, fibroids, etc.

- Diagnosis—gestational age of 20–37 weeks, >3 contractions in 30-minute period **and** cervical effacement or cervical dilation >2 cm

- Clinical presentation—lower abdominal/back heaviness or pain, increased vaginal discharge with or without a bloody show

- Management: tocolysis (maximum time gained is 2–7 days)
  - ▶ Goal of tocolysis is to allow time for fetal lung maturity to occur with administration of **IM betamethasone** and transportation of the mother to a facility with neonatal intensive care unit (NICU) facilities
    - ▷ Contraindications (allow labor to proceed or perform cesarean section): placental abruption, ruptured membranes, chorioamnionitis, fetal jeopardy, preeclampsia or eclampsia, or advanced cervical effacement/dilation
  - ▶ Tocolytic agents—there is no "drug of choice"; the preferred agent will depend on comorbid disease and clinician preference
    - ▷ IV beta-agonists (ritodrine or terbutaline)—contraindications are uncontrolled diabetes, severe cardiac disease, or hyperthyroidism; rarely used nowadays
    - ▷ IV magnesium sulfate—contraindication is myasthenia gravis and end-stage renal disease
    - ▷ Oral calcium-channel blockers (nifedipine)—contraindications are decreased systolic function or severe congestive heart failure (CHF)

7

▷ NSAIDs (indomethacin)—the least preferred of all agents; **do not** use if gestational age >32 weeks (causes premature closure of ductus arteriosus) and multiple other side effects, including oligohydramnios

Hypertension, Eclampsia, and Preeclampsia

Hypertensive States in Pregnancy

Disease	Clinical Signs/ Symptoms	Diagnosis	Management
Chronic HTN	Diagnosis of HTN preceded pregnancy or <20 weeks' gestation at diagnosis	BP >140/90 mm Hg with or without proteinuria; generally worsens as pregnancy progresses	• Drug therapy is indicated if diastolic is persistently >95–100 mm Hg or signs of end-organ damage • DOC: oral methyldopa; may use labetalol but higher rate of IUGR when used chronically
Gestational HTN	Asymptomatic elevation of BP >140/90 mm Hg and >20 weeks' gestation	All labs normal, including urine (*no* proteinuria)	• Close follow-up • No pharmacologic therapy
Preeclampsia	• Mild: excessive weight gain and new, rapid-onset peripheral edema • Severe: same as mild, plus complaints of headache, epigastric pain, and/or visual changes, oliguria	• Mild: BP >140/90 mm Hg and urine dipstick protein 1–2+ or >300 mg/24-hour urine • Severe: BP >160/100 mm Hg and urine protein dipstick 3–4+ or >5 g/24-hr urine	**All term gestations (>37 weeks with favorable cervix) should be delivered regardless of disease severity** (see Management of Mild and Severe Preeclampsia, page 330)

(continued)

7

Hypertensive States in Pregnancy (continued)

Disease	Clinical Signs/ Symptoms	Diagnosis	Management
Eclampsia	Equals pre-eclampsia **plus new-onset tonic-clonic seizures** in the absence of known CNS disease (e.g., trauma, tumor, etc.)	Any degree of HTN plus pro-teinuria and new onset seizures	• Status epilepticus: IV diazepam (or phenytoin) until initial seizures controlled • Seizure prophylaxis or initial seizure resolved: IV magnesium sulfate • Control blood pressure as for preeclampsia/eclampsia • **Board tip:** If patient has a history of MG, use diazepam (mag-nesium sulfate is contraindicated)
HELLP syndrome	Preeclampsia or eclampsia complicated by new-onset **abdominal epigastric/RUQ pain**	Peripheral smear shows **schisto-cytes**, liver func-tion tests are **elevated**, and platelet count is **<100,000/mm³**	**Delivery** as soon as possible; if <34 weeks' gestation and mother and baby are stable give IM betamethasone and deliver within 48 hours

Abbreviations: blood pressure, BP; central nervous system, CNS; drug of choice, DOC; hemolysis, elevated liver enzymes, and low platelets, HELLP; hypertension, HTN; intrauterine growth retardation, IUGR; myasthenia gravis, MG; right upper quadrant, RUQ

7

Management of mild and severe preeclampsia

• All pregnancies >37 weeks should be delivered regardless of severity; if cervix is unfavorable, cervical ripening agents are indicated

• Any signs and symptoms of maternal end-organ damage or fetal jeopardy are an indication to induce labor regardless of gesta-tional age; consider IM betamethasone for fetal lung maturity if maternal and fetal status allows

- Indications for antihypertensive therapy—**does not** alter fetal outcome; decreases maternal morbidity and mortality through **prevention of hemorrhagic stroke**
  - ▸ Initiate therapy when systolic blood pressure is >150 or diastolic is >100 mm Hg
  - ▸ DOC: labetalol
- If <34 weeks' gestation: give IM betamethasone
  - ▸ Is delivery, inpatient management, or outpatient management indicated?
  - ▸ Mild preeclampsia and remote from term: is the patient is able to comply with frequent follow-up?
    - ▹ If compliance ensured—monitor maternal blood pressure and fetal well-being with twice-weekly nonstress testing, daily fetal movement counts, and weekly CBC (follow platelets), chem 7 (monitor creatinine), and liver function tests (onset of HELLP [hemolysis, elevated liver enzymes, and low platelets])
    - ▹ If compliance not ensured—hospitalization, with above testing for emergent intervention if needed
  - ▸ Severe preeclampsia → **prompt delivery** of the fetus is indicated
    - ▹ If <32 weeks—admit to ICU, then give a loading dose of IV magnesium sulfate; lastly, control blood pressure with IV labetalol (plus hydralazine if indicated) and deliver as soon as possible

7

LABOR AND DELIVERY

Stages of Labor and Delivery

Stage	Phase	Clinical Findings/ Normal Progression	Disorders and Management
One	Latent	• Regular contractions and slow cervical dilation • Primipara: up to 20 hours • Multipara: up to 14 hours	Any longer than this: diagnosis is prolonged latent phase

(continued)

Stages of Labor and Delivery (continued)

Stage	Phase	Clinical Findings/ Normal Progression	Disorders and Management
	Active	• Rapid dilation of the cervix with fetal descent • Primipara: 1.2 cm/hour • Multipara: 1.5 cm/hour	• Any longer than this: diagnosis is either prolonged active phase or arrest of labor • Most common cause of arrest is **hypotonic uterine contractions**; next step in management is amniotomy (if membranes have not ruptured yet) with IV oxytocin
Two	N/A	• Cervix is completely dilated and fetus descends for delivery • Primipara: 2 hours • Multipara: 1 hour	• Any longer than this: diagnosis is prolonged second stage or arrest of fetal descent • If arrest of fetal descent: may observe, perform vaginal operative delivery (forceps or vacuum), or perform cesarean section
Three	N/A	• Fetus and placenta are delivered • Should last no longer than 30 minutes	Risk of maternal hemorrhage if prolonged (most common cause is hypotonic contractions); use IV oxytocin to speed up the process

Fetal Monitoring

• Normal fetal heart rate: 110–160 beats per minute (bpm)

• Accelerations—rapid increase in fetal heart rate due to **fetal movement** (unrelated to uterine contractions) and lasts less than 2 minutes; **always normal**

   ‣ <32 weeks' gestation—normal is acceleration ≥10 bpm lasting ≥10 seconds

   ‣ >32 weeks' gestation—normal is acceleration ≥15 bpm lasting ≥15 seconds

- Variable decelerations—rapid decrease in fetal heart rate by ≥15 bpm lasting ≥15 seconds due to **compression of the umbilical cord** (not related to uterine contractions); mild-moderate variable decelerations (drop of up to 60 bpm) are acceptable, but any drop ≥60 bpm is concerning for fetal jeopardy (severe variable deceleration)

- Early decelerations—gradual decrease in fetal heart rate due to fetal head compression during a normal uterine contraction; **exactly coincides** with uterine contraction and is always normal

- Late decelerations—gradual decrease in fetal heart rate due to uteroplacental insufficiency during a uterine contraction; onset is **delayed** in relation to the contraction and is **always abnormal**

Epidural Anesthesia

- Indications—allows **continuous infusion** of anesthetic; use for anesthetic relief **throughout labor**

- Used for surgical anesthesia (cesarean section) with high concentrations of local anesthetics

- Disadvantages—possible patchy block requiring high-dose infusions (therefore more likely to produce systemic toxicity) and slow onset

- Contraindications—hemodynamic instability, coagulopathy, and local site infection

- Relative contraindications—increased intracranial pressure and systemic maternal infection

- Complications
  - ► Hypotension (sympathetic blockade results in peripheral vasodilation and decreased venous return)
    - ▷ Management—volume expansion, maternal left lateral decubitus position and Trendelenburg position, phenylephrine, and/or ephedrine for pressure support
  - ► Patchy/failed block

7

- Anesthetic toxicity
  - ▷ Management—100% oxygen, IV barbiturate or benzodiazepam if convulsions, cardiopulmonary resuscitation as needed
- Total spinal block (dyspnea, hypotension, loss of consciousness)
  - ▷ Management—emergent intubation and hemodynamic support

Spinal Anesthesia

- Indicated if cervical dilation is at 8–9 cm and delivery is imminent (fast onset, wears off quickly)

- Not indicated earlier in labor since multiple spinal punctures would be required for continuous effect

- Preferred for scheduled surgical anesthesia

- Contraindications and complications—same as for epidural anesthesia

POSTPARTUM MANAGEMENT

- Normal postpartum period lasts 4–6 weeks after delivery
- Normal uterine involution
  - Lochia—lasts about 2–3 weeks; initially bright red (lochia rubra), then light pink (lochia serosa), then white (lochia alba)
- Postpartum mood
  - Postpartum blues ("baby blues")—moody, tearful, but **able to care for self and child**; no intervention
  - Postpartum depression—**hopeless, helpless**, and **neglects self and child**; DOC is a selective serotonin reuptake inhibitor (SSRI) even if breast-feeding
  - Postpartum psychosis—severe insomnia, **delusions**, and **hallucinations** with bizarre behavior and **neglect of self and child**; must admit to the hospital; most physicians prefer oral atypical antipsychotics as the DOC (olanzapine, risperidone)

- Postpartum breast-feeding
  - ► Ensure that patient's fluid intake and nutritional status are adequate (needs increase by 250–300 kcal/day)
  - ► Note contraindications for medical reasons (e.g., HIV, HCV, etc.) and advise **against** breast-feeding (these viruses are excreted in breast milk and may infect the fetus)
  - ► Breast-feeding is not contraindicated with most maternal medications (e.g., SSRI, lithium, coumadin, propylthiouracil [PTU], etc.)

Postpartum Hemorrhage

- Definition—excessive blood loss resulting in hemodynamic instability after delivery; blood loss >500 cc after vaginal birth or >1,000 cc after cesarean section
- Most common causes and management
  - ► Most common cause is uterine atony—multiple risk factors (multiple gestations, infection, some drugs); **large, boggy uterus** noted on physical examination; first step in management is **fundal massage**, followed by IV oxytocin; if oxytocin is insufficient, try IM methylergonovine only **if patient does not have HTN**
  - ► Second most common cause is vaginal lacerations—forceps or vacuum delivery most common risk factors; search for and repair any lacerations
  - ► Other causes include retained placenta—inspect delivered placenta and determine if intact; if not, perform manual removal or dilation and curettage
    - ▷ Rarely, disseminated intravascular coagulation (DIC) (from any cause of prolonged bleeding or retained, dead fetus) or uterine inversion (beefy-red protrusion from vagina) may occur

7

Postdural Puncture Headache

- May occur with epidural or spinal puncture
- Clinical—headache absent when supine, sitting up causes severe fronto-occipital headache, relieved by returning to the supine position
  - ▸ Management—conservative
    - ▹ Advise bed rest and analgesics with caffeine; usually resolves spontaneously within a week
    - ▹ If this fails or headache is severe → blood patch is first-line; relief within 24 hours in 90% of patients

7

PEDIATRICS

NEWBORNS

Apgar Score

- Assesses infant well-being at 1 and 5 minutes of life
- A low score at 1 minute may show that the neonate requires medical attention
- Five-minute score indicates how the neonate responded to initial management
- Does **not** predict neurologic outcome

Apgar Scoring System

Score	0	1	2
Heart rate	Absent	<100/min	>100/min
Respiratory rate	Absent	Shallow, irregular	Good, crying
Color	Pale or blue	Body pink, pale/blue extremities	Pink
Tone	Limp	Weak	Active
Reflex irritability	Absent	Facial grimacing	Active withdraws

Must-Know Birth Injuries

Birth Injury	Presentation/Severity	Outcome
Subconjunctival hemorrhage	Minor, resolves spontaneously	No permanent deficit
Duchenne-Erb paralysis	Affects **C5-C6**; failure to abduct the shoulder, externally rotate or supinate the forearm	• Most recover spontaneously with physical therapy • If no change in 6 months → neuroplasty
Klumpke paralysis	Affects **C7-8 ± T1**—total hand paralysis; may be associated with ipsilateral **Horner syndrome**	Same as above
Clavicular fracture	Most common with **difficult delivery**	Full recovery; occasionally needs immobilization
Caput succedaneum	Diffuse swelling **crossing** cranial sutures	Resolves in days
Cephalohematoma	Subperiosteal hematoma that **does not cross** suture lines	Resolves in weeks to months
Subcutaneous fat necrosis	Due to stress-induced injury to immature fat	Usually self-limited

Newborn Findings

Normal and abnormal physical examination

- Skin

Newborn Skin Findings

Diagnosis	Physical Findings	Treatment
Cutis marmorata	**Lacy, reticulated** pattern when baby is cold	None; improves with time
Erythema toxicum	Firm, **yellow-white papules** and pustules rich in **eosinophils**	Fades in a few days
Hemangioma	• Superficial lesions: bright-red and usually regress • Deep lesions with bluish undertone and may be permanent	• Pulsed laser • Steroids, if needed

(continued)

Newborn Skin Findings (continued)

Diagnosis	Physical Findings	Treatment
Milia	Firm, **white papules** due to inclusion cysts	Resolve spontaneously
Mongolian spot	Blue-to-gray macules most common in dark-skinned patients; **do not** confuse with physical abuse	Leave it alone; fades with time
Neonatal acne	Acne due to **maternal androgens**	Resolves spontaneously
Port-wine stain	Permanent vascular malformation seen on **face and neck**	**Pulsed laser**
Salmon patch	Symmetric, **pale-pink macule**	Facial macules resolve; posterior neck macules usually persist; no therapy needed

- Head/neck
  - ▸ Branchial cleft cyst—arises laterally from the midline and requires surgical removal
  - ▸ Thyroglossal duct cyst—arises from the midline; moves with swallowing
- Abdomen

Congenital Abdominal Malformations

Disease	Diagnosis	Treatment
Congenital diaphragmatic hernia	**Bowel sounds** in unilateral **chest**; chest x-ray shows bowel loops in chest	Immediate surgical repair
Omphalocele	Midline hernia **covered with sac**	Surgical
Gastroschisis	Midline hernia with **no sac**	Life-threatening; cover with **moistened laps immediately** → surgical repair
Umbilical hernia	Small reducible hernia at birth	None; resolves spontaneously

8

- Genitourinary

Congenital Genitourinary Malformations

Disease	Diagnosis	Treatment
Hypospadias	Urethra opens on **ventral surface**	**Do not circumcise**
Epispadias	Urethra opens on **dorsal surface**	Urology consult; urinary incontinence likely
Undescended testes	Unable to palpate testes in scrotal sac	• First, verify presence of testes in the scrotal sac with ultrasound • Second, if testes do not descend by **1 year of age** → surgery

Disease in the Newborn

Infant of diabetic mother (IODM)

- Pathophysiology—maternal hyperglycemia → neonatal hyper-insulinemia → growth of all bodily organs except the brain

- Labs—hypoglycemia after cord separation; other electrolyte disorders are hypocalcemia, hypomagnesemia, and hyper-bilirubinemia; follow electrolytes frequently after birth

- Physical exam— normal to plethoric infant, cardiomegaly (asymmetric septal hypertrophy), polycythemia, renal vein thrombosis (hypercoagulable), increased risk of atrial septal defect (ASD), ventricular septal defect (VSD); small left colon syndrome may be seen

Jaundice in the newborn

When you should worry about jaundice:

- If seen on the **first day of life**

- If total bilirubin rises **>5 mg/dL/day**

- If total bilirubin is **>12 mg/dL in a term infant**

- If direct bilirubin is **>2/mg/dL**

Neonatal sepsis

- Infants at increased risk of sepsis—prematurity, maternal infection, preterm premature rupture of membrane (PPROM)

- Most common causes (in descending order)—**group B *Streptococcus, Escherichia coli, Listeria***

- Diagnosis—**pan cultures** (urine culture, blood culture, cerebrospinal fluid [CSF] culture); CBC with differential; lumbar puncture if meningitis suspected

- Treatment—ampicillin plus an aminoglycoside, or ampicillin plus third-generation cephalosporin that will penetrate blood-brain barrier (BBB)

TORCH Infections

Disease	Transmission	Clinical Findings	Characteristic Features/ Diagnosis	Treatment/ Preventive Medicine
Toxoplasmosis	**Primary infection from cat feces; raw/ undercooked meat**	Multiple, including jaundice, HSM, thrombocytopenia, microcephaly, chorioretinitis, hydrocephalus, **intracranial calcifications**	**Serum IgM antibodies in neonate**	• Maternal: **spiramycin** during pregnancy • Neonate: **sulfadiazine or leucovorin** for 6 months, then **spiramycin**
Syphilis (**O** = other)	**Transplacental**	Two sets of findings based on age: • First 2 years: **snuffles, maculopapular rash, FTT, jaundice** • Older than 2 years: **Hutchinson teeth, mulberry molars, Clutton joints, saber shins, saddle nose, rhagades**	Darkfield examination of secretions (snuffles) or positive VDRL; most sensitive test is IgM–FTA-ABS	Penicillin for mother and neonate **Note:** If mother is penicillin-allergic you **must** desensitize.

(continued)

8

TORCH Infections (continued)

Disease	Transmission	Clinical Findings	Characteristic Features/ Diagnosis	Treatment/ Preventive Medicine
Rubella	**Transplacental during first trimester (80% risk); risk** decreases with gestational age	**Blueberry-muffin spots,** congenital heart defects, bilateral **cataracts, deafness**	• **Maternal rash in first** trimester; **incomplete vaccinations** • Diagnosis: pos-**itive maternal IgG antibody in prenatal labs excludes; if negative, get IgM antibodies**	Avoid anyone with a rash during first trimester; vaccinate only **after** delivery (live attenuated virus)
CMV	**Primary or reactivation infection**	HSM, jaundice, **periventricular calcifications,** IUGR, chorioretinitis, **sensorineural hearing loss**	• If history of HIV, HAART during pregnancy decreases risk • Diagnosis with **neonatal urine culture**	Ganciclovir
Herpes simplex	**Transvaginal during delivery with active maternal lesions**	Pneumonia, shock, general-ized **herpetic rash,** and other signs of systemic disease in first week; then kera-**toconjunctivitis** in second week, then **widespread CNS disease**	• Best initial test: Tzanck smear of lesions (mul-tinucleated giant cells) • Most sensitive test: PCR-DNA	• **Elective cesarean sec-tion if active lesions at time of labor and delivery;** many physi-cians will offer elective cesarean even without lesions • Neonates may receive acyclovir to suppress disease

Abbreviations: cytomegalovirus, CMV; central nervous system, CNS; fluorescent treponemal antibody absorption test, FTA-ABS; failure to thrive, FTT; highly active antiretroviral therapy, HAART; hepatosplenomegaly, HSM; intrauterine growth retardation, IUGR; polymerase chain reaction, PCR; Venereal Disease Research Laboratory, VDRL

8

TERATOGENIC DRUGS

- Angiotensin-converting enzyme (ACE) inhibitors → **renal anomalies**, craniofacial anomalies

- Diethylstilbestrol (DES) → **adenocarcinoma** or **clear cell carcinoma** of the **vagina**

- Ethanol → fetal alcohol syndrome, which includes poor physical and brain growth or malformations and specific dysmorphic facial features: **short palpebral fissures**, **thin vermillion border** of lip, smooth philtrum, and flat midface

- Isotretinoin → multiple congenital anomalies, including facial defects and congenital heart disease

- Lithium → **Ebstein anomaly**

- Phenytoin → hypoplastic nails; typical facies, including cleft lip/palate and widely spaced eyes, intrauterine growth retardation (IUGR)

- Tetracyclines → **grossly discolored teeth**, nail hypoplasia

- Warfarin → facial anomalies and **chondrodysplasia**

- Valproate and carbamazepine → mental retardation, **neural tube defects**

GENETIC DISORDERS

Angelman Syndrome

- **Maternal** deletion of 15q11q13 (versus Prader-Willi syndrome)

- Characteristic feature: **"Happy children who can't talk"**—loud, inappropriate laughter with failure to develop vocabulary; use sign language to communicate; walk like **puppets** (ataxia and jerky limb movements)

- Seizure disorders common

8

Achondroplasia

- Autosomal dominant inheritance
- Characteristic features include **short stature, prominent forehead, lumbar lordosis**; may have frequent **otitis media** and hearing loss

Alport Syndrome

- X-linked dominant form of hereditary nephritis
- Characteristic onset of gross and microscopic **hematuria** immediately **after** a recent **upper respiratory infection (URI)**; renal biopsy reveals **foam cells**; also have **bilateral sensorineural hearing loss**

Ehlers-Danlos Syndrome

- Autosomal dominant inheritance of defect in **elastin**
- Characteristic features include **hyperextensible skin, blue sclera, easy bruisability, poor wound healing, ectopia lentis**
- Increased risk of aortic root dilation and **dissecting aortic aneurysm, retinal detachment**, and **prolapsed mitral valve**

Fetal Alcohol Syndrome (FAS)

- Studies have never been able to predict a dose-related onset of FAS; therefore, **all** women should be advised to completely abstain from alcohol while pregnant
- Characteristic features include mental retardation (MR), attention deficit hyperactivity disorder, **cupid's-bow lip**, microcephaly, **maxillary hypoplasia**, cardiac anomalies (septal defects)

Fragile X Syndrome

- Most often affects males; fragile site on X chromosome with variable number of CGG repeats
- If repeat number >200, males fully affected and some females affected (usually milder)

- Variable degrees of **MR, large head and ears,** long face; **macroorchidism**

Galactosemia (vs) galactokinase def - bilat cataracts only

- Deficiency of G-1-phosphate (G-1-P) uridylyltransferase deficiency leads to accumulation of G-1-P in kidneys, liver, and brain

- Symptoms are **direct hyperbilirubinemia/jaundice; hypo-glycemia, cataracts, MR,** hepatomegaly, low BGL

- Predisposed to *E. coli* **sepsis**

- Treatment with lactose-free diet; does not reverse neurologic deficits

Klinefelter Syndrome (XXY)

- Males have characteristic physical features: **long limbs, slender, often tall**

- **Decreased androgens** leads to decreased body hair, small testes, small penis, gynecomastia

- Treatment—**testosterone replacement** at puberty

Marfan Syndrome (vs) homocystinuria - same physical sks - thrombosis

- Autosomal dominant inheritance of defective **fibrillin gene**

- Characteristic features are **tall stature, long limbs, slender, arachnodactyly (very long fingers),** pectus carinatum or excavatum

- Increased risk of **lens subluxation** and aortic root dilatation **coarctation of the aorta**

- Treat with **beta-blockers** to decrease risk of vascular sequelae

- Use **back brace** to prevent scoliosis in puberty if required

Osteogenesis Imperfecta

- Autosomal dominant inheritance defect in **type I collagen**

8

- Type I—**translucent teeth, blue sclera, transparent skin**, bowing of limbs, scoliosis and kyphosis, fractures (do not confuse with child abuse), **double-jointed**, otosclerosis

- Type II—**lethal**; growth deficiency with multiple fractures and callus formation even in utero

Phenylketonuria (PKU)

- Defect in **phenylalanine hydroxylase** with accumulation of phenylalanine in tissues

- Toxicity in central nervous system (CNS)—gradual onset of MR, seizures after birth

- Characteristic features—**fair hair, fair eyes, fruity smell** [musty written above "fruity"]

- Treatment with **low-phenylalanine diet** [handwritten: ↳ b/c no tyrosine for melanin] [handwritten: + replace tyrosine]

Potter Syndrome

- **Renal agenesis/dysgenesis** leads to **oligohydramnios** and **pulmonary hypoplasia**

- Characteristic features include **Potter facies** (hypertelorism, epicanthal folds, low-set ears, micrognathia); abnormally positioned hands and feet

- Death from **respiratory insufficiency**

Polycystic Kidney Disease

- Autosomal recessive type most severe—presents in **children**; bilateral polycystic kidneys are **palpable** in the abdomen; most have some form of **pulmonary hypoplasia** (similar to Potter sequence); may also have hepatic cysts

- Autosomal dominant type less severe—presents in adults between the age of 40 and 60 and are diagnosed with **hypertension (HTN)** and bilaterally enlarged and polycystic kidneys on renal ultrasound; usually have other systemic cysts (such as liver); increased risk of **berry aneurysms**. Usually history of first-degree relative affected. Only treatment is to control HTN.

Prader-Willi Syndrome

- Largely **paternal** deletion of 15q11q13
- **Obese, binge-eating children** with variable degrees of **MR**; small hands/feet, small genitals
  - ▸ Prune-belly syndrome

Trisomy Disorders

Diagnosis	Characteristic Features	Things to Remember
Trisomy 21—Down syndrome	Slanted palpebral fissures with inner epicanthal folds; Brushfield spots (speckled iris); tongue protrusion, simian crease, congenital heart defects	• Increased risk of multiple disorders: – Hypothyroidism – Duodenal atresia – ALL – Endocardial cushion defect is most common cardiac anomaly – Early-onset Alzheimer dementia
Trisomy 18—Edwards syndrome	Low-set ears, micrognathia, **clenched fist, rocker-bottom feet, hammer toe**	• Increased risk of **omphalocele** • Most do not survive past 1 year
Trisomy 13—Patau syndrome	Holoprosencephaly with severe MR, cleft lip/palate, **cutis aplasia**, polydactyly	75% **in utero death** rate; diagnosed most often with obstetrical ultrasound

Abbreviations: acute lymphoblastic leukemia, ALL; mental retardation, MR

Turner Syndrome (XO)

- Sporadic cases of missing paternal chromosome
- Characteristic physical findings—**short stature, webbed neck** due to **cystic hygroma** in utero, congenital lymphedema causes **puffy hands/feet**, wide-spaced nipples, low hairline, **streak ovaries**, and infertility
- Increased risk of **coarctation of the aorta, bicuspid aortic valves, HTN**

8

- Treatment with **estrogen supplementation at puberty**; add **growth hormone (GH) and steroids** to increase height if bone age (BA) is <13 years
- Major differential diagnosis (DDx): Noonan syndrome
  - ▶ Affects **males**
  - ▶ **Short stature; short, webbed neck**; pectus excavatum; pulmonary stenosis; **small penis**; and **cryptorchidism**

Williams Syndrome

- Characteristic features includes short stature, **friendly and talkative child with elfin facies** (prominent lips, depressed nasal bridge, blue eyes, and **pointed ears**)
- Predisposed to **hypercalcemia, renal artery stenosis, and aortic stenosis**

NORMAL PEDIATRIC DEVELOPMENT AND MILESTONES

Failure to Thrive (FTT)

- May be a manifestation of neglect, malnutrition, severe systemic disease
- Careful history-taking and physical examination are most important in narrowing down a DDx
- Should order a full workup: electrolytes, liver function tests (LFTs), CBC, urinalysis, sweat chloride test, stool studies, and calorie counting

Childhood Obesity and Metabolic Syndrome

- Risk factors include family history, excessive feeding, inactivity, poor source of food
- Body mass index (BMI) of 25–29.9 considered overweight; BMI of >30 considered obese

- Overweight babies at increased risk of becoming overweight adults
- Treat with exercise and balanced diet
- See Metabolic Syndrome, page 84

Kwashiorkor and Marasmus

- Most common in **impoverished** nations
- Inadequate caloric intake and protein deficiency from **starvation**
- Kwashiorkor children have generalized edema and distended abdomens from **severe protein deficiency**
- Marasmus children have severe **total caloric deprivation** with thin, wasted extremities and little to no body fat
- **Very slow refeeding** must be done or risk of severe electrolyte imbalance ("refeeding syndrome"); may cause death

CHILDHOOD MILESTONES

Important Primitive Reflexes

Reflex	Age of Appearance/Disappearance
Moro: extension of head causes extension and flexion of arms and legs	Should disappear by age 3–4 months
Grasp: infant should grasp your finger when you place it in his/her palm	Should disappear by age 4–6 months
Rooting: brushing your finger on infant's cheek causes him/her to turn the head to that side	Should disappear by age 4–6 months
Parachute: if you simulate a fall (pretend you are dropping the infant), his/her arms should extend	Appears by 6–8 months

8

Childhood Milestones

Age	What You Must Know
Newborn	Turns head and is alert to sound
3 months	Lifts head above plane of body, **social smile**, coos
6 months	Knows how to roll over, creeps and crawls, **stranger anxiety**, sleeps all night
9 months	Will walk with two-hand assistance, **pincer grasp**, alert to name
12 months	**Cruises**, walk with one-handed assistance, knows "Ma-ma" and "Da-da"
15 months	**Walks alone**, builds **three-cubed tower**, uses cup, **temper tantrums begin**
18 months	**Runs, but stiffly**; walks down stairs with assistance; builds **four-cubed tower**; knows 10 words; says "**No!**", knows body parts
24 months	**Runs well**, walks up and down stairs without assistance (one foot at a time), makes **two-word sentences**, makes **parallel play**
30 months	Goes up stairs with alternating feet, says "**I**," knows his/her own name
3 years	Goes down stairs with alternating feet, **three-word sentences, copies circle and cross**
4 years	**Hops on one foot, throws ball overhand, rides a tricycle**, can draw a **square**, participates in **group play**
5 years	**Copies triangle**

8

CARDIOLOGY

Childhood HTN

- Diagnosis of HTN → two readings on two separate occasions >95th percentile for age

- Secondary causes are the most common cause in children (versus primary being most common in adults)

  ▶ In children, think of intrinsic renal disease, endocrine disorders, or aortic coarctation; renal ultrasound warranted

  ▶ In adolescents, more likely to be essential HTN

- Treatment
  - ▸ Obese—weight loss
  - ▸ Drugs of choice (DOCs)
    - ▹ Diuretic or beta-blocker is initial DOC in children
    - ▹ Add calcium-channel antagonist if still uncontrolled
    - ▹ ACE inhibitor is the DOC if renal disease/causes present
    - ▹ Neural crest tumors—same treatment as adults; that is, an alpha-blocker, followed by beta-blocker

Congenital Heart Defects

Important points

- Children **do not** present with the typical signs and symptoms of cardiac disease that adults do

- Any infant or child with a murmur must have a 2-D echo (except innocent murmurs)—always the best next step in management after the ABCs
  - ▸ Other helpful tests include chest x-ray, ECG, MRI, or cardiac catheterization, but these are not as important as the echo

- Echocardiogram is **always** the gold standard for diagnosis of structural heart defects

- Innocent murmurs
  - ▸ More than 30% of children age **3–7 years** with **normal growth** and development will have one
  - ▸ Murmur is **always systolic** (i.e., diastolic murmurs in children are always pathologic)
  - ▸ **Never** >2 out of 6 in intensity

- Clinical findings of cardiac disease/anomalies are subtle
  - ▸ Neonates have nonspecific findings, including failure to feed, sleepiness, diaphoresis with feeding (only exertion a neonate has), and tachypnea
  - ▸ Older children usually only complain of dyspnea on exertion

8

Atrial septal defects (ASDs) and ventricular septal defects (VSDs)

- ASD
  - ▸ Defect of **ostium secundum** is most common presentation
  - ▸ Usually closes spontaneously in infancy, or presents in 20s
  - ▸ Physical exam reveals **loud S1, wide fixed-split S2 with systolic ejection murmur**
  - ▸ Diagnosis—chest x-ray shows cardiomegaly; ECG shows **right axis deviation** with right ventricular conduction delay; echo is gold standard
  - ▸ Surgical repair in symptomatic adults; 2:1 shunt; all females due to increased cardiovascular risk in pregnancy

- VSD
  - ▸ **Most common congenital heart defect**
    - ▹ Muscular VSD most likely to close spontaneously
    - ▹ Membranous (most common) less likely to close spontaneously
  - ▸ Degree of shunting determined by ratio between peripheral vascular resistance (PVR) and systemic vascular resistance (SVR); when PVR > SVR, **Eisenmenger syndrome** ensues
  - ▸ Physical exam reveals **harsh holosystolic murmur** over the left sternal border, heard best in **fourth left intercostals space**, loud S2
  - ▸ Treatment—surgery in first year of life indicated if FTT or evidence of pulmonary artery hypertension

Coarctation of the aorta

- 90% of cases occur in adults (most at origin of subclavian artery)
- The remaining 10% occur in infancy and usually start at site of head/neck artery extending into the ductus arteriosus
  - ▸ Decreased right ventricular output → **pink upper body and cyanosis of lower body** → total heart failure and acidosis when ductus arteriosus closes

- Diagnosis—chest x-ray shows nonspecific findings of pulmonary congestion and cardiomegaly; ECG shows right ventricular or biventricular hypertrophy; best test is echo; MRI also clearly defines severity

- Treatment—**prostaglandin E_1 (PGE$_1$) infusion** to maintain patency of patent ductus arteriosus (PDA) until surgery can be performed

Ebstein anomaly

- Most common risk factor is maternal use of **lithium**

- Associated with increased risk of **Wolff-Parkinson-White syndrome**

- Abnormal tricuspid valve divides right ventricle in two parts → regurgitation with dilation of right atrium → shunting of blood through foramen ovale (unable to close) → decreased right ventricular output and peripheral cyanosis

- Physical exam—**holosystolic murmur over left sternal border**; cyanosis

- Diagnosis—chest x-ray shows cardiomegaly (very large right atrium); ECG findings variable; echo is gold standard

- Treatment—PGE$_1$, followed by surgery

Endocardial cushion defect

- Most common congenital heart lesion in **Down syndrome**

- ASD and VSD with atrioventricular (AV) valve insufficiency

- Physical exam—**precordial lift; loud S1; wide, fixed-split S2; systolic ejection murmur and low-pitched diastolic rumble**

- Diagnosis—chest x-ray shows cardiomegaly, echo is gold standard

- Treatment—surgical correction as soon as possible before onset of heart failure

8

Hypoplastic left heart

- Underdeveloped mitral/aortic valve, left ventricle, and ascending aorta → right ventricle becomes responsible for all pulmonary and systemic blood flow → left atrial blood transfers to right atrium → mixing of venous and oxygenated blood

- Clinical—**dusky blue skin** when **PDA closes**, right parasternal lift

- Treatment—surgical repair, search for other major malformations (common; if present, surgery may not be worth it)

Patent ductus arteriosus (PDA)

- Increased risk in **females, congenital rubella syndrome, and prematurity**

- Clinical presentation—**"machinery"-like, to-and-fro murmur; bounding peripheral pulses and widened pulse pressure**

- Treatment—indomethacin

Tetralogy of Fallot

- Four components: pulmonary stenosis + VSD + overriding aorta + right ventricular hypertrophy

- Most common cyanotic heart lesion

- Clinical findings—older children exhibit characteristic behavior when not corrected
  - ▶ **"Tet spells"**—acute restlessness and panic, gasping, followed by syncope
    - ▷ Treatment—place in lateral knee-to-chest position; give O_2, morphine, and beta-blockers
  - ▶ Dyspnea on exertion—**squat to feel better**

- Physical exam findings—variable types of murmur; it is most important to know clinical findings described above

- Diagnosis—chest x-ray shows **boot-shaped heart**; ECG shows right axis deviation; echo is gold standard

- Treatment
  - PGE$_1$ to maintain PDA
  - Perform Blalock-Taussig shunt as soon as possible (systemic to pulmonary shunt)
  - Follow with elective valvulotomy, patching of VSD, and myomectomy at 4–12 months of age

Total anomalous pulmonary venous return

- All four pulmonary veins connect to systemic venous blood flow; **no survival unless ASD or patent foramen ovale** is present
- Cyanosis and tachypnea; confirm with echo
- Give immediate PGE$_1$, followed by surgery

Transposition of the great vessels

- Increased risk in infants of diabetic mothers
- Aorta arises from the right ventricle, and pulmonary artery enters the left ventricle; requires a PDA and patent foramen ovale for survival
- Clinical presentation—severe cyanosis with closure of PDA; may or may not have systolic ejection murmur
- Diagnosis—narrow base of heart with absence of main pulmonary artery segment gives an **"egg on a string"** appearance to the chest x-ray
- Treatment—PGE$_1$, followed by surgical correction

Truncus arteriosus

- Single arterial vessel sits over a VSD receiving left and right ventricular blood
- Clinical presentation—minimal cyanosis, wide pulse pressure, bounding pulses, and hyperdynamic precordium
- Diagnosis—echo is gold standard
- Treatment—surgical correction after medically stabilized

8

ENDOCRINOLOGY

Normal Growth: Chronological Age (CA) and Bone Age (BA)

Best evaluated by comparing chronologic age (CA, the child's actual age) with bone age (BA, determined from wrist x-ray) and growth velocity (either normal or abnormal)

Adrenal Disorders

Congenital adrenal hyperplasia (CAH)

- All are from autosomal recessive inheritance
- 21-hydroxylase deficiency
  - ▸ The most common of all CAH disorders
  - ▸ Accumulation of serum **17-hydroxy-progesterone** (best initial test is morning serum level); gold standard is to measure before and after a bolus of adrenocorticotropic hormone (ACTH) if initial serum screening is high
    - ▹ Shunting to androgen synthesis → pseudohermaphroditism in females
    - ▹ Decreased cortisol production → increased ACTH causes adrenal hyperplasia
      - – Salt loss → **hypotension and hyponatremia**
      - – Inability to excrete potassium from renal tubules → **hyperkalemia**
  - ▸ Treatment—hydrocortisone plus fludrocortisone (if salt-losing) supplementation; must **increase** dosages during stress (infection, surgery, etc.)
- 11-beta-hydroxylase deficiency
  - ▸ Clinical features—female pseudohermaphroditism or penile enlargement in neonates, postnatal virilization (usually in teenage years) in 50% of cases, **HTN, hypokalemia**
  - ▸ Diagnosis—increased random serum **11-deoxycortisol** (best initial test), **11-deoxycorticosterone**, dehydroepiandrosterone (DHEA), DHEA sulfate, androstenedione, and testosterone;

increased urinary concentrations of 11-deoxycortisol and 11-deoxycorticosterone

▷ Increased serum 11-deoxycortisol before and after ACTH stimulation is gold standard

▷ Increased urinary metabolites more helpful in neonatal diagnosis

- Treatment—hydrocortisone best initial therapy; spironolactone or amiloride if HTN persists

Cushing syndrome

- Most common cause of exogenous origin is glucocorticoid administration; endogenous causes include adrenal tumors or pituitary producing adenoma

  ▶ If due to adenoma secreting ACTH → termed **Cushing disease**

- Clinical—moon facies, abdominal striae, ecchymosis, buffalo hump and truncal obesity, delayed puberty and growth, hyperglycemia, and osteoporosis

- Diagnosis and treatment—the diagnostic algorithm is the same for both adults and children (see Cushing Syndrome, page 77) likewise, the treatment is also the same

Diabetes Mellitus

See the discussion of type 1 diabetes, type 2 diabetes, and metabolic syndrome starting on page 84.

Parathyroid Disorders

- Hypoparathyroidism

  ▶ Multiple etiologies from aplasia/hypoplasia to genetic to autoimmune

  ▶ Clinical presentation related to **hypocalcemia**, including muscle cramps, **perioral numbness**, tingling, positive Trousseau signs, **seizures**

8

▶ Labs—decreased serum calcium and increased serum phosphorus (best initial tests); follow with serum parathyroid hormone (will be low); vitamin D will also be low; **rule out** hypomagnesemia (exacerbates symptoms)

▶ Treatment—based upon severity of clinical presentation
  ▷ Tetany/seizures → IV calcium gluconate, followed by calcitriol
  ▷ Hypocalcemia without emergent signs/symptoms or maintenance therapy → calcitriol or vitamin D_2 plus calcium-rich, low-phosphate diet

Pituitary Disorders

● Hypopituitarism
  ▶ May be congenital or acquired
  ▶ Deficiency of growth hormone with or without other hormones
  ▶ Clinical presentation
    ▷ Congenital—severe growth failure in first year of life and dysmorphic features
    ▷ Acquired—more gradual onset with nonspecific findings including FTT, sensitivity to cold, hypoglycemia, etc.
      – If **craniopharyngioma** is present, will also have **headache, visual changes**, etc.
  ▶ Diagnosis—each hormone you think is deficient should be tested individually; for example, ACTH and thyroid-stimulating hormone (TSH) if you think there are components of adrenal insufficiency and hypothyroidism
  ▶ Treatment—based upon results of deficiencies, supplement as needed

Precocious Puberty

● Defined as onset of sexual development in girls <8 years old or boys <9 years old

Diagnosis and Management of Precocious Puberty

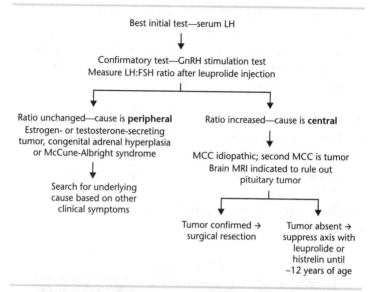

Best initial test—serum LH

Confirmatory test—GnRH stimulation test
Measure LH:FSH ratio after leuprolide injection

Ratio unchanged—cause is **peripheral**
Estrogen- or testosterone-secreting
tumor, congenital adrenal hyperplasia
or McCune-Albright syndrome

Search for underlying
cause based on other
clinical symptoms

Ratio increased—cause is **central**

MCC idiopathic; second MCC is tumor
Brain MRI indicated to rule out
pituitary tumor

Tumor confirmed →
surgical resection

Tumor absent →
suppress axis with
leuprolide or
histrelin until
~12 years of age

Abbreviations: follicle-stimulating hormone, FSH; gonadotropin-releasing hormone, GnRH; luteinizing hormone, LH; most common cause, MCC

- Incomplete precocious puberty is defined as early onset of either thelarche, adrenarche, or menarche (rare); most common cause is normal variant, and patients usually have positive family history
- In those without positive family history, follow up closely for onset of complete precocious puberty

Thyroid Disorders

Congenital hypothyroidism

- Mandatory neonatal screening in place in all U.S. states, so incidence of cretinism is rare
- Clinical presentation—prolonged jaundice, **macroglossia**, umbilical hernia, **edema, mental and developmental retardation**, widened anterior and posterior fontanels, generalized hypotonia

Acquired hypothyroidism

- For diagnosis and treatment, see Hypothyroidism, page 72
- Important points—most common age of onset is **adolescence**; increased incidence in Down syndrome, Klinefelter syndrome, Turner syndrome, congenital rubella syndrome, and other coexisting rheumatologic disorders

Hyperthyroidism

- Most common cause is Graves disease (same as adults), and most commonly presents in early teenage years
- For diagnosis and treatment, see Hyperthyroidism, page 73

Multiple Endocrine Neoplasia (MEN)

You must know these disorders.

MEN Syndromes

Type	Clinical Findings
MEN Type IIA	• Thyroid hyperplasia/malignancy • Adrenal hyperplasia/ pheochromocytoma • **Parathyroid hyperplasia**
MEN Type IIB	• Multiple **superficial neuromas** • Medullary thyroid cancer • Pheochromocytoma

GASTROENTEROLOGY

Newborn Gastrointestinal Disease

Meconium ileus

- Impacted meconium leads to intestinal obstruction; seen with **cystic fibrosis**
- Best initial test—abdominal x-ray shows bowel loop distention; may follow with barium enema revealing small colon distal to obstruction
- Treatment—**Gastrografin enema**

Meconium plug

- First passage of very hard and sticky meconium; associated with IODM, Hirschsprung disease, cystic fibrosis, and maternal opioid use

Necrotizing enterocolitis (NEC)

- Premature infants develop **transmural intestinal necrosis** soon **after introduction of food**; symptoms of **bloody stools, apnea, and abdominal distension** develop
- Best initial test—abdominal x-ray; **pneumatosis intestinalis pathognomic** (air bubbles within bowel wall) of NEC
- Treatment—**stop feeds**, IV antibiotics, supportive care; surgical removal of necrotic bowel

Hirschsprung disease

- Most common cause of bowel obstruction in neonates
- Aganglionic distal colon and rectum → failure to pass stool **48 hours** after birth
- Best initial test—**rectal manometry**
  - ▸ Barium enema may reveal **megacolon** proximal to obstruction
- Most accurate test—rectal suction biopsy confirms absence of neural ganglion
- Treatment—surgical resection of aganglionic bowel

Duodenal atresia

- **Bilious vomiting** after **first feeding**
- Best initial test—abdominal x-ray shows **"double-bubble sign"**
- Treatment—surgical correction

Imperforate anus

- **Failure to pass stool** after birth
- Physical exam reveals absence of anal canal (examiner is **unable to pass a cotton swab** into the rectum)

8

- No further diagnostic tests needed
- Treatment—surgical correction

Gastroesophageal reflux disease (GERD)

- Most common in first few months of age, and resolves by 1–2 years of age
- Clinical findings—**frequent "spit-ups" immediately after feeding**, irritability, cough, wheezing, episodes of apnea
- Diagnosis—history and physical adequate in most; best test is esophageal pH monitoring
- Management—**thicken feeds and give smaller, more frequent meals first**; education for parents on position of feeding
  - If this fails—H_2 blockers are first-line pharmacotherapy, then proton pump inhibitors (PPIs) if these fail; surgery is only for most severe cases (rarely required)

Pyloric stenosis

- Most common in **first-born males**, Northern European descent
- Clinical presentation—**nonbilious projectile vomiting** after feeding at approximately **2–8 weeks of age**, constant hunger and desire to feed; palpable **olive-shaped epigastric mass**
- Diagnosis—best test is **ultrasound** (hypertrophic pylorus looks **"target-like"** in cross-section)
- Treatment—**pyloromyotomy**

Childhood Gastrointestinal Disease

Celiac disease

- See also page 121
- Most are Caucasians age 6 months to 2 years with genetic predisposition to intolerance (HLA-DQ2) of **gluten**-containing products including rye, wheat, and barley
- Symptoms of **malabsorption** most prominent with symptoms of **select vitamin deficiencies**, especially **iron deficiency anemia**;

major clue to diagnosis is presence of **dermatitis herpetiformis**, an itchy, papulovesicular eruption located symmetrically on extensor surfaces

- Diagnosis
  - ▸ Best initial test—**antiendomysial** and **antigliadin** antibodies
  - ▸ Gold standard—small-intestine biopsy reveals flattened villi
- Treatment—complete abstinence of all gluten-containing products for **life**

Constipation

- Common in school-age children, due to voluntary withholding of stool
- Physical exam reveals stool palpable in cecum/suprapubic region; rectal exam reveals full rectal vault
- Treatment—manual disimpaction, enemas, and/or stool softeners
  - ▸ Education on bowel training and instruction not to withhold stool is important

Diarrhea

- See also Infectious Diarrhea, page 118
- First step is to determine acute (usually <5 days) vs. chronic (>1 month) diarrhea to narrow differential
- Epidemiology and history extremely important in narrowing the DDx
- Causes of diarrhea in children and adults are very similar and most organisms are the same
- Algorithmic management of acute diarrhea based on history
  - ▸ Febrile + nonbloody diarrhea → viral enteritis most common cause
  - ▸ Afebrile + nonbloody diarrhea → viral enteritis most common cause
  - ▸ Febrile + bloody diarrhea → infectious enteritis most common cause

8

► Afebrile + bloody diarrhea → most worrisome, think of intussusception, hemolytic uremic syndrome (HUS), and pseudomembranous colitis

- **Rotavirus** infection is the most common cause of acute viral enteritis in children (followed by enterovirus)

- Cases of infectious bacterial enteritis have the same epidemiology as adult diarrhea

  ► Consider antimicrobial therapy **only** when suspicion is very high and children appear **toxic** and are **acutely febrile** (antimicrobial therapy differs in children <17 years of age because fluoroquinolones cannot be used); base choice of parenteral versus oral therapy on clinical grounds

  ▷ Initial parental therapy—ceftriaxone

  ▷ Initial oral therapy—trimethoprim-sulfamethoxazole (TMP-SMX) plus ampicillin

Intussusception

- Ileocolic telescoping of bowel; Meckel diverticulum is a common lead-point

- Clinical presentation—age 3 months to 2 years (80% of cases); have sudden onset of **black, "currant jelly" stools; colicky abdominal pain**; usually **draw the feet up to the chest**; may have history of **recent URI**

- Physical exam—**sausage-shaped mass in right lower quadrant (RLQ)**

- Diagnosis—**ultrasound** is best initial test; abdominal plain film is second-line

- Treatment—pneumatic or hydrostatic enema reduces lesion in most; surgery if this fails

Meckel diverticulum

- Remnant of the yolk sac contains **gastric tissues**—secretion of acid causes **intermittent, painless rectal bleeding**

- Follow the "rule of 2's"—**2 years of age, 2% of the population, 2 types of tissue, 2 cm long, and 2 feet from the ileocecal valve**
- Diagnosis—**Meckel radionucleotide scan**
- Treatment—surgical removal

HEMATOLOGY

Anemia of Chronic Disease

- Most often seen in the setting of adult medicine but may be seen in those with juvenile rheumatoid arthritis (JRA), etc.
- Normocytic anemia with sequestration of iron stores in bone marrow
- Primary treatment and diagnosis are the same as in adults—treating the underlying cause is the most important factor

Blackfan-Diamond Syndrome

- Congenital **pure red blood cell aplasia** due to programmed cell death—exact mechanism not known
- Clinical presentation—**triphalangeal thumbs**, short stature, **tow-colored hair** (very fair to blond hair), **snub nose**, wide-set eyes, thick upper lip, and an "intelligent expression"
- Labs—**profound macrocytic anemia** by 2–4 months of age (hemoglobin often 4–6.5 mg/dL on CBC), normal bone marrow cellularity with **decreased red blood cell (RBC) precursors**; increased RBC adenosine deaminase (ADA) activity
- Treatment—**prednisone** is best initial therapy; if ineffective or too toxic, you must transfuse every 4–6 weeks instead
- Bone marrow transplantation may be curative

Beta-Thalassemia Major (Cooley Anemia)

- Absence of beta chains leads to formation of **alpha-chain tetramers**; physiologic increase in hemoglobin F (alpha + gamma chains)

8

- Presents around **second month of life** when hemoglobin A (alpha + beta chains) would normally increase → infants have **severe anemia (hemoglobin 3–4 mg/dL)** and hepatosplenomegaly
- Increase in medullary hematopoiesis leads to thickening of bones, especially in **face and skull**
- Diagnosis
  - ▸ Best initial test is peripheral smear—**profound microcytosis** (MCV often **60–65 µg/dL**; versus iron deficiency, which is usually in the 70 µg/dL range); hypochromia, **Heinz bodies**, teardrop and target cells
  - ▸ Gold standard is hemoglobin electrophoresis which shows presence of hemoglobin F **only**
- Treatment—**transfusions**, followed by **deferoxamine** to treat iron overload; bone marrow transplant is **curative**
- Mortality/morbidity—most will die of hemochromatosis or infection in adolescence
- More susceptible to infection with *Yersinia enterocolitica* (iron-loving organism—iron-overloaded patients), a major cause of sepsis

Alpha-Thalassemia (Hemoglobin H Disease)

- Absence of alpha chains leads to formation of **beta-chain tetramers**; causes formation of **hemoglobin H**
- Hemolysis occurs **throughout gestation and birth**, so infants have jaundice and hyperbilirubinemia at birth; some may die in utero of **hydrops fetalis**
- Clinical features—resembles beta-thalassemia, except **less severe**
- Diagnosis—peripheral smear is the best initial test; follow with hemoglobin electrophoresis to confirm (shows presence of hemoglobin H)
- Treatment—transfusions and splenectomy not required until second to third decade of life; transfusions most often needed during time of oxidant stress (infection, etc.) when hemolysis is more likely; treat iron overload with deferoxime

Fanconi Anemia (Congenital Pancytopenia)

- Pathophysiology—spontaneous chromosomal breaks during embryogenesis
- Clinical—usually diagnosed between 6 and 9 years of age
  - **Hyperpigmentation, café-au-lait spots, hypoplastic thumbs, short stature, hypogonadism**, with or without other major organ defects
- Diagnosis—**pancytopenia with macrocytosis**, increased **hemoglobin F** ("stress" erythropoiesis); bone marrow biopsy reveals **marrow hypoplasia; increased alpha-fetoprotein**
  - Gold standard—chromosomal breakage in cultured cells
- Treatment—**androgens (oxymetholone)** with or without **granulocyte colony-stimulating factor** until bone marrow transplant can be performed (curative); transfuse as needed
- Mortality/morbidity—**increased risk of leukemia** and bone marrow failure

Glucose-6-Phosphate Dehydrogenase (G6PD) Deficiency

- X-linked—males most severely affected
- Episodic hemolysis after exposure to oxidant stressors—aspirin, sulfa drugs, antimalarial drugs, fava beans, diabetic ketoacidosis, etc.
- Congenitally acquired form often more severe than acute hemolytic G6PD deficiency
- Diagnosis
  - Best initial test is peripheral smear showing **Heinz bodies and bite cells**
  - Most accurate test is the fluorescent spot test (measures G6PD activity)
- Treatment
  - Prevention and disease education is the most important step
  - Treat acute hemolysis with transfusion as needed

8

Hemophilia A and B

- Hemophilia A
  - ▸ X-linked deficiency of **factor VIII**
  - ▸ Clinical—easy bruisability with crawling first noted as toddlers; hallmark finding is **hemarthroses** with minimal trauma; may have intramuscular hemorrhage with hematoma formation
  - ▸ Diagnosis—**partial thromboplastin time (PTT) is 2–3 times the reference range**; all other lab values are **normal**; follow with a **mixing study**, which will correct the PTT
    - ▹ Gold standard—specific factor VIII assay
  - ▸ Treatment
    - ▹ Mild bleeding/surgical prophylaxis—desmopressin
    - ▹ Severe bleeding—factor VIII replacement
- Hemophilia B
  - ▸ X-linked deficiency of **factor IX**
  - ▸ Clinical—same as hemophilia A
  - ▸ Diagnosis—same as hemophilia A except specific factor IX assay done instead
  - ▸ Treatment—monoclonal or recombinant factor IX is the treatment of choice; next-best choice is plasma-derived factor concentrates
- Important points about hemophilia A and B
  - ▸ Avoidance of aspirin and other antiplatelet medications is paramount
  - ▸ If repeat hemarthroses ("target joint")—treat with joint aspiration as needed to relieve pain, and a short course of prednisone to relieve inflammation

Hereditary Spherocytosis

- Autosomal dominant deficiency of **spectrin** → loss of biconcave shape → early splenic phagocytosis

- Clinical—anemia/hyperbilirubinemia, hypersplenism, and gallstones in newborns/early childhood; wide variety of clinical severity

- Diagnosis—best initial test is peripheral smear showing **spherocytes**; confirm with **osmotic fragility test**

- Treatment—**splenectomy**; plus cholecystectomy if positive for gallstones

Immune Thrombocytopenic Purpura

- Autoimmune development of **IgG antibodies against platelets** leads to peripheral destruction and thrombocytopenia

- Most often follows an **acute viral illness**

- Clinical—sudden onset of **petechiae and purpura**, rare cases of intracranial hemorrhage

- Diagnosis—largely clinical and based on history and physical, peripheral smear, and CBC
  - ▸ Peripheral smear reveals normal to increased size of platelets
  - ▸ Bone marrow biopsy indicated only if chronic—increased megakaryocytes

- Treatment
  - ▸ Acute idiopathic thrombocytopenic purpura (ITP)— **intravenous immunoglobulin (IVIG) is the drug of choice (DOC)** (shown to increase platelet numbers better); may add or switch to corticosteroids if ineffective
  - ▸ Chronic ITP—supportive measures, most resolve spontaneously

8

Iron Deficiency Anemia

- Think of iron deficiency in the following:
  - ▸ Infants age 9–24 months who consume **cow's milk** and little iron-enriched food
    - ▹ Breast milk has the best bioavailability of iron
    - ▹ Formula should be enriched with iron

- ► Teenagers more susceptible during **growth spurt, menstruation**
- Lab—microcytic anemia
- Diagnosis
  - ► Best initial test—serum ferritin (will be **low**)
  - ► Gold standard—bone marrow biopsy (rarely used)
- Treatment—**oral ferrous sulfate**, increase dietary iron, use iron enriched formula

Lead Poisoning

- Normal blood lead level is zero; departments of health put their greatest effort into cases where the blood lead level exceeds 10 µg/dL
- Suspect in children of **low socioeconomic status, in inner-city housing, with "peeling paint" on walls, in families of painters** (more common in developing countries that do not use lead-free paint)
- Clinical—changes in pattern of normal behavior, stomach pain, constipation, **lead lines** on gums (bluish discoloration at the gum line), **conjunctival pallor**
- Diagnosis—initial tests can include x-rays (showing lead lines at metaphyseal plates), radiopacity in the GI tract on abdominal x-ray (from recent ingestion of paint)
- Treatment
  - ► Entirely dependent on blood level and **very high-yield** for the exam
  - ► In **all** children with an elevated blood level, mandatory parental education and evaluation for the possible source is required

Approach to Serum Blood Lead Levels

Blood Lead Level	Treatment
10–14 µg/dL	• Repeat at 1 month to confirm • Repeat at 3 months to monitor • Screen other household members
15–19 µg/dL	• Repeat at 1 month to confirm • Repeat at 2 months to monitor • Screen other household members • Refer to the Department of Health
20–44 µg/dL	• Repeat at 1 month • Provide lead hazard training • Consider starting oral DMSA (also called succimer) or oral penicillamine treatment
45–70 µg/dL	• Most should be hospitalized (remove from potentially hazardous environment) • Give parenteral EDTA therapy to ensure compliance if patient is very young • Give oral therapy with DMSA if compliance is not an issue
>70 µg/dL	• Considered a medical emergency • Immediate hospitalization is required • Treat with intramuscular dimercaprol *plus* parenteral EDTA

Abbreviations: dimercaptosulfuric acid, DMSA; ethylenediaminetetraacetic acid, EDTA

Macrocytic Anemia

- See also page 127
- Children are more likely to be deficient in folate than in B-12
- Folate deficiency—suspect in mothers feeding infants solely with **goat's milk**
- Vitamin B-12 deficiency—suspect in **vegans**; pernicious anemia rare in children
- Both folate-deficiency and B-12 deficiency are diagnosed with correspondingly decreased serum levels and treated with adequate supplementation

8

Physiologic Anemia

Intrauterine hypoxia stimulates erythropoietin; downregulation of erythropoietin after birth produces a progressive decline in serum hemoglobin within the first 2–3 months of life with gradual return to baseline.

Sickle-Cell Anemia

- Autosomal recessive—glutamic acid is replaced with valine
- "Sickling" during stress (infection, fever, hypoxia, acidosis)—microvascular occlusions
- Newborns asymptomatic until hemoglobin F is replaced with hemoglobin A at **2–4 months of age**
- Functional asplenia by 5–6 years of age
- Clinical—**acute dactylitis** (necrosis of small bones) is most common initial presentation; acute splenic sequestration is second most common presentation
    - ▸ Symptoms **progress more centrally with age**—chest (acute chest syndrome), head (stroke), back (vertebral infarction), abdomen, and penis (priapism)
- Most common cause of death—acute chest syndrome and sepsis
- Diagnosis
    - ▸ Best initial test is peripheral smear showing sickle cells
    - ▸ Best confirmatory test is hemoglobin electrophoresis
- Treatment
    - ▸ Hydroxyurea is the mainstay of treatment; add erythropoietin if this fails
    - ▸ Regular immunizations plus pneumococcal vaccination are important
        - ▹ Add penicillin prophylaxis starting at age 2 months to 5 years
    - ▸ Folate supplementation

- Recommended screening tests
  - ▸ Monitor cerebral blood flow with transcranial Doppler annually to assess stroke risk
  - ▸ Annual retinal examination

Shwachman-Diamond Syndrome

- Rare autosomal recessive disorder
- **Triad of exocrine pancreatic insufficiency, bone marrow failure, and skeletal abnormalities**
  - ▸ Second most common cause of pancreatic insufficiency in children, after cystic fibrosis
- Treatment—manage complications, no cure

INFECTIOUS DISEASE

Candidal Infection

The difference between diaper rash and candida is important.

Infant Dermatitis

Diagnosis	Candida Diaper Dermatitis	Irritant Diaper Dermatitis
Clinical findings	• Occurs when irritant dermatitis is left untreated for >3 days • **Involves intergluteal folds** • Clinically, presents with **beefy-red plaques,** papules, and **pustules** leaving a scale after rupture • Diagnosis: clinical; KOH prep not needed	• Wide range of severity, from erythema to papules to erosions • **Spares intergluteal folds** • Diagnosis: clinical
Treatment	Topical nystatin or clotrimazole	Topical petrolatum or zinc oxide paste; diaper "holidays"

8

Cat-Scratch Disease (*Bartonella henselae*)

- Transmission from scratch of **a kitten or a cat that is less than 1 year of age**
- Clinical—**red-white papules**, 3–5 mm, along the **scratch site** with local **lymphadenitis** and other nonspecific systemic signs of infection
  - ▸ Parinaud oculoglandular syndrome—occurs when scratch is near or in the eye
    - ▹ **Unilateral conjunctivitis**, conjunctival granuloma, and **preauricular lymphadenopathy**
- Diagnosis—confirm with *B. henselae* antibody titer (required due to difficulty of growing in routine culture media)
  - ▸ If titer is inconclusive—Warthin-Starry stain or polymerase chain reaction (PCR) analysis of tissue biopsy
- Treatment—antibiotic treatment highly debated (condition is usually self-limited) except in disseminated disease or the immunocompromised. Self–resolving in most by 2–4 months.
  - ▸ Drug of choice—**azithromycin**
  - ▸ Alternatives are clarithromycin, rifampin, TMP-SMX

Epstein-Barr Virus (Infectious Mononucleosis)

- "Kissing disease"; most commonly presents in teenagers/young adults
- Clinical—insidious onset of generalized **fatigue** and nonspecific findings; hallmark is **generalized adenopathy, splenomegaly**, and **exudative pharyngitis**
  - ▸ **Maculopapular rash** after taking **ampicillin or amoxicillin**
- Diagnosis—peripheral smear shows **atypical lymphocytosis** (Downey cells)
  - ▸ Approach to management
    - ▹ If heterophil antibody test (initial test of choice) positive → treat
    - ▹ If heterophil antibody test negative + high clinical suspicion → get IgM antibody to viral capsid antigen (most specific)

- Mortality/morbidity
  - ▸ Increased risk of malignancy: **Burkitt lymphoma** and **nasopharyngeal carcinoma**
  - ▸ **No** contact sports until splenomegaly resolves (~6 weeks)
- Treatment—supportive care; if impending airway obstruction or severe illness, give steroids and consult ear, nose, and throat specialist as soon as possible

Helminthic Infections

Organism	Transmission	Clinical Findings	Diagnosis	Treatment
Ascariasis (*Ascaris lumbricoides*)	Soil contamination (with feces) leading to cutaneous entry of larvae	• Travels to lungs: **Loeffler syndrome** • Triad of cough, blood-tinged sputum, eosinophilia; possible intestinal obstruction	Fecal smear	• DOC: mebendazole • Alternatives: albendazole, ivermectin, or nitazoxanide
Hookworms (*Ancyclostoma and Necator*)	As above	• Intense pruritus at site of cutaneous entry; hook into intestine and feed off host blood → anemia, eosinophilia, abdominal pain • Chlorosis: green-yellow skin in chronic infection	Fecal smear	Albendazole, mebendazole, and pyrantel pamoate all acceptable
Enterobiasis; "pinworms" (*Enterobius vermicularis*)	Ingestion of eggs from contaminated sources (fingernails, bedding, etc.)	Inhabits the colon; deposition of eggs around rectum at night leads to **severe perianal pruritus** (kids scratch their anal areas); **no** eosinophilia	**Scotch-tape test** on rectum at night shows eggs	Albendazole, mebendazole, and pyrantel pamoate all acceptable

8

(continued)

Helminthic Infections (continued)

Organism	Transmission	Clinical Findings	Diagnosis	Treatment
Trichinosis (*Trichinella spiralis*)	Ingestion of raw or under-cooked pork	• Travel to **striated muscle** and **encyst** • Triad of **periorbital edema, myositis, and eosinophilia;** may cause CNS disease (multifocal small white lesions in cortex/white matter)	• Best initial test: serology (ELISA most common) • Gold standard: muscle biopsy	• Supportive **unless** positive CNS, cardiac, or pulmonary disease • DOC: mebendazole or albendazole
Trichuriasis; "whip-worm" (*Trichuris trichiura*)	Soil contamination	• Loves the **cecum** • **Right lower quadrant or periumbilical pain; rectal prolapse; no** eosinophilia • May mimic inflammatory bowel disease	Fecal smear	• Mebendazole is first-line • Albendazole or ivermectin are also effective

Abbreviations: central nervous system, CNS; drug of choice, DOC; enzyme-linked immunosorbent assay, ELISA

Influenza

- Types A and B responsible for epidemic disease; attacks occur in fall and winter months

- Clinical—abrupt onset of **coryza, conjunctivitis, pharyngitis**, nonproductive cough, and moderate-to-severe systemic signs/symptoms (fatigue, **myalgias**, headache, and **fever**)

- Diagnosis—best initial test is **reverse transcriptase PCR (RT-PCR)** testing of **nasopharyngeal swab**; if negative and clinical suspicion is high, do a viral culture or serologic testing with ELISA

- Treatment—DOC is **neuraminidase inhibitors** (such as oseltamivir) ideally administered orally during the first 48 hours of symptoms; supportive care
  - ▸ Amantadine and rimantadine are **not** first-line therapy due to the high rate of resistance of influenza A viruses
  - ▸ Mortality/morbidity—pneumonia most feared; also otitis media, secondary bacterial infection, etc.; drug therapy highly recommended in those at risk of severe disease

Ophthalmia Neonatorum and Conjunctivitis

- Ophthalmia neonatorum
  - ▸ For the boards, knowing the **onset of symptoms** is most important in determining cause (see the Newborn Conjunctivitis table)
  - ▸ **Gram stain and culture** of discharge is required for diagnosis of suspected gonococcal or chlamydial infection, and the patient must be hospitalized and monitored for response to treatment

Newborn Conjunctivitis

Diagnosis	Clinical Findings	Treatment
Chemical conjunctivitis	Onset in first 24 hours after birth (from topical erythromycin or silver nitrate given after birth); **conjunctival injection with serous discharge**	Supportive
Gonococcal conjunctivitis	Onset **within 1 week** of birth; **purulent discharge**	• **IM or IV ceftriaxone** and copious saline irrigation • Complications if left untreated: **corneal ulceration,** iridocyclitis
Chlamydial conjunctivitis	Onset **within 2 weeks** of birth; **purulent discharge**	• **Oral erythromycin** and copious saline irrigation • Complications: **corneal ulceration/scarring, blindness**

8

Childhood Conjunctivitis

Diagnosis	Clinical Findings	Treatment
Bacterial conjunctivitis	**Unilateral purulent discharge** with **conjunctival injection**	• **Topical** ciprofloxacin ophthalmic drops + warm compresses • **Highly contagious**; keep child home from school until treatment started
Viral conjunctivitis	**Bilateral serous discharge** and conjunctival **injection; systemic** symptoms of URI	Supportive (adenovirus and enteroviruses most common causes)

Allergic conjunctivitis	**Bilateral serous discharge** and conjunctival **injection** and **rhinorrhea, sneezing; seasonal onset**	• **Avoidance** most important
		• For symptomatic relief:
		  – Topical vasoconstrictor/ antihistamine such as naphazoline (Visine®) is first-line
		  – More refractory symptoms: topical antihistamine/mast cell stabilizer such as olopatadine (Patanol®)

Chemical conjunctivitis	**Acute, extensive tissue damage** from exposure to cleaners, smoke, etc.	**Copious saline irrigation** with initial contact; ophthalmology consult

Abbreviations: upper respiratory infection, URI

Otitis Externa and Otitis Media

8

- Otitis externa/"swimmer's ear"
  - ► Causes—excessive moisture (swimming), dryness, **diabetes** (more common in adults)
  - ► Etiology (in descending order of frequency)—***Pseudomonas aeruginosa*** → *Staphylococcus aureus* → *Staph. epidermidis*
  - ► Clinical—**severe pain** with **manipulation of outer ear** with or without conductive hearing loss, **otorrhea, edema, erythema**
    - ▷ **Malignant otitis externa (beware of in immuno-compromised children)**—extension into temporal bone and base of skull; diagnosis with CT scan (plus cultures); requires hospitalization, **IV ciprofloxacin (add amphotericin B if *Aspergillus* is suspected) for 6–8 weeks**

> ► Treatment—simple otitis externa is treated with combination of topical ciprofloxacin, steroid, and antiseptic eardrops
>> ▷ If severe edema—use soaked **wick** three times daily for 2 days and follow with cleaning/drops as above

- Otitis media
  - ► Most common in children due to straighter eustachian tube alignment—easier entry for bacteria
  - ► Etiology (in descending order of frequency)—*Streptococcus pneumonia* → *nontypeable Haemophilus influenzae* → *Moraxella catarrhalis*
  - ► Clinical—must distinguish between acute otitis media and otitis media with effusion
  - ► Treatment—see the Treatment of Otitis Media table

Treatment of Otitis Media

Acute Otitis Media	Otitis Media with Effusion
DOC: **amoxicillin** (In penicillin-allergic patient: If type I rxn: macrolide; if non-type I rxn: cephalosporin) ↓	Monthly follow-up with hearing test in 3 months if no improvement ↓
No improvement in 2–3 days—use second-line drug ↓	Tympanostomy tubes if: • 6–12 months of bilateral OME • 4 months of OME with evidence of hearing loss
Oral amoxicillin-clavulanate or IM ceftriaxone (if not taking oral meds) ↓	
If no improvement: tympanocentesis for culture and sensitivity	

Abbreviations: otitis media with effusion, OME; reaction, rxn

Complications of otitis media

- Acute mastoiditis—suspect when **pinna is displaced** inferior and anterior; **pain with percussion of mastoid process**; get immediate **CT scan of temporal bone**

- ► Treatment based on CT findings
  - ▷ Evidence of inflammation without bone destruction → myringotomy + IV antibiotics
  - ▷ Evidence of bone destruction → mastoidectomy + IV antibiotics

- • Cholesteatoma—cystic growth in middle ear or temporal bone with possible expansion intracranially
  - ► Clinical findings—**localized white opacity of tympanic membrane (TM)**, polypoid growth from TM with or without malodorous discharge; confirm diagnosis with **CT scan** of temporal bone
  - ► Treatment—surgical resection

Osteomyelitis and Septic Arthritis

- • Etiology
  - ► Osteomyelitis—***Staph. aureus*** most common cause overall; Group B *Strep.*, *Strep. pneumoniae*, and *Kingella* are also common
    - ▷ In **sickle-cell** disease—increased incidence of ***Salmonella*** (*Staph. aureus* still most common cause)

Diagnosis and Management of Osteomyelitis

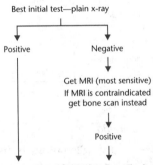

Best initial test—plain x-ray

Positive   Negative

Get MRI (most sensitive)
If MRI is contraindicated
get bone scan instead

Positive

Get bone biopsy, then start empiric therapy until cultures available
Best choice—third-generation cephalosporin + vancomycin

Note: If therapy cannot be delayed (soft tissue infection, sepsis), it may skew culture results.

▷ **Puncture wounds** as portal of entry—increased incidence of *Pseudomonas aeruginosa* infection

▸ Septic arthritis—*Staph. aureus* most common cause

- Clinical—same for both diseases, so children have erythema, decreased movement, refusal to walk, with variable degrees of systemic features of infection

- Diagnosis and management—see Diagnosis and Management of Osteomyelitis algorithm on the preceding page

Bacterial Meningitis

- Key concepts

  ▸ Any child suspected of having *H. influenzae* meningitis should receive a dose of dexamethasone 1 hour prior to starting antibiotics → proven to decrease mortality

  ▸ If no evidence of focal neurologic deficits and child is not toxic-appearing—get a lumbar puncture first, then start antibiotics

  ▸ If child is toxic-appearing with focal neurologic deficits or with known immune deficiency—give stat dose of antibiotics → get stat CT scan of the head → then get a lumbar puncture

  ▸ Obtain lumbar punctures every 24–48 hours until CSF is documented to be sterile

Epidemiology of Meningitis in Children

Age	Most Common Cause	Empiric Treatment
<1 month	Group B *Streptococcus* → *Escherichia coli* → *Listeria*	• 0–7 days of age: ampicillin plus gentamicin • >7 days of age: ampicillin, gentamicin, and cefotaxime (extend gram-negative coverage)
1 month–2 years	*Strep. pneumoniae* → *Neisseria meningitidis*	Third-generation cephalosporin (cefotaxime, ceftriaxone) plus vancomycin

(continued)

8

Epidemiology of Meningitis in Children (continued)

Age	Most Common Cause	Empiric Treatment
2 years–18 years	*N. meningitides* → *Strep. pneumoniae* → *Haemophilus influenzae* type B	Third-generation cephalosporin (cefotaxime, ceftriaxone) plus vancomycin
Adults	*Strep. pneumoniae*	Third-generation cephalosporin (cefotaxime, ceftriaxone) plus vancomycin

Organism specific therapy of bacterial meningitis

- Group B *Streptococcus*—penicillin G
- *Listeria*—continue treatment with ampicillin and gentamicin
- Gram-negative bacteria—use an extended-spectrum cephalosporin such as cefotaxime or ceftazidime plus gentamicin
- Coagulase-negative *Staphylococcus*—vancomycin

Pediatric HIV and AIDS

In the United States, vertical transmission is the most common mode of transmission (see The First Prenatal Visit, page 322).

- Romania and Africa have the highest pediatric HIV infection per capita
- Suspect diagnosis if any of the following are present: recurrent bacterial infections, FTT, opportunistic infections, invasive fungal infections, and thrush
- Diagnosis
  - All infants <18 months of age will have positive HIV screen due to circulating **maternal** antibodies (if acquired vertically). Use HIV viral load to diagnose infection instead
  - For children >18 months of age, a positive screen is, by definition, acquired HIV infection (positive ELISA → confirm with Western blot)

- Treatment
  - ► All infants born to HIV-positive mothers should recieve zidovudine (ZDV) syrup at birth and add TMP-SMX at 6 weeks of age (*Pneumocystis jiroveci* pneumonia [PCP] prophylaxis)
  - ► In all infants/children with confirmed HIV infection → triple antiretroviral therapy

Pharyngitis

Clinical Presentation of Pharyngitis

Disease	Presentation	Diagnosis	Management
Streptococcal pharyngitis	Rapid onset of fever, adenopathy, sore throat, plus **exudative tonsillitis**	Rapid strep test, then: • If positive, treat • If negative, throat culture to confirm	• Penicillin is first-line • Azithromycin or clindamycin if allergic • Treatment prevents rheumatic fever
Coxsackie virus pharyngitis	• Herpangina = small ulcers in the oropharynx; no exudates • Hand, foot, and mouth disease = gradual onset of fever, with **painful oral ulcers, ulcers of the hands and feet**	Clinical	Supportive; self-resolving
Pharyngocon-junctival fever (adenovirus)	Pharyngitis, conjunctivitis, and generalized URI symptoms	Clinical	Supportive; self-resolving

Abbreviations: upper respiratory infection, URI

8

Complications of Acute Pharyngitis

Complication	Presentation	Diagnosis	Treatment
Retropharyngeal abscess	• Peak age **2–4 years** • Constitutional symptoms plus **muffled "hot-potato" voice, torticollis, refusal to move head/turn neck, drooling/ salivation**	**Posterior-lateral pharyngeal wall** bulge	• Empiric IV **ampicillin-sulbactam or clindamycin** (use vancomycin if MRSA suspected) • Surgical drainage if signs of airway compromise
Peritonsillar abscess	Usually children **>4 years of age**; constitutional symptoms plus severe sore throat, dysphagia, change in voice	**Lateral deviation of tonsil and uvula** away from side of infection	• Same as above • For surgical therapy, may use either needle aspiration, I&D, or tonsillectomy, depending on patient circumstance

Abbreviations: incision and drainage, I&D; methicillin-resistant Staphylococcus aureus, MRSA

Indications for Tonsillectomy and Adenoidectomy (T&A) in Children

- Tonsillectomy
  - ≥7 documented streptococcal infections in 1 year **or** ≥5 per year for 2 years **or** ≥3 per year for 3 years
  - Airway obstruction from enlargement
- Adenoidectomy
  - Nasal obstruction
  - Chronic sinusitis failing medical therapy
  - Recurrent otitis media where tympanostomy tubes have **failed**

Rheumatic Fever

- Most common **from 4 to 9 years of age**; recent history of **streptococcal pharyngitis** (skin infection does **not** cause rheumatic fever)

- Clinical presentation—**migratory arthritis**, carditis, CNS involvement, **rash**

- Use **Jones criteria** for diagnosis—evidence of preceding infection (positive rapid strep test or culture, or elevated antistreptolysin O antibody titer) plus two major or one major plus two minor criteria (see the Jones Criteria table)

- Treatment—three main goals of therapy
  - ▸ Symptomatic relief—aspirin
  - ▸ Eradication of Group A *Strep.*—penicillin (azithromycin if allergic)
  - ▸ Long-term prophylaxis—penicillin V or sulfadiazine
  - ▸ **Note:** Treat congestive heart failure (CHF) if symptoms of heart failure are present

Jones Criteria

Major Criteria	Minor Criteria
Migratory polyarthritis	Fever
Pancarditis	Increased ESR
Subcutaneous nodules	Arthralgia
Erythema marginatum	Long PR interval
Sydenham chorea (face, tongue, arms)	

Abbreviations: erythrocyte sedimentation rate, ESR

Neonatal Exposure to Tuberculosis

- Suspected maternal tuberculosis at time of delivery → separate mother from infant and get chest x-ray
  - ▸ Chest x-ray negative → maternal isoniazid (INH) prophylaxis for 9 months with return to baby

8

► Chest x-ray positive → separate mother from neonate with respiratory isolation of mother until sputum results return (2–12 weeks)

  ▷ Maternal sputum results positive → INH for 9 months in baby plus treatment with antitubercular therapy for mother, return baby to mother

    – Neonates with active pulmonary tuberculosis (Tb)— INH, rifampin, pyrazinamide, and streptomycin for 2 months; then INH plus rifampin for 10 months

    – No active pulmonary disease (purified protein derivative [PPD] testing in the neonate)

      - PPD test positive → continue INH for 9 months

      - PPD test at 3 months and 6 months → if negative after second PPD at 6 months, stop INH and repeat PPD testing at 12 months

Whooping Cough (Pertussis)

- Transmission of *Bordetella pertussis* by aerosol droplets
- Three phases
  ► Catarrhal phase—"common cold" for first 2 weeks
  ► Paroxysmal phase—episodes of **severe, uncontrollable coughing** with **inspiratory "whoop"** (while trying to catch their breath); may last weeks
  ► Convalescent phase—resolution
- Diagnosis
  ► Clinical; look for history of incomplete immunizations
  ► May perform **PCR** of nasopharyngeal aspirates; gold standard is culture
- Treatment—**for patients and all close contacts, azithromycin is the drug of choice**

Viral Exanthems

- Postexposure prophylaxis for varicella
  - ► Immunocompromised/pregnant patients
    - ▷ First 96 hours of exposure—varicella zoster immune globulin (VariZIG®)
    - ▷ >96 hours from exposure—IVIG
  - ► Healthy adults 3–5 days after exposure—test for antibodies; if negative, give varicella vaccine

Diagnosis and Management of Viral Exanthems

Disease	Clinical Presentation	Diagnosis	Treatment
Chickenpox	• **Pruritic** rash in **various stages of development** • Macules → papules → vesicles → pustules	**Clinical;** PCR-DNA or DFA testing of scrapings if unsure of diagnosis (atypical presentation)	• Children <12: no treatment • Children >12 or adults: oral acyclovir if uncomplicated; IV acyclovir if complicated (immunosuppression, dissemination) • Diphenhydramine for symptomatic relief of pruritus
Erythema infectiosum (fifth disease, parvovirus B19 infection)	Mild constitutional illness, **arthritis, intense red "slapped cheeks"** plus **lacy rash**	Clinical except when diagnosing hydrops fetalis (PCR-DNA testing of fetal blood)	• Supportive • Watch for **aplastic crisis** in those with sickle-cell disease
Measles	**Cough, coryza,** and **conjunctivitis** with onset of generalized maculopapular rash; **Koplik spots**	Clinical	Supportive, plus **vitamin A** (proven to reduce morbidity and mortality)

8

(continued)

Diagnosis and Management of Viral Exanthems (continued)

Disease	Clinical Presentation	Diagnosis	Treatment
Mumps	Constitutional symptoms plus **salivary gland swelling**; parotids most common— so-called **"chip-munk cheeks"**; orchitis	Clinical; **elevated serum amylase**	• Supportive • Bed rest for severe orchitis • Complications: sterility only if **bilateral** orchitis
Rubella	**Retroauricu-lar, posterior and occipital lymphadenitis/ adenopathy** with generalized **maculopapular rash** starting on the **face** and spreading downward; **arthralgia**	Clinical	Supportive
Roseola (HHV-6 infection)	**High fever** (up to 106°F [41.1°C]) plus adenopa-thy, followed by generalized **rose-colored** papular **rash when fever breaks**	Clinical	Supportive

Abbreviations: direct fluorescent antibody, DFA; human herpesvirus, HHV; polymerase chain reaction, PCR

8

IMMUNOLOGY

Childhood Immunodeficiencies

Disease	Pathogenesis	Clinical Presentation	Diagnosis	Treatment
Ataxia-telangiectasia	Autosomal recessive chromosomal defect	• Widespread telangiectasias and ataxia when infant begins to walk • Increased risk of **lymphoreticular malignancy**	Clinical; confirm with genetic testing	Supportive; death by age 20 years in most
Bruton agamma-globulinemia	• X-linked; affects males	• Multiple, recurrent infections starting around age 6 months • Little to no tonsillar/adenoid tissue; absence of adenopathy (unable to mount lymphoid response)	• **All** immunoglobulins decreased; **absence** of B cells	IVIG
Chédiak-Higashi syndrome	Autosomal recessive	Albinism, increased bleeding time, recurrent infections	**Giant granules** in peripheral leukocytes	• Treatment of choice: bone marrow transplant • Second-line: high-dose vitamin C
Chronic granulomatous disease	• Variable inheritance • Susceptible to **catalase positive organisms**	Recurrent pneumonia, abscess formation	NBT or DHR test	• Treatment of choice: bone marrow transplant • Second-line: prophylactic TMP-SMX

8

(continued)

Childhood Immunodeficiencies (continued)

Disease	Pathogenesis	Clinical Presentation	Diagnosis	Treatment
DiGeorge syndrome	• Congenital absence of the **third and fourth pharyngeal pouches** • Absent thymus, parathyroids • Wide-set eyes and low-set ears with or without cleft palate	• Severe **hypo-calcemia →** infantile tetany and seizures • Absence of T cells: **opportunistic infections**	Clinical	Thymic or bone marrow transplant
Selective IgA deficiency	• Not completely understood • At increased risk of other **autoimmune disease and malignancy**	Recurrent respiratory, skin, GI and GU infections (i.e., any **mucosal surface**)	Absence of serum IgA	• Supportive care • **Must have** IgA removed from blood products **→ fatal anaphylaxis** (intrinsic IgA antibodies)
Severe combined immuno-deficiency	Recessive form due to **adenosine deaminase deficiency**	Congenital **absence of all immunity →** multiple viral, bacterial and fungal infections	Absent thymus, absent lymph nodes, etc.	Bone marrow transplant or death by age 1 year
Wiskott-Aldrich syndrome	• X-linked: affects males • Affects protein synthesis	• Triad of **throm-bocytopenia, atopic der-matitis, and encapsulated infections** • **Look for** persis-tent **bleeding after circum-cision**, purpura, and atopy	Clinical picture should prompt genetic testing	Treatment of choice: bone marrow transplant

Abbreviations: dihydrorhodamine, DHR; gastrointestinal, GI; genitourinary, GU; intravenous immunoglobulin, IVIG; nitroblue tetrazolium, NBT; trimethoprim-sulfamethoxazole, TMP-SMX

NEPHROLOGY

Urinary Tract Infections (UTIs)

- Diagnosis and symptoms the same as adults

- Males—increased risk if uncircumcised

- Females—if <5 years of age, rule out sexual abuse; risk factors: improper wiping (back to front)

- Treatment

  ▸ Cystitis—PO amoxicillin, TMP-SMX, or nitrofurantoin

  ▸ Pyelonephritis—IV gentamicin with or without ampicillin; or a third-generation cephalosporin

- Indications for voiding cystourethrogram (VCUG)—all males, all females <5 years during first episode or >5 with second episode; fever

- **Renal ultrasound** indicated in all cases of **febrile UTI**

Nephritic and Nephrotic Syndromes

Nephritic	Pathophysiology	Diagnosis/ Clinical Features	Treatment
Acute post-streptococcal glomerulo-nephritis	Immune-mediated deposits in glomerular basement membrane after infection with group A beta-hemolytic streptococci (approximately 10 days after strep throat or 21 days after impetigo)	• **Triad** of edema, hematuria, and hypertension • UA shows **RBC casts and smoky-colored urine** • Decreased serum C3 • Best initial test: **ASO or anti-hyaluronic acid test** • Most accurate test; renal biopsy shows **"lumpy-bumpy"** deposits of IgG and C3 in glomerular basement membrane	• Penicillin × 10 days • Antihyperten-sives: CCA, ACE inhibitors

8

(continued)

Nephritic and Nephrotic Syndromes (continued)

Nephritic	Pathophysiology	Diagnosis/ Clinical Features	Treatment
Berger disease (IgA nephropathy)	Multiple causes; increased risk in celiac disease	• **Gross hematuria plus upper respiratory symptoms** • Normal serum C3 • Biopsy (gold-standard): mesangial IgA deposits on immunofluorescence	• ACE inhibitors + fish oils if HTN or proteinuria • Second-line: steroids if no improvement
Alport syndrome	X-linked dominant	• Triad of ocular, hearing, and renal abnormalities: 1. **Hematuria** after upper respiratory infections 2. Bilateral **sensorineural hearing loss** 3. **Extrusion of lens** into anterior chamber • **Foam cells** seen in renal biopsy	• Renal transplant first-line • ACE inhibitors second-line until transplant available
Hemolytic uremic syndrome	Immune-mediated destruction after infection with *Escherichia coli* 0157:H7	Triad of microangiopathic **hemolytic anemia, uremia,** and **thrombocytopenia** occurring after bout of bloody diarrhea	• **No antibiotics** • Symptomatic treatment: early dialysis, control HTN, correct electrolytes, etc.

Nephrotic	Pathophysiology	Diagnosis/ Clinical Features	Treatment
Minimal change disease (lipoid nephrosis)	Unknown	• Criteria for diagnosis: proteinuria >50 mg/kg/day; serum albumin < 3.0 mg/dL, edema, hyperlipidemia • **Diffuse edema** most common presenting symptom	• Oral **prednisone** • Infections common: beware of spontaneous bacterial peritonitis • Increased risk of **thromboembolic events**

Abbreviations: angiotensin-converting enzyme, ACE; anti-streptolysin O, ASO; calcium-channel antagonist, CCA; hypertension, HTN; red blood cell, RBC; urinalysis, UA

PEDIATRICS

Obstructive Uropathy

- Most common cause—posterior urethral valves
- Clinical—most diagnosed on prenatal ultrasound; if not → male infant with distended, palpable bladder and weak urinary stream
- Management—transurethral ablation first-line; vesicostomy second-line

Vesicoureteral Reflex

- Retrograde flow of urine from bladder → ureteral dilation → kidneys → hydronephrosis and renal fibrosis → nephropathy → end-stage renal disease (ESRD) in severe cases
- Diagnosis—VCUG is first-line test (shows grade of reflux); renal scan for scarring/atrophy if high-grade
- Management—medical (majority resolve with age)
  - **Prophylactic** TMP-SMX, trimethoprim, or nitrofurantoin
  - Surgical intervention if bilateral grade IV and V (five grades of severity), severe scarring, or recurrent UTI despite prophylaxis

NEUROLOGY

Cerebral Palsy

- Risk factors—intrauterine asphyxia, periventricular leukomalacia, low birth weight
- Impaired motor and/or speech development
- Diagnosis with MRI of brain and/or spine
- Treatment—multidisciplinary team, antispastic drugs (baclofen, dantrolene)

Friedreich Ataxia

Abnormal **frataxin** gene → ataxia and dysarthric speech before age 10 years → cardiomyopathy → death

Hydrocephalus

- Obstructive (noncommunicating) → abnormal cerebral aqueduct or lesions in/around 4th ventricle

  ▸ Arnold-Chiari type II—**hydrocephalus + myelomeningocele**

  ▸ Dandy-Walker malformation—**agenesis of cerebellar vermis** (ataxia) + expansion of fourth ventricle (prominent occiput)

- Nonobstructive (communicating) → abnormal arachnoid villi or loss of subarachnoid cistern

- Clinical features—increased head circumference, bulging anterior fontanels, headache, papilledema, irritability

- Treatment—**shunt**

Inherited CNS Disease

Adrenoleukodystrophy

X-linked → CNS disease plus primary adrenal insufficiency

Metachromatic leukodystrophy

- Autosomal recessive → deficient aryl sulfatase A → myelin breakdown → widespread neurologic deterioration

- Keyword—look for **metachromatic** staining pattern on biopsy

Lesch-Nyhan syndrome

X-linked → abnormal purine metabolism → increased serum uric acid → gout, self-mutilation (hand-biting), dystonia

Tay-Sachs disease

Autosomal recessive deficiency of beta-hexosaminidase A → Ashkenazi Jews, cherry-red macula, neurologic deterioration around 1 year of age

Neural tube defects

Deficiency of folic acid in early fetal development; requirements are 1 mg/day for pregnant women → increase to **4 mg/day** in those with history of affected children

Meningocele

Fluctuant spinal mass **covered with skin** → surgery

Myelomeningocele

Midline spinal mass covered with **thin membrane** with or without hydrocephalus (80%) → most have significant deficits, including paralysis from the waist down → surgery

Spina bifida

Defect of vertebral body but **no bulging neural tissue,** usually with overlying **patch of hair** → asymptomatic, no treatment needed

Neurofibromatosis—Autosomal Dominant

- Type I—**predominantly skin findings** → café-au-lait patches, freckles, Lisch nodules, neurofibromas

- Type II—**predominantly hearing loss** → bilateral acoustic neuromas, gait disturbance

- Treatment of types I and II—supportive, annual ophthalmologic exams, increased risk of malignancy

Seizure Disorders

Newborn seizures

- Multiple etiologies; occurs in first 24 hours of birth

- Most common cause is hypoxic encephalopathy, but **must rule out** electrolyte abnormalities; others are drug withdrawal, hemorrhage, etc.

Childhood seizures

- Febrile seizures—rapid increase in temperature usually results in generalized tonic-clonic seizure; new studies show slightly increased risk of future epileptic disorder; no testing indicated; treatment—control fever

8

Diagnosis and Treatment of Seizure Disorders

Type	Features	Diagnosis	Treatment
Simple partial	Unsynchronized tonic to clonic movements with or without aura; never postictal	EEG: spike, sharp waves	DOC: carbamazepine
Complex partial	Lip-smacking or increased salivation plus altered consciousness	• EEG: temporal lobe spikes or sharp waves • MRI to rule out organic brain disease	DOC: carbamazepine
Absence (petit mal)	Classic "stare" with complete unresponsiveness; no aura and no postictal state	EEG: spike and wave 3-second activity	DOC: ethosuximide
Tonic-clonic (grand mal)	Eyes roll back → unresponsive → rhythmic contractions → long postictal state (hours)	EEG: generalized seizure activity	DOC: carbamazepine or valproic acid
Myoclonic	Muscle contraction → complete loss of tone → fall forward	EEG: varied	DOC: valproic acid

Abbreviations: drug of choice, DOC

Sturge-Weber Syndrome

- Port-wine stain and seizure disorder develops into hemiparesis and retardation
- Diagnosis—skull x-ray shows intracranial occipital and parietal calcifications
- Need measurement of intraocular pressure—most have glaucoma
- Treatment—control seizures, supportive

Tuberous Sclerosis

- Autosomal dominant → bulging tubers calcify inside ventricular cavity → outflow obstruction → hydrocephalus
- Diagnosis—CT scan plus characteristic skin lesions
  - ▸ Ash-leaf macule—hypopigmented lesion intensifies with Wood lamp
  - ▸ Sebaceous adenoma—erythematous facial nodules resemble cystic acne
  - ▸ Shagreen patch—lumbosacral "orange-peel" lesion

Wilson Disease

- Autosomal recessive defect in **copper** metabolism → buildup in liver, then in CNS
- Development of acute or chronic liver failure, then multiple CNS abnormalities
- Ocular Kayser-Fleischer rings are **pathognomonic**
- Diagnosis
  - ▸ Best initial test → serum ceruloplasmin (increased)
  - ▸ Gold standard is liver biopsy (cirrhosis and increased copper content)
- Treatment—**penicillamine**

ONCOLOGY

Must-Know Brain Tumors

Craniopharyngioma

- **Supratentorial tumor**
- Clinical—panhypopituitarism and visual deficits from mass effect on chiasm; keyword → calcification of sella turcica on x-ray
- Treatment—surgery and radiation

8

Medulloblastoma

- **Infratentorial tumor** of the cerebellar vermis
- Clinical—outflow obstruction in fourth ventricle causing hydrocephalus; CT scan shows homogenous mass in the posterior fossa
- Treatment—radiation + chemotherapy

Important Pediatric Malignancies

Wilms tumor—nephroblastoma

- Most common presenting symptom is **asymptomatic** abdominal mass
  - ▸ Other findings—hemihypertrophy and aniridia
- Diagnosis—best test is abdominal/pelvic CT scan
- Treatment—nephrectomy → vincristine + dactinomycin + radiation

Neuroblastoma

- Most common presenting symptom is **painful** abdominal mass, and most metastasize by diagnosis
- Diagnosis
  - ▸ Best initial test is serum homovanillic acid (HVA) and vanillylmandelic acid (VMA) (elevated)
  - ▸ Gold-standard test is biopsy
- Treatment—resection → cyclophosphamide + doxorubicin + radiation

Rhabdomyosarcoma

- Botryoid type—classic presentation of **"grapelike"** masses **protruding from vagina**
- Increased incidence with neurofibromatosis
- Treatment—surgical resection

ORTHOPEDICS

Congenital Torticollis

- Malpositioning in utero → head tilted to one side with chin deviation

- Treatment—passive stretching exercises

Must-Know Orthopedic Disorders

Diagnosis and Age Affected	Risk Factors and Pathogenesis	Diagnosis	Treatment
Developmental dysplasia of the hip in **infants**	Breech position, LGA infant	• Best initial test: Barlow test causes dislocation, which is easily palpated • Best test: hip ultrasound	Pavlik harness
Legg-Calvé-Perthes disease in child **5–9 years old**	• Male • Avascular necrosis of femoral head	• **Characteristic antalgic gait** (painless limping) • **Do frog-leg** x-rays → compression and necrosis	Casting and rest
Osgood-Schlatter disease in **teenager**	Overuse injury (active, sports) of the **tibial tubercle**	Entirely clinical: swelling, tenderness of the tibial tubercle (x-ray only if atypical history)	Rest, knee immobilization
Slipped capital femoral epiphysis in **teenager**	Obesity	• Sudden onset of extreme pain with external rotation at hip • Do frog-leg x-rays; show classic **"ice-cream cone sign"** i.e., slippage of acetabulum off the femoral head	Surgical pinning; otherwise avascular necrosis will occur

Abbreviations: large for gestational age, LGA

8

Scoliosis

- Asymmetry of posterior chest wall with >20 degrees deviation of the norm during Adams test (bending forward)

- Diagnosis—anteroposterior (AP) and lateral spinal x-rays

- Treatment—brace if 30–40 degrees and skeletally immature; surgery if >40 degrees and skeletally immature

Talipes Equinovarus (Clubfoot)

- Stiff, medially rotated foot that is **unable to flatten** on exam surface

- Treatment—serial casting and splints; if not corrected by 3 months of age → surgery

PULMONOLOGY AND EAR, NOSE, AND THROAT

Newborn Pulmonary Disease

Must-Know Newborn Respiratory Diseases

Disease	Cause	Diagnosis	Treatment
Respiratory distress syndrome	Surfactant deficiency → cannot maintain alveolar volume	• **Hypoxemia is hallmark** • Best initial test: CXR showing **ground-glass appearance**, atelectasis, air bronchograms • Most accurate test: lecithin-to-sphingomyelin ratio (<2:1)	• First-line: inhaled surfactant plus CPAP • Second-line: intubation and mechanical ventilation if decreased responsiveness • Preventive measures: antenatal corticosteroids in premature labor
Transient tachypnea of the newborn	• Decreased absorption of lung fluids • Increased risk with **cesarean section or rapid second stage of labor**	Tachypnea after birth with **minimal need for O_2 supplementation**	Resolves spontaneously over hours to a few days

(continued)

Must-Know Newborn Respiratory Diseases (continued)

Disease	Cause	Diagnosis	Treatment
Meconium aspiration syndrome	Hypoxia results in fetal BM during labor; aspiration with first breath → airway obstruction	History and CXR showing **patchy infiltrates**, increased AP diameter, and diaphragmatic flattening	First: start supplemental oxygen ↓ Second: CPAP if persistent hypoxemia ↓ Third: high-frequency mechanical ventilation ↓ Last resort: extracorporeal membrane oxygenation

Abbreviations: anteroposterior, AP; bowel movement, BM; continuous positive airway pressure, CPAP; chest x-ray, CXR

Sudden Infant Death Syndrome (SIDS)

- Defined as death of an infant not explained by organic findings at autopsy

- Risk factors: low socioeconomic status, African American, smoking, winter, low birth weight, large family

- Prevent with supine sleeping and pacifier, avoid soft bedding, avoid overheating environment

- Autopsy may show **petechial hemorrhages** and pulmonary edema (thought to be due to chronic asphyxia)

8

Tracheoesophageal Fistula (TEF) and Esophageal Atresia

- Classic presentation—coughing, choking, and gagging with **first feeding**

- Most common type—proximal esophageal atresia and distal fistula → x-ray shows large amount of **air in stomach**

- Treatment—surgical; rule out **cardiac anomalies**

Childhood Pulmonary Disease

Upper respiratory system

Allergic rhinitis

- Increased risk from exposure to smoke, heavy allergens, family history

- Classic clinical triad—rhinorrhea, conjunctivitis, postnasal drip with cough at night

- Physical findings—dark circles under eyes, **pale nasal mucosa** with hypertrophied turbinates, **cobblestoning** of posterior pharynx and conjunctiva

- Diagnosis—best test is smear showing eosinophilia of naso-pharyngeal secretions
  - ▸ Isolation of allergy: RAST (radioallergosorbent) or skin-prick testing

- Treatment—**avoid allergen**, then management based on age:
  - ▸ <3 years: intranasal cromolyn sodium
  - ▸ >3 years: mild/episodic symptoms, give oral antihistamine; moderate/persistent symptoms, give intranasal glucocorticoids

Croup

- Due to parainfluenza virus infection

- Upper respiratory illness → characteristic **barking cough, followed by inspiratory stridor** → may lead to hypoxia

- Diagnosis—clinical; if x-ray is done, look for **steeple sign**

- Treatment—cool or warm mist → nebulized epinephrine if no improvement → steroids if severe inflammation

Epiglottitis

- Most common causes: *Strep. pyogenes, Strep. pneumoniae, Staph. aureus,* and *Mycoplasma* (*Haemophilus* is no longer common secondary to vaccination)

- Upper respiratory illness → high fever → hoarseness → **drooling, tripod** sitting position → accessory muscle usage → expiratory stridor

- Diagnosis—clinical exam will show **bright-red epiglottis**; x-ray not required, but if done, look for **thumb sign**

- Treatment—early intubation, followed by broad-spectrum antibiotics

Epistaxis (nosebleed)

- Most common cause is picking the nose; may be initial sign of leukemia

- Initially, use pressure → nasal packing if pressure unsuccessful

Foreign-body aspiration

- Most common in **toddlers** → choking, coughing, wheezing after putting something in the mouth (most common object is peanuts) → severity depends on site in which object is lodged (anything from wheezing to respiratory distress)

- Diagnosis—chest x-ray may or may not show object; air-trapping distal to obstruction

- Treatment—**rigid bronchoscopy**

Sinusitis

- May be viral or bacterial, but toxic history (fever, severe symptoms) more likely to be bacterial; symptoms of persistent upper respiratory symptoms for >10 days

- Diagnosis—clinical; CT scan of sinuses is gold standard (x-rays not reliable)

- Treatment
  - ▸ DOC—amoxicillin-clavulanate is now recommended due to rising antimicrobial resistance patterns in *Haemophilus influenzae*
  - ▸ Doxycycline or a respiratory fluoroquinolone can be used in those with severe penicillin allergy

8

> ▸ If treatment fails to improve symptoms in 3–5 days, consider formal sinus imaging (CT or MRI) with maxillary sinus aspirates for culture

Lower respiratory system

Asthma

- Airway inflammation is **reversible** (contrast to chronic obstructive pulmonary disease [COPD], which is irreversible)
- Most childhood asthma resolves by adulthood
  - ▸ Intrinsic asthma **not** due to prior sensitization—cold air, exercise, infection, extreme emotional distress
  - ▸ Extrinsic asthma due to **sensitization**—increased **IgE** in response to provoking factors, family history, atopy, eczema
  - ▸ Most common cause of exacerbation is **infection**
- Clinical—diffuse wheezing, initially expiratory then inspiratory; decreased air movement and accessory muscle usage; common initial presentation is **persistent coughing** (especially exercise-induced)
  - ▸ Poor prognostic indicators in acute exacerbation—pulsus paradoxicus, respiratory fatigue, cyanotic appearance
- Diagnosis—clinical; gold standard is pulmonary function tests (PFTs)
  - ▸ PFTs
    - ▹ Initial test of choice—give beta-agonist and measure forced expiratory volume in 1 second (FEV1) → >12% improvement diagnostic
    - ▹ If negative (attack resolved at time of testing)—give provocation challenge with cold air or methacholine (cholinergic agonist) → decrease in FEV1 >20% diagnostic
  - ▸ Chest x-ray
    - ▹ Acute exacerbations—no change, or positive for infiltrate
    - ▹ Chronic—diaphragmatic flattening, peribronchial thickening

8

- ▸ Acute exacerbation—follow arterial blood gas (ABG)
  - ▹ Early → decreased PCO_2 with increased pH (respiratory alkalosis); near normal PO_2
  - ▹ Later → increased PCO_2 with decreased pH (respiratory acidosis); decreased PO_2
  - ▹ Impending failure → near-normal ABG (normal PCO_2)
- Home monitoring—use peak flow meter, divided into zones (green 80–100%; yellow 50–80%; red <50% of personal best)

Management of Acute Asthma Exacerbation

Start supplemental oxygen, maintain sat >90%, and check ABG

↓

Give albuterol via nebulizer
(Ipratropium if + h/o heart disease—most important in elderly with COPD)

↓

Stat dose of IV steroids (salumedrol)

↓

Chest x-ray

Admit if:
1. PEF <50% of personal best
2. Failure to respond to treatment with beta-agonists
3. Infiltrate on chest x-ray

Intubate if:
1. Confusion
2. Hypotension
3. Silent chest
4. Severe hypercapnea
5. Impending respiratory failure
6. Paradoxical respiration

8

Abbreviations: arterial blood gas, ABG; chronic obstructive pulmonary disease, COPD; history of, h/o; peak expiratory flow, PEF; saturation, sat

- While inpatient—give high-dose IV steroids and taper down to oral dose for 10–14 days total treatment
- Outpatient management—tiered approach to treatment, with increasing severity; additional agents are added to control symptoms (see Diagnosis and Management of Chronic Asthma, following page)

Diagnosis and Management of Chronic Asthma

Type	Day Symptoms	Night Symptoms	PFTs	Drug of Choice
Mild intermittent	Once/week	Once/month	FEV1 >80% of predicted	Short-acting, inhaled beta-agonist PRN
Mild persistent	More than twice/week	More than twice/month	FEV1 >80% of predicted	Add an inhaled corticosteroid
Moderate persistent	Daily	More than once/week	FEV1 60–80% of predicted	Add an inhaled long-acting beta-agonist
Severe persistent	Continuous	Often	FEV1 <60% of predicted	• Add oral leukotriene modifier • If not controlled, then add oral corticosteroids

Abbreviations: forced expiratory volume in 1 second, FEV1; pulmonary function tests, PFTs; as often as needed, PRN

- Common asthma medications (must know)
  - ▸ Short-acting inhaled beta-agonists—albuterol, levalbuterol
  - ▸ Long-acting inhaled beta-agonists—salmeterol and formoterol
  - ▸ Inhaled corticosteroids
    - ▹ First generation—beclomethasone, flunisolide, triamcinolone
    - ▹ Second generation (**preferred, less systemic effects**)— budesonide, fluticasone, mometasone
  - ▸ Oral medications
    - ▹ Leukotriene modifiers—zafirlukast, montelukast
    - ▹ Nonsteroidal anti-inflammatory drugs (NSAIDs)— cromolyn sodium, nedocromil sodium
      - – First-line add-on for **exercise-induced asthma** not controlled with beta-agonist

8

▷ Theophylline—used in steroid-dependent asthma as sparing agent; has narrow therapeutic window and high incidence of side effects

Bronchiolitis

- Majority due to respiratory syncytial virus (RSV) infection

- Young children → small airway inflammation → air-trapping and hyperinflation

- Clinical—upper respiratory symptoms plus **paroxysms of wheezy cough; apnea in infants**

- Diagnosis—clinical; gold standard is RT–PCR testing of naso-pharyngeal swab

- Treatment—respiratory isolation, nebulized beta-agonists; ribavirin used only in severe cases (respiratory distress)

- Prevention in high-risk, exposed children—RSV IVIG or RSV monoclonal antibody

Cystic fibrosis

- Autosomal recessive defect in cystic fibrosis transmembrane conductance regulator (CFTR) gene on chromosome 7 → more than 100 known mutations → if genetic testing negative, must perform sequencing of CFTR gene locus for confirmation of diagnosis

- Pathophysiology—unable to secrete chloride ions into secretions → failure of water molecules to thin out secretions → thickened, obstructing mucus and GI tract secretions

- Clinical
    - ▸ Signs according to age
        - ▷ Newborns: meconium ileus; x-ray shows dilated loops of small bowel with air–fluid levels and "ground-glass" appearance; treatment with diatrizoic acid (Gastrografin®) enema
        - ▷ Infants: bulky, greasy stools and FTT; fat-soluble vitamin deficiency; pancreatitis; diabetes; rectal prolapse; infertility; vast pulmonary findings include hyperresonance to percussion, bronchiectasis, recurrent pneumonia; **salty taste of sweat**

8

- Diagnosis—best test is the sweat test
  - If equivocal—test potential difference across nasal epithelium
  - Genetic testing confirmatory but not required if positive family history and typical symptoms

- Treatment—symptomatic control
  - Pulmonary obstruction—chest physiotherapy, nebulized albuterol/saline
  - Infection—inpatient DOC is intravenous (1) tobramycin plus pipercillin or (2) ceftazidime plus piperacillin for pulmonary infection
  - Pancreatic enzyme and fat-soluble vitamin replacement
  - Force fluids (encourage aggressive fluid intake)
  - Long-term ibuprofen shown to slow progression

Pneumonia

- Incidence by age:
  - <1 month: beta-hemolytic streptococci most common cause
  - 1 month–15 years: streptococcus pneumonia most common cause
  - >15 years: mycoplasma pneumonia most common cause

- Keywords in certain infections:
  - Chlamydia trachomatis: infant with history of **conjunctivitis** at birth, interstitial findings on chest x-ray, **staccato cough** (deep inspiration between each cough), and **eosinophilia**
  - *Staph. aureus* pneumonia: very toxic-appearing, chest x-ray shows focal infiltrate with **cavitation** and air–fluid levels (abscesses), empyema common
  - *Mycoplasma* pneumonia: gradual onset of cough and dyspnea over 2–3 weeks, chest x-ray with diffuse interstitial infiltrates looks worse than the patient appears

- Treatment of pneumonia
  - ▸ Outpatient care—DOC is amoxicillin if typical bacterial pneumonia is suspected (e.g., lobar infiltrates). Add azithromycin or use alone if interstitial pneumonia is obvious or suspected.
  - ▸ Inpatient care—initial DOC is cefuroxime
    - ▹ If staph suspected, add vancomycin
    - ▹ If atypical (chlamydia or mycoplasma) suspected, add macrolide

RHEUMATOLOGY

Henoch-Schönlein Purpura

- Pathophysiology—**IgA**-mediated vasculitis of small vessels (skin, GI, and renal deposits) seen after **URI**
  - ▸ Most common cause of purpura in children (with normal platelets)
- Clinical symptoms/signs
  - ▸ Rash: pink maculopapular rash below the waist → petechiae and purpura
  - ▸ GI: abdominal pain, bloody stools, may develop **intussusception**
  - ▸ Renal: **glomerulonephritis → red-cell casts**
- Labs: Elevated erythrocyte sedimentation rate (ESR), anemia, increased serum IgA and IgM
- Diagnosis—clinical; gold standard is **skin biopsy** and is indicated only if diagnosis is uncertain
- Treatment—symptomatic; if GI symptoms severe, give course of steroids

Juvenile Rheumatoid Arthritis (JRA)

- Three subtypes:
  - ▸ Pauciarticular (HLA-DR8 and DR5) involves <5 joints
  - ▸ Polyarticular (HLA-DR4) involves >5 joints and **rheumatoid nodules**

8

> ► Systemic onset involves joint + intraabdominal organs + **daily fever** + **effervescent rash**

- Clinical—morning stiffness lasting >**15 minutes**, fatigue, joint pain, and decreased mobility in the absence of joint erythema
- Criteria for diagnosis—age <16, more than one joint affected, duration >6 weeks, exclude other causes of arthritis
- Other diagnostic findings:
  - ► Most are antinuclear antibody (ANA)-positive
  - ► Positive **rheumatoid factor** associated with **poor prognosis**
- Treatment
  - ► First-line: **NSAIDs**
  - ► Add methotrexate if disease not controlled (safest)

Kawasaki Disease

- Vasculitis affecting medium-size arteries, common in Japanese ancestry, majority of patients are <5 years of age
- Diagnosis
  - ► Fever for >5 days **plus** any five of the following: bilateral bulbar conjunctivitis, oral erythema, desquamation of fingertips, erythema and edema of hands, rash, cervical lymphadenitis, myocarditis, coronary artery aneurysms
  - ► After diagnosis suspected, must get **2-D echocardiogram**, check labs (various anomalies)
- Treatment—DOC in acute disease is **IVIG plus high-dose aspirin**
  - ► Add warfarin if platelets >1 million (hypercoagulable state)

PSYCHIATRY

Note: The diagnostic criteria in this chapter are written according to DSM-IV criteria. DSM-V was not yet published at press time.

ANTIDEPRESSANTS

The most important concept in answering test questions and distinguishing psychiatric disorders is knowing the DSM criteria and side-effect profiles of psychotropic medications.

Selective Serotonin Reuptake Inhibitors (SSRIs)

- Includes paroxetine, sertraline, citalopram, and fluoxetine
- Most common side effects—"jitteriness," headaches, restlessness, agitation, GI symptoms (diarrhea and nausea), and insomnia
- **Preferred** in **diabetics** and **post-myocardial infarction** patients
- When to use alternate agent—**weight gain** (paroxetine) and **sexual dysfunction** (citalopram, escitalopram) (impotence/decreased sexual appetite) may be troublesome for some patients. Can try on alternate SSRI or change class.

Serotonin-Norepinephrine Reuptake Inhibitors (SNRIs)

- Includes venlafaxine and duloxetine
- Side-effect profile similar to SSRIs except with increased diaphoresis and dizziness, **delayed orgasm**, and worsened glycemic control
- **Preferred** in patients with **neuropathic pain**

Tricyclic Antidepressants (TCAs)

- Most common side effects due to anticholinergic effects—dry mouth, blurry vision, constipation, urinary retention, tachycardia, confusion/delirium, orthostasis
- When to use alternate agent—**avoid** in the **elderly** and/or with significant **weight gain**; prolongs QT interval

Monoamine Oxidase Inhibitors (MAOIs)

- Most common side effects due to enhanced sympathetic tone—hypertension with potential to become malignant when ingested with **tyramine-containing foods** (cheese, wine, beer, bananas, any smoked or aged food products)
- Used as a last resort

Other Antidepressants

It is very important to know these.

- Bupropion—low incidence of weight gain, sexual dysfunction; aids in **smoking cessation**
- Mirtazapine—a mixed antagonist with **sedating qualities**; helpful for those with bothersome **insomnia**; causes **significant weight gain**

ANTIPSYCHOTICS

Atypicals

- First-line for treatment of schizophrenia
- Must-know profiles of specific atypical antipsychotics
  - ▶ Aripiprazole—no cardiac side effects; **minimal weight gain**
  - ▶ Clozapine—**agranulocytosis; lowers the seizure threshold**; rarely used
  - ▶ Olanzapine—significant weight gain and **glucose intolerance**
  - ▶ Quetiapine—low incidence of extrapyramidal side effects (preferred for those with movement disorders); very sedating

- Risperidone—least sedating of all atypicals; elevates serum prolactin
- Ziprasidone—causes **QT prolongation; minimal weight gain**

D₂ Antagonists

Includes haloperidol, thioridazine, and chlorpromazine; usually avoided long-term since side-effect profile is extensive; good for short-term management of agitation (e.g., haloperidol)

ADVERSE EFFECTS OF PSYCHOTROPIC MEDICATIONS

- Tardive dyskinesia
  - May present as akathisia, generalized dystonia, localized dystonia, and others
  - Akathisia—patients have "motor restlessness" causing frequent change of bodily position and inability to remain still; treat by stopping the offending drug and add a benzodiazepine
  - Choreoathetosis and involuntary movements
    - ▷ Exact etiology unknown; occurs with prolonged treatment with typical (first-generation) antipsychotics or metoclopramide
  - Management—**discontinue** the offending drug and switch to a second-generation antipsychotic
    - ▷ Symptomatic treatment with local botulinum injections, tetrabenazine (drug of choice), trihexyphenidyl, or benztropine
- Acute dystonia
  - Pathophysiology—may be primary (etiology unknown) or secondary (genetic or tardive dyskinesia)
  - Clinical—**acute, nonsustained, and involuntary** muscle contractions of various muscle groups; may be generalized or localized

9

> Diagnosis and management—start with a levodopa trial (rules in or rules out dopamine responsive dystonia)
  ▷ If positive response, then continue
  ▷ If no response—use either anticholinergics such as trihexyphenidyl or benztropine (best choice if generalized) or intramuscular botulinum injection (best choice if localized)

- Neuroleptic malignant syndrome
  - Due to **dopamine blockade**
  - **Tetrad** of mental status change, muscular **"lead-pipe" rigidity**, hyperthermia, and autonomic instability with **bradykinesia**
  - Diagnosis—clinical presentation with or without rhabdomyolysis; occurs within **days to weeks** of administering drug
  - Management—first, **discontinue** the offending drug; then use dantrolene, bromocriptine, or amantadine
    ▷ Resolves in **days to weeks**

- Serotonin syndrome
  - Due to **excessive serotonergic activity**
  - **Tetrad** of mental status change, muscular **clonus**, hyperthermia, and autonomic instability with **hyperkinesias**
  - Diagnosis—clinical presentation with or without rhabdomyolysis; occurs within **hours** of administering drug
  - Management—first, **discontinue** the offending drug; then use benzodiazepines plus cyproheptadine
    ▷ Resolves within **24 hours**

ADJUSTMENT DISORDER

- Cause—an environmental stressor or change in life circumstances causes significantly more stress than would be reasonably expected for the person's age
- Diagnosis—occurs **within 3 months** of the stressor and **resolves within 6 months** of the event (e.g., divorce or peer problems)
- May be with overwhelming feeling of anxiety, sadness, or turmoil resulting in erratic and withdrawn behavior

- Management—remove the stressor, if possible; use benzodiazepines for anxiety or an SSRI for depression

ANXIETY DISORDERS

Overwhelming anxiety occurring in the absence of a provoking factor or in excess of what would be expected in a specific circumstance.

Anxiety Disorders

Diagnosis	Symptoms	Criteria	Management
Acute stress disorder	An identifiable, traumatic event results in excessive fear and/or helplessness	Experience of **flashbacks** and frequent **revisiting of the trauma**; lasts **<1 month** after the event	Counseling is first-line to prevent evolution into PTSD
PTSD	The same as acute stress disorder	All of the above but lasts **>1 month** after the event	• Psychosocial therapy long-term • Benzodiazepines for short-term symptomatic relief
Phobia	Extreme anxiety or fear of certain things or situations	Symptoms must be severe enough to **disrupt daily life**	• Cognitive-behavioral therapy is first-line • Stage fright: beta-blockers are first-line
Generalized anxiety disorder	Excessive anxiety, dizziness, and worry about life in general	Must last for **>6 months**	• Cognitive-behavioral therapy is first-line • SSRIs or SNRIs are also helpful
Panic disorder	Intense anxiety with sympathetic symptoms lasting a few minutes **without** any identifiable stressor	Clinical symptoms • Without agoraphobia: not afraid to leave home • With agoraphobia: **avoidance** of public places for fear of embarrassment	• Psychotherapy is first-line • SSRIs may be helpful long-term • Benzodiazepines for short-term symptomatic relief

9

(continued)

Anxiety Disorders (continued)

Diagnosis	Symptoms	Criteria	Management
Obsessive-compulsive disorder	Obsessions and compulsions are recognized by the patient as unreasonable and provoke intense anxiety	**Interferes with daily life** and causes **extreme stress to the patient**	SSRIs are first-line; psychotherapy helpful

Abbreviations: posttraumatic stress disorder, PTSD; serotonin-norepinephrine reuptake inhibitor, SNRI; selective serotonin reuptake inhibitor, SSRI

DISSOCIATIVE DISORDERS

Disruption of consciousness, memory, identity, or perception, causing significant distress for the individual

Dissociative Disorders

Disorder	Symptoms	Diagnosis	Management
Depersonalization/derealization	Feeling of being "detached" from one's own body or thoughts	Clinical history and identifiable stress	Psychotherapy
Dissociative fugue	Sudden travel with complete amnesia and formation of a new identity	Identifiable stress and clinical history	Resolves spontaneously
Dissociative amnesia	Patients complain of episodes where they cannot recall important events	Identifiable stress and clinical history	Usually resolves with time; remove stressor
Dissociative identity disorder (multiple-personality disorder)	Several distinct personalities control the patient's behavior	Strongly associated with **childhood abuse**; clinical history	Very hard to treat; intense psychotherapy required

AUTISM VS. ASPERGER DISORDER

"Autistic spectrum disorders" is used to describe a spectrum of autistic findings including Asperger disorder and autism; management includes counseling and behavior modification therapy.

- **Asperger disorder:** Criteria for diagnosis—impaired social interaction, impaired communication **with preservation of speech**, repetitive and stereotypical patterns of behavior including purposeless rituals **before 3 years of age**

- **Autism:** Criteria for diagnosis—impaired social interaction, impaired communication including **lack of speech development**, repetitive and stereotypical patterns of behavior including purposeless rituals **before 3 years of age**

ATTENTION DEFICIT HYPERACTIVITY DISORDER (ADHD)

- Clinical—children have **short attention span**, constantly **fidget**, are **disruptive** in class, do not obey commands, have **poor relationships** with peers and siblings, and display **poor academic performance**

- Diagnosis—must be **<7 years of age**; symptoms must last for **>6 months**, must be present in **multiple settings** (e.g., school and home), and must interfere with the normal environment

- Management—stimulants including methylphenidate or dextroamphetamine are first-line; atomoxetine is the best choice if the patient is high-risk for substance abuse and age is >6 years

9

OPPOSITIONAL DEFIANT DISORDER (ODD) AND CONDUCT DISORDER

Diagnosis	Symptoms	Management
ODD	Recurrent hostile and defiant behavior with frequent **arguing, vindictiveness**, and deliberately negative actions for **>6 months; interferes with home, work, and/or school**	• Reward good behavior • If no early intervention, will progress to conduct disorder
Conduct disorder	Recurrent aggression, **destruction of property**, violation of rules, **theft, animal torture**, and bullying for **>6 months; interferes with home, work, and/or school**	• Highly structured living environment • Punishment/incarceration often not helpful

Abbreviations: oppositional defiant disorder, ODD

ENURESIS

- Primary enuresis—the child has never achieved continence of urine

- Secondary enuresis—the child was previously continent for at least 6 months before enuresis resumed; new stressors (especially divorce, new sibling, new school, etc.) play a primary role

- Timing of symptoms
  - ▶ Isolated nocturnal enuresis is extremely common; related to delayed bladder maturation, etc.
  - ▶ If both nocturnal and daytime incontinence, have a higher level of suspicion for organic abnormalities

- Management—rule out urinary tract infection (UTI) and organic anomalies if reasonable level of suspicion exists
  - ▶ Otherwise, management based on age
    - ▷ If <7 years, parental reassurance of spontaneous resolution is the best step

▷ If >7 years or able to participate in feedback, the first step is **behavioral modification** (e.g., give child a sticker or other reward for "dry days"); if this fails after 3–6 months, the next step is an **enuresis alarm**

MUNCHAUSEN SYNDROME BY PROXY

- Clinical—the deliberate affliction of disease, illness, or abuse on a child by the parent for the parent's personal gain of sympathy or psychological fulfillment ("Munchausen syndrome" proper refers to deliberate self-harm for the same psychological fulfillment and/or sympathetic gain)
- Diagnosis—videotape surveillance or direct eyewitnesses in presence of high clinical suspicion
- Treatment—involve child protective services and social services

MENTAL RETARDATION

- IQ 20–35 = severe retardation; little speech, requires significant care
- IQ 35–50 = moderate retardation; able to perform activities of daily living (ADLs); works and lives in assisted-living environment, but is not able to conform to social norms
- IQ 50–70 = mild retardation; able to live independently and with little supervision; will have self-esteem issues with or without conduct disorders
- IQ 70–100 = borderline intellect

9

SLEEP AND SLEEP DISTURBANCES

Sleep Stages

- Stage 1—presence of theta waves; lightest sleep stage
- Stage 2—presence of sleep spindles and K complexes; longest stage of sleep (benzodiazepines increase stage 2 sleep)

- Stages 3 and 4—deep sleep with high-amplitude delta waves; restores alertness and energy

- REM (rapid eye movement) sleep—characterized by complete atonia except the extraocular muscles; important for consolidation of memory

Nighttime Phenomena

Diagnosis	Symptoms	Occurs During	Management
Nightmare	"Bad dream"; person **remembers the dream** after awakening	REM sleep	None
Night terror	Awakens screaming; **does not recall the dream**	Stage 3 and 4 sleep	None
Sleepwalking	Low-level awareness with **blank facial expression**; decreased responsiveness to stimulation; **awakens confused**	Stage 3 and 4 sleep	Benzodiazepines

STRANGER ANXIETY AND SEPARATION ANXIETY

- Stranger anxiety—children age 8 months–2 years cry in presence of strangers and unfamiliar environments

- Separation anxiety—children age 7 months–3 years become anxious, cry, and cling when separated from the primary caregiver

  ► Separation anxiety disorder—occurs in older age groups (school-age children is a common presentation) and is characterized by excessive worry when separated from the primary caregiver; often experience "stomach aches," insomnia, self-mutilatory behavior, etc.; manage with behavioral modification

TOURETTE SYNDROME

- Clinical—onset of motor and vocal tics during childhood; may have component of echolalia (repetitive words/phrases), coprolalia (repetitive obscene or foul language), or grunting

- Management—therapy indicated only when tics interfere with daily function or are bothersome to the patient
  - ▸ Localized—botulinum toxin injection
  - ▸ Generalized motor and vocal tics—pimozide, fluphenazine, or tetrabenazine; all are effective

EATING DISORDERS

Anorexia Nervosa

- Criteria include **weight <85% of ideal body weight (IBW)**, purposeful dieting for fear of being "fat," distorted body image, and **amenorrhea** from severe malnutrition; may be restricting-type or binge/purging-type

- Management—nutritional rehabilitation and cognitive behavioral therapy

- Hospitalization required if <75% of IBW or if large amount of weight has been lost in a short period of time and are at increased risk of **refeeding syndrome** → hypophosphatemia, hypokalemia, hypomagnesemia → fatal cardiac arrhythmias and/or heart failure

- Hospitalization also indicated if patient flatly refuses to eat

Bulimia Nervosa

- Binge eating with sense of **loss of self-control**, followed by purging (vomiting/laxative use) or nonpurging (exercise, caloric restriction) behavior; occurs at least 2 times per week for >3 months, and is dissatisfied with weight and body; usually **normal to slightly overweight**

- Management—combination of antidepressants and cognitive behavioral therapy has the best outcome

9

IMPULSE CONTROL DISORDERS

Failure to control impulses despite the knowledge of a potentially negative outcome

Impulse Control Disorders

Diagnosis	Symptoms	Management	Important Points
Intermittent explosive disorder	Extreme anger leading to assault or property destruction out of proportion to the identifiable stressor; resolves in minutes to hours	Cognitive-behavioral therapy and psychotropic medications	Usually history of marital problems and/or **divorce**, poor job compliance and/or history of getting **fired**
Kleptomania	Irresistible urge to steal items (especially during times of **stress**) with an overwhelming feeling of **gratification**	Behavior modification and insight-oriented therapy	Patient knows actions are wrong but just **cannot resist the impulse**
Pyromania	Deliberate fire-setting on **at least two separate occasions** with gratification and relief afterwards	As with kleptomania	Often evolves into **antisocial personality disorder**
Trichotillomania	Recurrent pulling of hair; results in patchy hair loss	As with kleptomania	Usually in **college students**

MOOD DISORDERS

- Definitions
  - ▶ Depressive episode—daily to almost-daily symptoms for at least 2 weeks; must have 5 of the following 9 symptoms to meet diagnostic criteria
    - ▷ Depressed mood, loss of interest and pleasure, change in sleep patterns, change in appetite and/or weight, change in psychomotor activity, fatigue, difficulty concentrating, feelings of worthlessness or guilt, thoughts of death or suicide

▶ Mania—symptoms of heightened sensation, insomnia, and feeling of invincibility for at least 1 week; or any episode requiring hospitalization

▶ Hypomania—symptoms of mania that last at least 4 days but are not severe enough to interfere with normal social functioning

Mood Disorders

Diagnosis	Diagnostic Criteria	Management
MDD	At least one depressive episode	• SSRI or SNRI is first-line • TCAs are second-line • MAOIs are third-line • Order of above is based on side-effect profiles, not on therapeutic efficacy, and is preferred by most clinicians • Choice should always take into account individual patient circumstances
Bipolar disorder	• Type I—at least one episode of mania with or without a depressive episode • Type II—at least one episode of hypomania followed by a depressive episode • Rapid-cycling bipolar disorder: four or more mood episodes within a 1-year period	• Mood stabilizers are first-line; usually **lithium** is the DOC • If no response, may switch to or add another mood stabilizer (valproic acid, lamotrigine, or carbamazepine) or switch to an atypical antipsychotic • **Note:** Lithium should be avoided in renal failure and pregnancy (associated with **Ebstein anomaly**).
Cyclothymic disorder	**Hypomania plus** episodes of **depressive symptoms** for a minimum of **2 years**	Treat as bipolar disorder; or psychotherapy alone is indicated if symptoms are mild and not disruptive to the patient's life
Dysthymic disorder	Multiple episodes of **depressive symptoms** with a maximum of 2 months of no symptoms within a **2-year period**	Psychotherapy plus antidepressants (see Management of MDD, above)

9

(continued)

Mood Disorders (continued)

Diagnosis	Diagnostic Criteria	Management
Seasonal depression	Recurrent depressive syndrome with **predictable onset and remission**; usually occurs in **fall/winter**	Light therapy (or something similar such as sunshine or other light source) is first-line, unless patient is severely suicidal

Abbreviations: drug of choice, DOC; monoamine oxidase inhibitor, MAOI; major depressive disorder, MDD; serotonin-norepinephrine reuptake inhibitor, SNRI; selective serotonin reuptake inhibitor, SSRI; tricyclic antidepressant, TCA

GRIEF

Normal Grief

- Feelings of sadness, numbness, shock, anger, disbelief, anxiety, frequent recollection of past events, and insomnia related to the loss of a loved one; symptoms may occur in any order and tend to resolve in stages over several months

- Resolution begins around 6 months after the death and resolves completely by 1 year

Pathologic Grief

- Evidence of severe depression, suicidal ideations, or complete social withdrawal; in other words, these people are not just sad, they have complete maladjustment after the loss

- Risk factors for pathologic grief—sudden death of a loved one, extreme dependence, poor social support, or previous psychiatric history

- Management—cognitive-behavioral therapy appears most useful (teach patient how to survive without the loved one); if patient meets criteria for MDD and it has been >6–8 weeks after the loss of a loved one, antidepressants are first-line

9

PERSONALITY DISORDERS

Symptoms are pervasive, constant, and have been present for a long period of time and can be traced back to early adulthood; they cause significant distress and have a negative impact on the patient's life.

Most Commonly Tested Personality Disorders

Diagnosis	Common Associations/ Risk Factors	Symptoms	Treatment
Borderline personality disorder	• **Childhood abuse;** concomitant with other psychiatric disorders • **Predominantly** affects **females**	• **Volatile** interpersonal relationships • **Intense fear of abandonment** • Views others as **"all good or all bad"** (splitting) • **Mood swings** and difficulty with anger control and impulsivity	• **Cognitive-behavioral therapy** is first-line • Pharmacotherapy is helpful as an adjunct
Schizotypal personality disorder	Family history of schizophrenia, and patients may go on to develop it themselves	• Have **"odd"** and **"eccentric"** personalities • Have **paranoid ideas** but **no** evidence of delusions • Have **social anxiety**	Aid in development of social skills; administer antipsychotics; both are first-line
Narcissistic personality disorder	—	• **Grandiosity, self-admiration,** and sense of **entitlement** • Becomes angry when someone else "steals the spotlight"	• Very difficult, since most patients lack insight into their problem • Insight-oriented therapy appears to be best
Antisocial personality disorder	• History of childhood **conduct disorder** • Predominantly affects **males**	Recurrent **violation of laws, violence,** lack of remorse and extreme outbursts of anger **after age 15**	• Very difficult to treat; many patients die from overdose or violence • Some studies suggest **insight-oriented therapy** may be useful

9

PSYCHOTIC DISORDERS

Diagnosis	Symptoms	Diagnostic Criteria	Management
Brief psychotic disorder	Extremely stressful event/trauma causes acute onset of psychosis	Lasts >1 day but <1 month, and usually interferes with functioning	Antipsychotics and benzodiazepines; hospitalize if necessary
Delusional disorder	**Nonbizarre*** delusions that are greatly exaggerated or do not exist	Lasts ≥1 month and does not interfere with level of functioning	Insight-oriented therapy is first-line
Schizophrenia	Delusions, hallucinations, disorganized behavior and speech; dresses "oddly"	Lasts ≥**6 months** and interferes with daily function and perception of what is reality	• Atypical antipsychotic is first-line • Benzodiazepines for acute agitation
Schizophreniform disorder	As for schizophrenia	As for schizophrenia, except lasts <**6 months**	As for schizophrenia
Schizoaffective disorder	Combination of psychosis and mood disorder symptoms (depression)	Meets criteria for MDD or mania **plus** delusions/hallucinations for ≥2 weeks	Antipsychotics or mood stabilizers, depending on predominance of symptoms

Abbreviations: major depressive disorder, MDD

*Nonbizarre delusions are defined as delusions that could be true but are not (e.g., being poisoned or robbed). Bizarre delusions are defined as those that could not be true (e.g., "someone cut out my intestines" or "aliens took me to their spaceship last night").

SOMATOFORM DISORDERS

- **Cognitive-behavioral therapy** is the management of choice for all patients with somatoform disorders
- Body dysmorphic disorder—preoccupation with an imagined or physical bodily defect that causes significant stress to the patient

- Conversion disorder—typically seen in a young female with sudden onset of paralysis, seizures, and/or blindness or deafness, with complete, spontaneous resolution; associated with some type of inner conflict

- Factitious disorder—the voluntary and knowledgeable manufacturing of disease for some type of personal or monetary gain (e.g., Munchausen syndrome)

- Hypochondriasis—preoccupation with having a disease on the basis of normal bodily functions or misinterpretation of symptoms

- Malingering—purposely faking signs and symptoms for some type of personal gain

- Somatization disorder—presence of multiple physical complaints, usually before the age of 30, with no medical explanation; patients usually have multiple diagnostic tests and surgeries with completely normal findings. Includes at least four pain symptoms, two GI tract symptoms, one sexual symptom, and one pseudoneurologic symptom.

SUBSTANCE ABUSE/DEPENDENCE

- Substance abuse—recurrent use of a drug leads to significant impairment in functioning with possible harm to self or others, legal problems due to abuse, and/or continued use despite awareness of the problem the substance is causing; social support systems are most effective

- Substance dependence—abuse **plus** physical dependence (symptoms of withdrawal and tolerance to the substance); requires inpatient detoxification and rehabilitation followed by social support systems (e.g., Alcoholics Anonymous)

9

OPHTHALMOLOGY AND OTOLARYNGOLOGY

OTOLARYNGOLOGY

Hearing Loss

Presbycusis

- Pathophysiology—due to effects of normal aging and is the most common cause of hearing loss in the elderly (>50% of all adults over age 75 have some degree of presbycusis!)
- Clinical—progressive hearing loss starting at the higher frequencies (4,000–2,000 hertz)
- Management—hearing aids restore hearing for almost everyone; cochlear implants only for severe cases

Otosclerosis

Pathophysiology—autosomal dominant and seen in 10% of Caucasians; 1% will become symptomatic due to overgrowth of the stapes footplate. Can perform surgical stapedectomy for cure.

Acute sensorineural hearing loss

- Pathophysiology
  ▸ Cochlear (sensory) damage from viral infections, ototoxic drugs, meningitis, aging, Ménière disease, or cochlear otosclerosis
  ▸ Neural damage from cerebellar angle tumors

▷ Acoustic neuromas—benign, slow-growing tumors of the eighth cranial nerve resulting in tinnitus, unilateral hearing loss, and gait imbalance
  – Diagnosis—MRI
  – Management—radiosurgery or surgical resection

Diagnosis of Hearing Loss

- Otoscopy—used to directly visualize processes such as cerumen impaction, infection, tympanic membrane perforation

- Weber test—place tuning fork (256 Hz) on patient's forehead and evaluate where patient hears the "hum"
  ▸ Normal—heard equally in both ears
  ▸ Abnormal—localizes to one ear
    ▷ Conductive hearing loss—localizes to the deaf ear
    ▷ Sensorineural hearing loss—localizes to the normal ear

- Rinne test—ask the patient which side is louder when the base of the tuning fork is placed on the mastoid (method #1) or when the tuning fork is placed alongside the ear (method #2)
  ▸ Normal—#2 is louder than #1
  ▸ Conductive hearing loss—#1 is louder in the deaf ear
  ▸ Sensorineural hearing loss—#2 is louder in the deaf ear

Management of Sudden Sensorineural Hearing Loss

- An acute, unexplained unilateral loss of hearing, usually over ≤3 days
- Place on prednisone 1 mg/kg/day early; it may improve outcome
- Etiology not well understood (viral-related injury, rheumatologic, microvascular)
- Most regain a good amount of hearing (≥50%) within 2 weeks

Mastoiditis

- Clinical—ear pain, swelling behind the ear, erythema, hearing loss, fever, and headache; most commonly seen in children as an extension of middle ear infection

10

- Diagnosis—tender, swollen area above or behind the ear
  - ► CBC shows leukocytosis with left shift
  - ► CT scan shows congestion of **air cells** and possible **loss of septation**
- Microbiology—*Strep. pneumoniae, Strep. pyogenes, Staph. aureus; Pseudomonas* if history of recurrent infections
- Management—empiric antimicrobial therapy (see below) *plus*:
  - ► Myringotomy with tube placement will be required if there is abscess or bone involvement or if intracranial extension is evident on imaging
  - ► Mastoidectomy may also be performed depending on extent of disease
  - ► Empiric antimicrobial therapy
    - ▷ Vancomycin
    - ▷ Add Gram-negative coverage if either history of acute otitis in preceding 6 months or recent use of antibiotics with IV ceftazidime, cefepime, or piperacillin-tazobactam

OPHTHALMOLOGY

Sudden Loss of Vision

Diagnosis and Management of Sudden Loss of Vision

Disorder	Cause	Diagnosis	Treatment
Retinal detachment	• Laser procedures • High O_2 treatment as a child	• **No pain** • Floaters and flashes • **"Curtain falling"** • Retinal separation	Immediate retinal reattachment or laser surgery
Retinal artery occlusion	Atherosclerosis, emboli, or temporal arteritis	• **No pain** • Gradual onset • Retinal hemorrhage	• Intra-arterial thrombolysis, azetazolamides, or anterior chamber paracentesis can be attempted • Emergent ophthalmologic evaluation is warranted

(continued)

431

Diagnosis and Management of Sudden Loss of Vision (continued)

Disorder	Cause	Diagnosis	Treatment
Retinal vein occlusion	Glaucoma, DM, HTN	• **No pain** • **Gradual** onset • Retinal hemorrhage	Treat only if macular edema or revascular-ization is present
Occipital cor-tex infarct	CVA	• **No pain** • CT or MRI is diagnostic • Normal eye exam	Manage as CVA
Endophthal-mitis	• Infection of vitreous • Cataract surgery • Penetrating injury • Hematog-enous spread	• **Pain** • Decreased red reflex • Conjunctival infection • Hypopyon	Intravitreal antibiotics and vitrectomy

Abbreviations: cerebrovascular accident, CVA; diabetes mellitus, DM; hypertension, HTN

Glaucoma

Due to increased intraocular pressure

Diagnosis and Management of Glaucoma

Type	Cause	Features/Diagnosis	Treatment
Open-angle	• 90% of cases • Risk factors: DM, HTN, elderly, African American, myopia, family history	• **Painless** • **Gradual** loss of vision • Abnormal cup-to-disc ratio (>50%) • IOP >20–30 mm Hg	• Goal is to decrease IOP • Topical prostaglandins (first-line) • Topical beta-blockers • Adrenergic agonists • Cholinergic agonists • Carbonic anhy-drase inhibitors

(continued)

Diagnosis and Management of Glaucoma (continued)

Type	Cause	Features/Diagnosis	Treatment
Closed-angle	Caused by sudden dilation of pupils from medications to dilate pupils, or by sitting in a darkened movie theater	• **Painful** • **Sudden change** in vision • Halos around lights • Nausea • Conjunctival hyperemia • Fixed, mid-dilated pupil	• Immediate treatment with topical pilocarpine (causes pupillary constriction), plus topical apraclonidine, topical timolol, and acetazolamide PO or IV • Immediate expert ophthalmologic evaluation • Laser iridotomy

Abbreviations: diabetes mellitus, DM; hypertension, HTN; intraocular pressure, IOP

Macular Degeneration

- Clinical—painless loss of vision, often with visual distortion when looking at straight lines

- Risk factors—age, Caucasian, smoking, hypertension (HTN), vascular disease, ultraviolet (UV) light exposure, fatty diet

  ▸ Decrease the risk by risk factor modification

  ▸ **Tip:** Macular degeneration is the leading cause of adult blindness in developed countries.

- Diagnosis—abnormal pigmentation or hemorrhaging in the macular area, "drusen" deposits

  ▸ Fluorescein angiography—shows a neovascular membrane beneath the retina

- Management

  ▸ Dry type—quit smoking! Antioxidants may help.

  ▸ Wet type—intravitreous injection of a vascular endothelial growth factor (VEGF) inhibitor (ranibizumab, bevacizumab) or thermal laser photocoagulation

10

Orbital Cellulitis

- Considered an **ophthalmologic emergency**
- Often the results of extension of rhinosinusitis
- Usually bacterial; consider fungal etiologies if history suggestive of impaired cell-mediated immunity (immunosuppression, DM, leukemia, etc.)
- Clinical—**pain** worsens with **eye movement**, plus eye movement is limited
  - ► Swelling, **proptosis**
  - ► Conjunctival hyperemia and edema, fever, malaise
  - ► Decreased visual acuity or color vision
- Diagnosis
  - ► **CT scan** shows diffuse orbital infiltrate, with or without sinus opacity or orbital abscess
  - ► May or may not have intracranial extension, cavernous sinus thrombosis
- Management
  - ► Surgical (ENT) evaluation is warranted
  - ► Empiric antibiotics should be started as soon as cultures are obtained—IV vancomycin plus ceftriaxone or cefotaxime; add metronidazole IV if suspected intracranial extension

Corneal Abrasion

- Clinical—severe eye pain (as if a foreign body is present)
  - ► Excessive tearing, hyperemia, and photophobia
- Diagnosis—**fluorescein** staining with **Wood lamp**, then slit-lamp exam
- Management
  - ► Topical anesthetic application with irrigation if chemical exposure or foreign body seen on exam
  - ► Then give erythromycin ointment (helps prevent excessive abrasion to regenerating tissue); alternatives: polymyxin, sulfacetamide

► If abrasion is from contact lens wear, you **must** cover *Pseudomonas* with ofloxacin, ciprofloxacin, or tobramycin ointment or drops. **No** use of lenses until cleared by an ophthalmologist.

Visual Field Defects

Defect	Location
Bitemporal hemianopsia	Optic chiasm
Left homonymous hemianopsia	Right optic tract
Right upper quadrant anopsia	Optic radiations in the left temporal lobe
Right lower quadrant anopsia	Optic radiations in the left parietal lobe
Right homonymous hemianopsia with macular sparing	Left occipital lobe from posterior cerebral artery occlusion

Retinitis Pigmentosa

- Pathophysiology—a group of genetic disorders (at least 35 different genes) resulting in abnormalities of photoreceptors (rods and cones) or the retinal pigment epithelium

- Clinical—night blindness occurs first, usually over years to decades, and eventual "tunnel vision"
  ► Legally blind by age 40s or 50s
  ► Positive family history in 70% of patients

- Diagnosis—progressive loss of photoreceptor function through electroretinography
  ► Visual field testing
  ► Gene testing (over 50 genes have been found)
  ► Mottling of the retinal pigment epithelium with black bone-spicule pigmentation. Electroretinography is key to diagnosis.

- Management
  ► There is no cure
  ► If evidence of macular edema, give acetazolamide; if evidence of cataracts, extraction should be performed
  ► Routine use of high-dose vitamin A or E is not recommended
  ► May recommend a diet high in omega-3 fatty acids

10

Cataract

- Clinical—painless, progressive loss of vision due to opacification of the lens
- Risk factors—aging, female sex, estrogen exposure, diabetes mellitus (DM), trauma
  - ▸ Can be congenital
- Diagnosis—loss of red reflex
  - ▸ Opacification of the lens seen on slit-lamp exam
  - ▸ **Tip:** Cataracts are the #1 cause of blindness worldwide.
- Management—surgical replacement with an artificial implant

HERBAL REMEDIES AND SUPPLEMENTS

HERBAL REMEDIES AND SUPPLEMENTS

Aloe Vera

- Used as a topical aseptic and anti-inflammatory agent for burns, minor cuts and wounds; may **prolong** wound healing time

- Used orally as a laxative; caution when taking **zidovudine** → increases drug levels

Black Cohosh (*Cimicifuga racemosa*)

- Used orally for treatment of **premenstrual syndrome** and **menopausal symptoms**

- Clinically proven estrogenic effects from phytoestrogens and natural anti-inflammatory compounds resembling acetylsalicylic acid (ASA)

- Contraindicated in estrogen-dependent tumors, endometrial cancer, and pregnancy (may stimulate uterine contractions)

> The primary problem with herbal supplements is the substantial variability in both quality and potency from one brand or preparation to another.

Burdock

- Mild **diuretic** properties; used as a blood cleanser/purifier and in the treatment of renal stones

- No known contraindications; used as an ingredient in many Asian dishes

Cranberry Juice and Extract

- Contains a high quinic acid content—alters bacterial adhesion to urinary epithelium and decreases urinary pH
- Used for **urinary tract infection (UTI)** prevention and **renal stones**

Dong Quai

- Strong phytoestrogen concentration; has vasodilatory properties; inhibits platelet aggregation
- Used for estrogen-deficiency states, most importantly **menopause**; mild **antihypertensive** effect
- Contraindicated with known history of bleeding or when taking warfarin and other platelet inhibitors

Echinacea

- Increases white blood cell (WBC) phagocytosis and production of tumor necrosis factor (TNF), interleukin (IL)-1
- Has demonstrated antimicrobial effects; useful topically for wound infections, cuts, burns
- Despite the above, trials have not consistently demonstrated efficacy over placebo; however, it does not appear to be harmful in most
- Contraindications—inhibitors CYP3A4, prolonged use associated with immunosuppression, and use not advised when taking immunosuppressive medications

Ephedra

- Contains naturally occurring ephedrine and pseudoephedrine → **sympathomimetic activity**
- Used for **asthma** and **chronic obstructive pulmonary disease (COPD)**

- Contraindicated in hypertension, myocardial infarction, history of arrhythmias, and use of monoamine oxidase inhibitors (MAOIs)

Garlic (*Allium sativum*)

- Shown to lower total and LDL cholesterol while increasing HDL cholesterol
- Increases glycemic control
- Fibrinolytic activity inhibits platelet aggregation
- Mild antihypertensive effects
- Caution with warfarin use and platelet inhibitors (potentiates effect) and with lipid-lowering agents

Ginkgo Biloba

- Enhances **memory**; popular supplement for students and those with **Alzheimer disease**
- Improves symptoms of peripheral vascular disease (**claudication**)
- Used for erectile dysfunction; several trials have shown benefit
- Improves vision in elderly patients with macular degeneration
- Contraindicated with warfarin use, bleeding disorders, or ASA use (has fibrinolytic activity and potentiates bleeding); do not use with MAOIs

Ginger (*Zingiber officinale*)

- Antiemetic properties make this herb popular for treatment of **morning sickness and hyperemesis**

Hawthorn Berries (*Crataegus oxyacantha*)

- Hawthorn bioflavonoids cause coronary and peripheral vasculature vasodilation; useful in **angina** and **claudication**
- Inhibits angiotensin-converting enzyme (ACE) → diuresis for mild congestive heart failure (CHF) and antihypertensive properties

11

- Used in Europe to **decrease need for digoxin** in CHF
- A large metaanalysis showed significant symptomatic improvement in NYHA class I–III

Kava Kava (*Piper methysticum*)

- Acts on the amygdala in the limbic system; used for **fibromyalgia, attention deficit hyperactivity disorder (ADHD)**, and menopausal symptoms
- Contraindicated in pregnancy, in Parkinson disease, and with use of central nervous system (CNS) depressants
- May cause severe **hepatitis**
- In 2002, the FDA issued a consumer advisory due to reports of fulminant hepatitis and liver failure

Licorice (*Glycyrrhiza glabra*)

- Used for adrenal insufficiency, as an antitussive agent, and as a tea for infant colic
- Prolonged use associated with syndrome of **mineralocorticoid excess syndrome** (hyperaldosterone state)
- Avoid use with digoxin and other potassium-depleting meds → **hypokalemia**

Saw Palmetto (*Serenoa repens*)

- Exact mechanism of action is not known; thought to alter dihydrotestosterone effect
- Used for treatment of BPH
- Large metaanalysis in 2010 failed to show significant benefit

St. John's Wort (*Hypericum perforatum*)

- Used for treatment of **mild to moderate depression;** European studies have shown some benefit

- Also used to decrease menopausal symptoms

- Alters the cytochrome P450 system; may cause hypertensive crisis; use is **not advised** in conjunction with other antidepressants

- May cause photosensitivity reactions

- May cause serotonin syndrome, especially when combined with **SSRIs**

Bearberry (*Uva ursi*)

- Antiseptic and analgesic urinary properties; used in **UTIs** and **nephrolithiasis**

- Contraindicated in pregnancy and renal failure

11

ABBREVIATIONS

5-FU, 5-fluorouracil
AAA, abdominal aortic aneurysm
ABG, arterial blood gas
ABO, acute bowel obstruction
ABVD, chemotherapy regimen of Adriamycin® (doxorubicin), bleomycin, vinblastine, and dacarbazine
ACE, angiotensin-converting enzyme
ACE-I, angiotensin-converting enzyme inhibitor
ACL, anterior cruciate ligament
ACOG, American College of Obstetricians and Gynecologists
ACS, acute coronary syndrome
ACTH, adrenocorticotropic hormone
ADA, adenosine deaminase
ADH, antidiuretic hormone
ADHD, attention deficit hyperactivity disorder
ADLs, activities of daily living
A-fib, atrial fibrillation
AFP, alpha-fetoprotein
AICD, automatic implanted cardiac defibrillator
ALL, acute lymphocytic/lymphoblastic leukemia
ALS, amyotrophic lateral sclerosis
AML, acute myelocytic leukemia
AMS, altered mental status

ANA, antinuclear antibody
AP, anteroposterior
AR, aortic regurgitation
ARB, angiotensin receptor blocker
ARDS, adult respiratory distress syndrome
ARF, acute renal failure
ARR, aldosterone-renin ratio
AS, aortic stenosis
ASA, acetylsalicylic acid
ASCA, anti–*Saccharomyces cerevisiae* antibodies
ASCUS, atypical squamous cells of undetermined significance
ASD, atrial septal defect
ASO, anti-streptolysin O
AT, angiotensin
ATRA, all-trans-retinoic acid
AV, atrioventricular
BA, bone age
BAL, bronchoalveolar lavage
BBB, blood–brain barrier
BCR-ABL, breakpoint cluster region-Abelson
BMI, body mass index
BMT, bone marrow transplant
BNP, B-type natriuretic peptide
BPH, benign prostatic hypertrophy
bpm, beats per minute
BSA, body surface area
C&S, culture and sensitivity

CA, chronological age

CABG, coronary artery bypass graft

CAD, coronary artery disease

CAH, congenital adrenal hyperplasia

CA-MRSA, community-acquired methicillin-resistant *Staphylococcus aureus*

CBC, complete blood count

CBD, common bile duct

CCA, calcium-channel antagonist

CCB, calcium-channel blocker

CCP, citrulline-containing peptide

CFTR, cystic fibrosis transmembrane conductance regulator

CHD, cardiovascular heart disease

CHF, congestive heart failure

CHOP, cyclophosphamide, hydroxy-Adriamycin® (doxorubicin), Oncovin® (vincristine), and prednisone

CIN, cervical intraepithelial neoplasia

CKD, chronic kidney disease

CLL, chronic leukocytic leukemia

CML, chronic myeloid leukemia

CMV, cytomegalovirus

CN, cranial nerve

CNS, central nervous system

COMT, catechol-O-methyltransferase

COPD, chronic obstructive pulmonary disease

CPAP, continuous positive airway pressure

CPK, creatinine phosphokinase

CPPD, calcium pyrophosphate deposition disease

CPR, cardiopulmonary resuscitation

CRF, chronic renal failure

CRH, corticotropin-releasing hormone

CRP, C-reactive protein

CSF, cerebrospinal fluid

C-spine, cervical spine

CVA, cardiovascular accident

D&C, dilation and curettage

DDx, differential diagnosis

DES, diethylstilbestrol

DFA, direct fluorescent antibody

DHEA, dehydroepiandrosterone

DHR, dihydrorhodamine

DI, diabetes insipidus

DIC, disseminated intravascular coagulation

DIP, distal interphalangeal

DKA, diabetic ketoacidosis

DLCO, carbon monoxide diffusion in the lung

DLV, delavirdine

DM, diabetes mellitus

DMARD, disease-modifying antirheumatic drug

DOC, drug of choice

DPL, diagnostic peritoneal lavage

DTRs, deep tendon reflexes

DVT, deep venous thrombosis

EDH, epidural hematoma

EF, ejection fraction

EFV, efavirenz

EG, esophagogastric

EGD, esophagogastroduodenoscopy

ELISA, enzyme-linked immunosorbent assay

EPO, erythropoietin

ERCP, endoscopic retrograde cholangiopancreatography

ESR, erythrocyte sedimentation rate

ESRD, end-stage renal disease

ETEC, enterotoxigenic *Escherichia coli*
ETOH, ethanol
EUS, endoscopic ultrasound
FAB, French-American-British
FAS, fetal alcohol syndrome
FAST, focused assessment with sonography in trauma
FBS, fasting blood sugar
FEV1, forced expiratory volume in 1 second
FFP, fresh frozen plasma
FHH, familial benign hypocalciuric hypercalcemia
FNA, fine-needle aspiration
FSH, follicle-stimulating hormone
FTA-ABS, fluorescent treponemal antibody absorption test
FTT, failure to thrive
FVC, forced vital capacity
G-1-P, G-1-phosphate
G6PD, glucose-6-phosphate dehydrogenase
GAD, glutamic acid decarboxylase
GAS, group A *Streptococcus*
GBS, group B *Streptococcus*
GCS, Glasgow Coma Scale
GERD, gastroesophageal reflux disease
GGT, gamma-glutamyl transferase
GH, growth hormone
GI, gastrointestinal
g/kg, gram per kilogram of patient body weight
GLP, glucagon-like peptide
GN, glomerulonephritis
GnRH, gonadotropin-releasing hormone
GP, glycoprotein
GSW, gunshot wound

HAART, highly active antiretro-viral therapy
HAV, hepatitis A virus
HbS, hemoglobin S
HBsAg, hepatitis B surface antigen
hCG, human chorionic gonadotropin
Hct, hematocrit
HCV, hepatitis C virus
HD, heart disease or hemodialysis
HELLP, hemolysis, elevated liver enzymes, and low platelets
HF, heart failure
Hgb, hemoglobin
HHV, human herpesvirus
HIT, heparin-induced thrombocytopenia
HOCM, hypertrophic obstructive cardiomyopathy
HONC, hyperosmolar nonketotic coma
HPL, human placental lactogen
HPV, human papillomavirus
HSIL, high-grade squamous intraepithelial lesions
HSM, hepatosplenomegaly
HSV, herpes simplex virus
HTN, hypertension
HUS, hemolytic uremic syndrome
HVA, homovanillic acid
I&D, incision and drainage
IBD, inflammatory bowel disease
IBS, irritable bowel syndrome
IBW, ideal body weight
ICU, intensive care unit
IDDM, insulin-dependent diabetes mellitus
IFN, interferon
IGF, insulinlike growth factor
IHD, ischemic heart disease
IL, interleukin

INH, isoniazid

INR, international ratio

IO, intraosseous

IODM, infant of diabetic mother

IPV, inactivated polio vaccine

ITP, idiopathic thrombocytopenic purpura

IUD, intrauterine device

IUGR, intrauterine growth retardation

IVDA, IV drug abuser

IVIG, IV immunoglobulin

JRA, juvenile rheumatoid arthritis

JVD, jugulovenous distention

LAD, left anterior descending

LADA, latent autoimmune diabetes of adulthood

LBBB, left bundle branch block

LDH, lactate dehydrogenase

LES, lower esophageal sphincter

LFT, liver function test

LGA, large for gestational age

LH, luteinizing hormone

LLQ, left lower quadrant

LLSB, left lower sternal border

LMWH, low molecular-weight heparin

LOC, loss of control

LP, lumbar puncture

LSIL, low-grade squamous intra-epithelial lesions

LUQ, left upper quadrant

LV, left ventricular

LVH, left ventricular hypertrophy

MAC, *Mycobacterium avium* complex

MAOI, monoamine oxidase inhibitor

MCC, most common cause

MCL, midclavicular ligament

MCP, metacarpophalangeal

MCV, mean cell volume

MDD, major depressive disorder

MDR, multidrug-resistant

MEN, multiple endocrine neoplasia

MG, myasthenia gravis

MGUS, monoclonal gammapathy of unknown significance

MI, myocardial infarction

MM, multiple myeloma

MMA, methylmalonic acid

MMR, measles, mumps, rubella

MODY, maturity-onset diabetes of youth

MR, mental retardation or mitral regurgitation

MRA, magnetic resonance angiography

MRCP, magnetic resonance cholangiopancreatography

MRKH, Mayer-Rokitansky-Küster-Hauser

MRSA, methicillin-resistant *Staphylococcus aureus*

MS, multiple sclerosis

MSH, melanocyte-stimulating hormone

MSM, men who have sex with men

MSSA, methicillin-sensitive *Staphylococcus aureus*

MVP, mitral valve prolapse

NAC, N-acetylcysteine

NBT, nitroblue tetrazolium

NEC, necrotizing enterocolitis

NICU, neonatal intensive care unit

NIDDM, non-insulin dependent diabetes mellitus

NNRTI, non-nucleoside (and -nucleotide) reverse transcriptase inhibitor

NPO, nothing by mouth (nil per os)

NRTI, nucleoside (and nucleotide) reverse transcriptase inhibitor

NSAID, nonsteroidal anti-inflammatory drug

NSTEMI, non-ST elevation myocardial infarction

NVP, nevirapine

OB-GYN, obstetrics and gynecology

OCP, oral contraceptive pill

ODD, oppositional-defiant disorder

OME, otitis media with effusion

OR, operating room

OSM, osmolality

p-ANCA, perinuclear antineutrophilic cytoplasmic antibody

PAS, periodic acid-Schiff

PCI, percutaneous coronary intervention

PCL, posterior cruciate ligament

PCOS, polycystic ovarian syndrome

PCP, *Pneumocystis jiroveci* (formerly *Pneumocystis carinii*) pneumonia

PCR, polymerase chain reaction

PDA, patent ductus arteriosus

PE, pulmonary embolism

PEA, pulseless electrical activity

PEEP, positive end-expiratory pressure

PFT, pulmonary function test

PGE$_1$, prostaglandin E$_1$

PI, protease inhibitor

PICA, posterior inferior cerebellar artery

PICC, percutaneous inserted central catheter

PID, pelvic inflammatory disease

PIP, posterior interphalangeal

PKU, phenylketonuria

PMH, past medical history

PMN, polymorphonuclear cell

PNH, paroxysmal nocturnal hemoglobinuria

PPD, purified protein derivative

PPI, proton pump inhibitor

PPROM, preterm premature rupture of membrane

PRL, prolactin

PRN, as needed (pro re nata)

PSA, prostate-specific antigen

PSC, primary sclerosing cholangitis

PT, prothrombin time

PTC, percutaneous transhepatic cholangiogram

PTH, parathyroid hormone

PTT, partial thromboplastin time

PTU, propylthiouracil

PUD, peptic ulcer disease

PVC, premature ventricular contraction

PVD, peripheral vascular disease

PVR, peripheral vascular resistance

RA, rheumatoid arthritis

RAIU, radioactive iodine uptake

RAST, radioallergosorbent test

RBBB, right bundle branch block

RBC, red blood cell

REM, rapid eye movement

RF, rheumatoid factor

RLQ, right lower quadrant

RMSF, Rocky Mountain spotted fever

RPGN, rapidly progressive glomerulonephritis

RPR, rapid plasma reagin

RSV, respiratory syncytial virus

RTA, renal tubular acidosis

RUQ, right upper quadrant

RV, right ventricular

RVH, right ventricular hypertrophy

SAAG, serum ascites albumin gradient

SAH, subarachnoid hemorrhage

SBO, small-bowel obstruction

SBP, spontaneous bacterial peritonitis

SCD, sequential compression devices

SDH, subdural hematoma

SIADH, syndrome of inappropriate antidiuretic secretion

SJS, Stevens-Johnson syndrome

SLE, systemic lupus erythematosus

SNRI, serotonin-norepinephrine reuptake inhibitor

SSRI, selective serotonin reuptake inhibitor

SSSS, staphylococcal scalded-skin syndrome

STD, sexually transmitted disease

STEMI, ST-elevation myocardial infarction

SVR, systemic vascular resistance

SVT, supraventricular tachycardia

T&A, tonsillectomy and adenoidectomy

Tb, tuberculosis

TBSA, total body surface area

TCA, tricyclic antidepressant

TEE, transesophageal echocardiogram

TEF, tracheoesophageal fistula

TEN, toxic epidermal necrolysis

TFT, thyroid function test

TIA, transient ischemic attack

TIBC, total iron-binding capacity

TIPS, transjugular intrahepatic portosystemic shunt

TLC, total lung capacity

TLCs, therapeutic lifestyle changes

TM, tympanic membrane

TMP-SMX, trimethoprim-sulfamethoxazole

TNF, tumor necrosis factor

TPA, tissue plasminogen activator

TPN, total parenteral nutrition

TSH, thyroid-stimulating hormone

TSS, toxic shock syndrome

TTE, transthoracic echocardiogram

TTP, thrombotic thrombo-cytopenic purpura

UA, urinalysis

URI, upper respiratory infection

USPSTF, U.S. Preventative Services Task Force

UTI, urinary tract infection

UV, ultraviolet

V/Q, ventilation-perfusion

VAL, valproic acid

VATS, video-assisted thoracic surgery

VCUG, voiding cystourethrogram

VDRL, Venereal Disease Research Laboratory

VEGF, vascular endothelial growth factor

V-fib, ventricular fibrillation

VMA, vanillylmandelic acid

VSD, ventricular septal defect

vWF, von Willebrand factor

WBC, white blood cell

WHO, World Health Organization

WPW, Wolff-Parkinson-White syndrome

ZDV, zidovudine

ZES, Zollinger-Ellison syndrome

CONTRIBUTORS

CONTRIBUTING AUTHORS OF EMERGENCY MEDICINE AND SURGERY

Alex Ordonez, MD

Samuel Morales, MD

The authors would like to extend their sincerest gratitude to the following contributors:

George T. Martin, MD,
Chairman of Medicine, Lutheran Medical Center, Brooklyn, NY

David C. Tompkins, MD,
Vice-Chairman of Medicine, Lutheran Medical Center

Tom-Meka Archinard, MD,
Vice-Chairman of Emergency Medicine, Lutheran Medical Center

Fausto Vinces, MD,
Director of Trauma Surgery, Lutheran Medical Center

Robert Zaloom, MD,
Director of Cardiac Catheterization Laboratory, Lutheran Medical Center

Iffath Hoskins, MD,
Chair of Obstetrics and Gynecology, Lutheran Medical Center

Jayanth Rao, MD,
Chair of Radiology, Lutheran Medical Center

Rami Daya, MD,
Chief of Hematology and Oncology, Lutheran Medical Center

Dimitri Kirpichnikov, MD,
Chief of Endocrinology, Lutheran Medical Center

Basel Alhaddad, MD,
Faculty Physician, Lutheran Medical Center

Vasilos Sierros, MD
Faculty Physician, Lutheran Medical Center

Dorcas Morgan, MD,
Faculty Physician, Lutheran Medical Center

Manzur Sheikh, MD,
Faculty Physician, Lutheran Medical Center

Reynaldo Tan, MD,
Attending Physician, Lutheran Medical Center

Alexander Vidershayn, MD,
Deparment of Radiology, Lutheran Medical Center

Fred Nenner,
Director of Social Services, Lutheran Medical Center

Angela McWilliams, MD,
University of Arkansas Medical Center, Little Rock, AR

Marco Gonzalez, MD,
St. Vincent's Medical Center, New York, NY

INDEX

ABOUT THE AUTHORS

Carla McWilliams, MD, is an attending physician for the Internal Medicine Residency Program and consultant for the Department of Infectious Disease at Lutheran Medical Center in Brooklyn, NY. She formerly was Associate Director of Medical Curriculum for Kaplan Medical in New York City and has extensive experience in developing USMLE board review materials.

Daniel Giaccio, MD, FACP, is the program director of the Internal Medicine Residency Program and vice chair of the Department of Medicine at Lutheran Medical Center in Brooklyn, NY. His more than 28 years of teaching residents and medical students and 18 years of private practice have given him a great depth of understanding in clinical medicine.